Biosensors and Cancer

Biosensors and Cancer

Editors

Victor R. Preedy PhD DSc

Professor of Nutritional Biochemistry
School of Medicine
King's College London
and
Professor of Clinical Biochemistry
King's College Hospital
UK

Vinood B. Patel

Department of Biomedical Science
School of Life Sciences
University of Westminster
London
UK

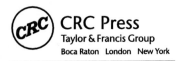

CRC Press
Taylor & Francis Group
Boca Raton   London   New York

CRC Press is an imprint of the
Taylor & Francis Group, an **informa** business

A SCIENCE PUBLISHERS BOOK

CRC Press
Taylor & Francis Group
6000 Broken Sound Parkway NW, Suite 300
Boca Raton, FL 33487-2742

© 2012 Copyright reserved
CRC Press is an imprint of Taylor & Francis Group, an Informa business

Cover Illustrations: Reproduced by kind courtesy of the undermentioned authors:
- Figure provided by author of Chapter 4, Mònica Mir
- Figure No. 3 from Chapter 8 by Dai-Wen Pang and Er-Qun Song
- Figure Nos. 1 and 7 from Chapter 16 by Seokheun Choi and Junseok Chae
- Figure No. 1 from Chapter 19 by Sigen Wang and Ruili Wang

No claim to original U.S. Government works

Printed in the United States of America on acid-free paper
Version Date: 20120327

International Standard Book Number: 978-1-57808-734-1 (Hardback)

Library of Congress Cataloging-in-Publication Data

Biosensors and cancer / editors, Victor R. Preedy, Vinood Patel.
       p. ; cm.
  Includes bibliographical references and index.
  ISBN 978-1-57808-734-1 (hardcover)
  I. Preedy, Victor R. II. Patel, Vinood B.
  [DNLM: 1. Biosensing Techniques--methods. 2. Neoplasms--diagnosis.
3.   Neoplasms--drug therapy. 4.   Tumor   Markers,   Biological.   QZ
241]
  LCclassification not assigned
  616.99′400284--dc23

                                                              2012008701

Visit the Taylor & Francis Web site at
http://www.taylorandfrancis.com

CRC Press Web site at
http://www.crcpress.com

Science Publishers Web site at
http://www.scipub.net

Preface

Biosensors have a simplistic concept but a great deal of sophistication in design, manufacture and application. They essentially have biological components within them and are used to detect, monitor or quantify substances. They use a variety of physical platforms and technologies. The biological components may include enzymes, membranes and cells or any other naturally occurring biological product. Some have artificial biological components such as modified molecules or polymers. Biosensors may be used to detect single or groups of molecules and have wide applicability to the life sciences. Each chapter in **Biosensors and Cancer** has an abstract, key facts, applications to other areas of health and disease and a "mini-dictionary" of key terms and phrases within each chapter. Finally, each chapter has a series of summary points. In this book focussing on cancer we have chapters on biosensors based on or utilizing optical imaging, surface plasmon resonance, microcantilevers, electrochemistry, aptamers, fluorescence, electrochemistry, nanobiosensors and nanowires. There are also chapters on oxidative damage to DNA, miRNA, leukemia, breast cancer, BCR-ABL activity, single living cells and thyroid cancer. Drug discovery, cancer diagnosis, anticancer drugs, and cancer detection identifying marker molecules for prostate cancer are also covered. Contributors to **Biosensors and Cancer** are all either international or national experts, leading authorities or are carrying out ground breaking and innovative work on their subject. The book is essential reading for oncologists, cancer workers and scientists, medical doctors, health care professionals, pathologists, biologists, biochemists, chemists and physicists, general practitioners as well as those interested in disease and sciences in general.

The Editors

Contents

Section 2: Blood, Molecules and Cells

Section 3: Treatments and Organs Specific Applications

List of Contributors

Carlo Bertucci
Department of Pharmaceutical Sciences, University of Bologna, Via
Belmeloro 6, 40126–Bologna, Italy.
E-mail: carlo.bertucci@unibo.it

Norman D. Brault
Department of Chemical Engineering, at the University of Washington,
USA.
E-mail: ndb16@u.washington.edu

Ana Maria Oliveira Brett
Departamento de Química, Faculdade de Ciências e Tecnologia,
Universidade de Coimbra, 3004-535 Coimbra, Portugal.
E-mail: brett@ci.uc.pt

Riccardo Castagna
Politecnico di Torino, Applied Science and Technology, Department, Corso
Duca degli Abruzzi 24, 10129 Torino, Italy.

Junseok Chae
School of Electrical, Computer, and Energy Engineering, Arizona State
University, Tempe, Arizona, USA.
E-mail: Junseok.Chae@asu.edu

Chia-Chen Chang
Institute of Biomedical Engineering, National Taiwan University, Taipei,
Taiwan.
E-mail: ccchang.ibme@gmail.com

Seokheun Choi
School of Electrical, Computer, and Energy Engineering, Arizona State
University, Tempe, Arizona, USA.
E-mail: shchoi2@asu.edu

Yang-Kyu Choi
Department of Electrical Engineering, KAIST, 335 Gwahangno, Yuseong-gu,
Daejeon 305-701, Republic of Korea.
E-mail: ykchoi@ee.kaist.ac.kr

Jose A. Costoya
Molecular Oncology Laboratory MOL, Departmento de Fisioloxia, Facultade de Medicina, Rua San Francisco s/n, 15782 Santiago de Compostela, Galicia, Spain.
E-mail: josea.costoya@usc.es

Stephanie Darmanin
Laboratory of Pathophysiology and Signal Transduction, Hokkaido University Graduate School of Medicine, N15W7, Kita-ku, Sapporo 060-8638, Japan. *Current Affiliation*: Centre for Infectious Medicine F59, Department of Medicine, Karolinska Institutet, Karolinska University Hospital Huddinge, Stockholm 14186, Sweden.
E-mail: stephanie.darmanin@ki.se

Victor Constantin Diculescu
Instituto Pedro Nunes, Laboratório de Electroanálise e Corrosão, Rua Pedro Nunes, 3030-199 Coimbra, Portugal.
E-mail: victorcd@ipn.pt

Seung Yong Hwang
Division of Molecular and Life Science, College of Science & Technology Hanyang University & GenoCheck Co. Ltd., Ansan, Gyeonggi-do, Korea.
E-mail: syhwang@hanyang.ac.kr

Pablo Iglesias
Molecular Oncology Laboratory MOL, Departmento de Fisioloxia, Facultade de Medicina, Rua San Francisco s/n, 15782 Santiago de Compostela, Galicia, Spain.
E-mail: pablo.iglesias@usc.es

Shaoyi Jiang
Department of Chemical Engineering, at the University of Washington, USA.
E-mail: sjiang@u.washington.edu

Chang-Hoon Kim
Department of Electrical Engineering, KAIST, 335 Gwahangno, Yuseong-gu, Daejeon 305-701, Republic of Korea.
E-mail: chkim@nobelab.kaist.ac.kr

Takeshi Kondo
Department of Hematology & Oncology, Hokkaido University Graduate School of Medicine, N15W7, Kita-ku, Sapporo 060-8638, Japan.
E-mail: t-kondoh@med.hokudai.ac.jp

Kuldeep Kumar
Biosensor Technology Lab, Department of Biotechnology, Punjabi University, Patiala-147 002, India.
E-mail: kuldeepbio@rediffmail.com

Seung Yong Lee
Department of Bio-Nano Technology, Hanyang University, Ansan, Gyeonggi-do, Korea.
E-mail: three2k@hanmail.net

Chii-Wann Lin
Institute of Biomedical Engineering, National Taiwan University, Taipei, Taiwan.
E-mail: cwlinx@ntu.edu.tw

Marco Mascini
Dipartimento di Chimica Ugo Schiff, Università degli studi di Firenze, Via della Lastruccia 3, Sesto Fiorentino (Fi), Italia.
E-mail: Marco.mascini@unifi.it

Ray Mernaugh
Department of Biochemistry, School of Medicine, Vanderbilt University, Nashville, TN 37232, USA.
E-mail: r.mernaugh@vanderbilt.edu

Chang Ming Li
School of Chemical and Biomedical Engineering, Center for Advanced Bionanosystems Nanyang Technological University, 70 Nanyang Drive, Singapore 637457.
E-mail: ecmli@ntu.edu.sg

Mònica Mir
Nanobioengineering Laboratory, Institute for Bioengineering of Catalonia (IBEC), Barcelona Science Park, Baldiri i Reixac, 10, 08028, Barcelona, Spain.
E-mail: mmir@ibec.pcb.ub.es

Tatsuaki Mizutani
Laboratory of Pathophysiology and Signal Transduction, Hokkaido University, Graduate School of Medicine, N15W7, Kita-ku, Sapporo 060-8638, Japan.
Current Affiliation: Ludwig Boltzmann Institute for Cancer Research, Waehringerstrasse 13A, A-1090, Vienna, Austria.
E-mail: Mizutani.Tatsuaki@lbicr.lbg.ac.at

May C. Morris
CRBM-CNRS-UMR 5237, University of Montpellier-IFR122, 1919 Route de
Mende, 34293 Montpellier, France.
E-mail: may.morris@crbm.cnrs.fr

Maria Teresa Neves-Petersen
Nanobiotechnology Group, Department of Biotechnology, Chemistry and
Environmental Sciences, University of Aalborg, Sohngaardsholmsvej 57,
DK-9000 Aalborg, Denmark.
E-mail: tnp@bio.aau.dk

Yusuke Ohba
Laboratory of Pathophysiology and Signal Transduction, Hokkaido
University, Graduate School of Medicine, N15W7, Kita-ku, Sapporo 060-
8638, Japan.
E-mail: yohba@med.hokudai.ac.jp

Ilaria Palchetti
Dipartimento di Chimica Ugo Schiff, Università degli studi di Firenze,
Via della Lastruccia 3, Sesto Fiorentino (Fi), Italia.
E-mail: ilaria.palchetti@unifi.it

Dai-Wen Pang
Key Laboratory of Analytical Chemistry for Biology and Medicine
(Ministry of Education), College of Chemistry and Molecular Sciences,
Research Center for Nanobiology and Nanomedicine, (MOE 985 Innovative
Platform), State Key Laboratory of Virology, Wuhan University, Wuhan
430072, People's Republic of China.
E-mail: dwpang@whu.edu.cn

Wilmer Alfonso Pardo
Nanobioengineering Laboratory, Institute for Bioengineering of Catalonia
(IBEC), Barcelona Science Park, Baldiri i Reixac, 10, 08028, Barcelona,
Spain.
E-mail:

Antonietta Parracino
Nanobiotechnology Group, Department of Physics and Nanotechnology,
University of Aalborg, Sohngaardsholmsvej 57, DK-9000 Aalborg,
Denmark.
E-mail: m.parracino@yahoo.it

Steffen B. Petersen
Nanobiotechnology Group, Department of Health Science and Technology,
Aalborg University, Frederik Bajers Vej 7 D2, Aalborg, Denmark.
E-mail: sp@hst.aau.dk

Carlo Ricciardi
Politecnico di Torino, Applied Science and Technology, Department, Corso Duca degli Abruzzi 24, 10129 Torino, Italy.
E-mail: carlo.ricciardi@polito.it

Josep Samitier
Nanobioengineering Laboratory, Institute for Bioengineering of Catalonia (IBEC), Barcelona Science Park, Baldiri i Reixac, 10, 08028, Barcelona, Spain.
E-mail:

Angela De Simone
Department of Pharmaceutical Sciences, University of Bologna, Via Belmeloro 6, 40126–Bologna, Italy.
E-mail: angela.desimone2@unibo.it

Er-Qun Song
Key Laboratory of Luminescence and Real-Time Analysis of the Ministry of Education, College of Pharmaceutical Sciences, Southwest University, Chongqing, 400715, People's Republic of China.
E-mail:eqsong@swu.edu.cn

Masumi Tsuda
Laboratory of Pathophysiology and Signal Transduction; Hokkaido University Graduate School of Medicine, N15W7, Kita-ku, Sapporo 060-8638, Japan.
E-mail: tsudam@med.hokudai.ac.jp

Neelam Verma
Biosensor Technology Lab, Department of Biotechnology, Punjabi University, Patiala-147 002, India.
E-mail: neelam_verma2@rediffmail.com

Ruili Wang
Division of Pharmacotherapy and Experimental Therapeutics, School of Pharmacy, University of North Carolina, 311 Pharmacy Lane, CB# 7569, Chapel Hill, NC 27599-7569, USA.
E-mail: rlwang@email.unc.edu and wangruili@hotmail.com

Sigen Wang
Department of Radiation Oncology& Department of Physics and Astronomy, University of North Carolina, 101 Manning Drive, CB# 7512, Chapel Hill, NC 27599-7512, USA.
E-mail: sgwang@email.unc.edu and sgwang88@yahoo.com

Qiuming Yu
Department of Chemical Engineering at the University of Washington, USA.
E-mail: qyu@u.washington.edu

Rosa Letizia Zaffino
Nanobioengineering Laboratory, Institute for Bioengineering of Catalonia (IBEC), Barcelona Science Park, Baldiri i Reixac, 10, 08028, Barcelona, Spain.
E-mail:

Xiangqun Zeng
Department of Chemistry, Oakland University, Rochester, MI 48309, USA.
E-mail: zeng@oakland.edu

Guo-Jun Zhang
Institute of Microelectronics, A*STAR (Agency for Science, Technology and Research), 11 Science Park Road, Singapore Science Park II, Singapore 117685.
E-mail: zhanggj@ime.a-star.edu.sg

Xin Ting Zheng
Institute for Clean Energy and Advanced Materials, Southwest University, Chongqing 400715, P.R. China.
E-mail: zhen0012@hotmail.com

SECTION 1: GENERAL

Functional Optical Imaging-based Biosensors

Pablo Iglesias[1,a] and Jose A. Costoya[1,b,*]

ABSTRACT

In vivo fluorescence and bioluminescence imaging are the most common techniques used in optical imaging. These methods, especially those based on fluorescent light emission, are provided with a high number of fluorescent tracers, either small organic dyes such as ICG or fluorescent proteins as in the case of GFP. Although tissue autofluorescence seems to be a major drawback of the technique when applied to imaging in living animals, the development of novel tracers able to emit in near-infrared wavelengths has given a boost to this method. On the other hand, bioluminescent light is emitted upon the chemical reaction of the enzyme luciferase with its substrate producing an emission peak between 560 and 580 nm. Both of these techniques have been commonly employed in cell biology as reporter assays that usually apprise on cell compartmentalization of gene products, transcriptional activity of interest genes or pathophysiological processes of diseases such as cancer. In the case of cancer, the transcription factor HIF-1α is a major regulator of the cell response to hypoxia by eliciting formation of neovessels. With all of these in mind, we have designed and characterized a BRET-based genetically encoded biosensor able to detect variations in the concentration of HIF-1α. Here we review our work in the field along

[1]Molecular Oncology Laboratory MOL, Departmento of Fisioloxia, Facultade de Medicina, Rua San Francisco s/n, 15782 Santiago de Compostela, Galicia, Spain.
[a]E-mail: pablo.iglesias@usc.es
[b]E-mail: josea.costoya@usc.es
*Corresponding author

List of abbreviations after the text.

with some remarkable examples of the application of optical imaging, either fluorescence and bioluminescence or BRET, to the development of biosensors.

INTRODUCTION

Classes of Imaging Methods

Traditionally, imaging methods applied to medicine would be separated in two broad categories, anatomical and functional imaging. Thus, anatomical imaging makes use of tissue contrast differences to locate affected organs, bones or detect tumours when applied to oncology. In this category, the most popular examples are magnetic resonance imaging (MRI) and X-ray computed tomography (CT), which have been successfully established as reference techniques in the clinic, playing a prominent role in the last decades since their debut as diagnostic tools. However, the limitations of these techniques are their inability to give any relevant information other than size or location of the pathophysiological features of the disease (Seaman et al. 2010). Unlike these, a second category comprises of imaging methods that are able to give more precise and detailed information about physiological processes such as oxygenation rate, perfusion and alterations of blood flow. In this regard, a variation of the MRI technique, functional MRI (fMRI) is currently being employed as a non-invasive method to preoperatively map functional cerebral cortex and to identify eloquent areas of the cerebral cortex in relation to brain cancers (Torigian et al. 2007). A third category could be added to these two traditional categories, molecular imaging methods, which are rapidly gaining popularity due to the better understanding of the molecular bases of disease. Formally, they can be defined as "the visualization, characterization, and measurement of biological processes at the molecular and cellular levels in humans and other living systems" (Mankoff 2007), i.e. these techniques inform on the molecular mechanisms underlying the biological processes of interest (Dunn et al. 2001; Alavi et al. 2004; Torigian et al. 2007).

Molecular Imaging: Optical Methods Overview

However, some of these techniques rely on ionizing radiation, such as CT and SPECT, involving higher doses than common X-ray imaging procedures, increasing exposure to radiation in the population that might be considered a public health issue in the future (Brenner 2007). And while the resolution of MRI and its ability to confer anatomic detail are difficult to match, it also requires extremely expensive instrumentation and is time-consuming, giving a poor throughput performance. On the other hand, optical methods such as fluorescence and bioluminescence rely on the emission of visible light that, unlike the former ones do not display the harming effects of ionizing radiations on living organisms or require high-budget equipment to monitor the overall process (Sampath et al. 2008).

Fluorescence has risen to a distinguished position in molecular and cell biology thanks to the widespread use of the *Aequoerea victoria* green fluorescent protein (GFP) that as of today remains one of the most common fluorescent reporters. Since then, it has developed a whole array of new fluorescent proteins with diverse excitation and emission wavelengths that comprises almost the whole visible spectrum, making this technique very versatile for a wide range of applications (Shaner et al. 2005). In addition, these novel fluorescent proteins display interesting features such as NIR-shifted emission wavelengths that permit avoiding overlapping emissions from tissue and/or organic compounds (Ntziachristos et al. 2003; Weissleder and Ntziachristos 2003).

In bioluminescence, luciferase enzymes are commonly employed as reporter genes in cell and molecular biology. Sources of luciferases are insects such as the firefly *Photynus pyralis*, marine invertebrates such as the sea pansy (*Renilla reniformis*), plants (*Gaussia princeps*) and several species of vibrionaceae (Hastings 1983). Unlike fluorescence where electron excitation and subsequent photon emission is mediated by a physical phenomenon (light absorption), bioluminescence light is chemically produced by decaying singlet state species that emit photons of visible light. These "light-emitting" reactions are catalyzed by luciferase enzymes when their chemical substrates such as D-luciferin or coelenterazin are present and subsequently oxidized. Although fluorescent light is usually brighter, with less light scattering and photon attenuation that makes fluorescence more suitable for 3D reconstruction, bioluminescent light lacks the problem of cell and tissue auto-luminescence, fluorescent photobleaching and in general facilitates quantitative imaging in deeper localizations than fluorescence. Besides, the substrate D-luciferin becomes readily available upon administration, able to cross the blood-brain barrier upon intraperitoneal or intravenous administration and lacking any harmful effect on living organisms when regularly administered (Edinger et al. 2002).

Bioluminescence Resonant Energy Transfer (BRET)

Transference of resonant energy is a well-known phenomenon on which proteomic and biochemical procedures rely on to determine protein-protein interactions (Pfleger and Eidne 2006). In a similar way as FRET where a donor fluorochrome is able to excite a second fluorochrome acting as an acceptor, in BRET a luminescent donor (Luc) excites a fluorochrome. As Fig. 1.1 shows, when the FLuc substrate, D-luciferin is present this is

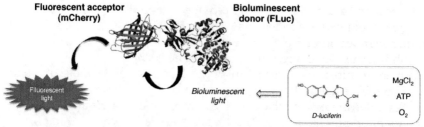

Figure 1.1. Outline of BRET occurring in a fusion protein where FLuc is the bioluminescence donor and a NIR fluorochrome is the fluorescence acceptor. The luciferase requires the presence of its substrate D-luciferin plus ATP, magnesium chloride and ATP to emit light. This light when close enough is able to excite the fluorochrome when the signal is registered.

oxidized by the luciferase emitting light as a by-product. This light is emitted high enough to excite a red fluorescent protein such as mCherry, a derivative of DsRed from *Discosoma* sp. (Shaner et al. 2004).

The efficiency of energy transfer is strongly dependent on Förster distance (R_0), the distance between the donor and acceptor generating 50% of the maximum possible energy transfer, which typically falls into the range of 1–10 nm. The orientation and freedom of movement of both proteins, in the case of fused pairs, can also be empirically tuned by inserting flexible linkers in between both proteins of appropriate length (Michelini et al. 2004; Dacres et al. 2010; Prinz et al. 2006). Although the choice of the suitable donor/acceptor pair is usually determined empirically, one of the most popular pairs is RLuc/GFP since this pair exhibits a spectral overlap of donor emission and acceptor excitation, which is one of the critical steps on the overall performance of the system.

Examples of Optical Methods Applied to Functional Imaging Biosensors

To illustrate the application of optical imaging methods to functional imaging biosensors we chose several outstanding examples. Bioluminescent imaging has been largely employed as transcription reporter *in vitro* assays by fusing response elements of target transcription factors to luciferase genes. These constructs may also be used to monitor the formation of grafted tumours *in vivo* and measure cell numbers during tumour progression and response to therapy. One of the best examples of applications of this type of biosensors is the E2F1-Luc transgenic mouse (Uhrbom et al. 2004). In this study, the authors report the construction of a chimeric construct formed by several response elements for E2F1, a master regulator of cell cycle progression that appears up-regulated in a high proportion of tumours, fused to a FLuc gene. Upon generating the transgenic mouse harbouring this biosensor they generated brain tumours by injecting intracranially

DF-1 cells, in order to recreate a PDGF-driven glioma model. Once the tumours were established and detected by BLI output, they submitted those mice affected with bioluminescent tumours with PTK787/ZK222584, an inhibitor of PDGF receptor and the rapamycin analog CCI-779. This treatment resulted in reduced light production that evidenced inhibition of cell proliferation of the tumour masses.

A similar strategy involves the use of tissue specific promoters coupled to a reporter gene. Bhang and colleagues (Bhang et al. 2011) report that the progression elevated gene-3 (PEG-3) promoter can be used to detect micrometastases in mice models of human melanoma and breast cancer either by BLI or employing radionuclides-based imaging techniques. The authors injected cells from either breast or human melanoma cells and then the pPEG-Luc (BLI) and pPEG-HSV1tk (PET) constructs along with linear polyethylenimine (l-PEI) polyplexes, as a means of gene delivery. Several masses were successfully detected and upon histological examination identified as micrometastasis. The accuracy of localization and size of these tumoural masses was further confirmed by whole-body acquisitions of SPECT-CT.

BRET may also be used as a basis of a biosensor as the self-illuminating quantum dots conjugated with luciferase reported by So and colleagues (So et al. 2006). Quantum dots are semiconductor nanocrystals with different optical properties depending on its size and its composition (Medintz et al. 2005). In this case, the authors conjugated several copies of RLuc8, an engineered red-shifted variant of *R. reniformis* luciferase designed to excite several polymer-coated ZnS/CdSe core shell quantum dots that emit fluorescent light at 655, 705 and 800 nm. Also in order to increase the cell uptake of these nanostructures, these functionalized quantum dots were conjugated with a polycationic peptide. The system proved to be highly effective in all cases (655, 705 and 800 nm) producing a quantifiable BRET signal thus demonstrating the possibilities of BRET-based biosensors modulated by specific biological interactions.

Applications to Areas of Health and Disease

These techniques are expected to fully develop in the forthcoming years as a prognostic tool for the clinical environment and more specifically for cancer treatment. In this context, to minimize the risk of recurrence it is desirable that the entire tumour is removed before metastasis takes place. In this regard, several cancer hallmarks can been used to design targeted molecular probes such as increased growth (augmented production of growth factor and growth factor receptors), unrestricted replicative potential, sustained angiogenesis and invasiveness of neighbouring tissues and/or metastatic abilities (Keereweer et al. 2010). One good example of this approach are the activatable probes developed by Weissleder and colleagues (Wunderbaldinger et al. 2003; Mahmood et al. 2003) and currently commercialized by VisEn Medical (ProSense and AngioSense), which target metalloproteinases abundant in the surroundings of the tumour. These probes are administered in a quenched state, only displaying a basal emission until cleaved by its target protease.

The first steps for translation of this technique to the clinic have been made in sentinel lymph node mapping. The presence of cancer cells in regional lymph nodes indicates metastasis and necessitates more aggressive, systemic treatment, such as chemotherapy. In this regard, several studies report the use of intraoperative near-infrared fluorescence monitoring employing low weight molecular ligands (peptides and small molecules) able to target tumoural cells in their niches. This approach is currently being assessed as prospective intraoperatory assistance to surgeons (Soltesz et al. 2006; Tanaka et al. 2006) with NIR-emitting derivatives of indocyanine green (ICG).

Bioluminescence Resonance Energy Transfer (BRET)-based Biosensors and the Transcription Factor HIF-1alpha

In this chapter, we describe the design, construction and characterization of a novel hypoxia genetic biosensor with near-infrared fluorescence (NIR-F) and bioluminescent properties. This genetic biosensor comprises a regulatory moiety activated by the hypoxia inducible factor HIF-1α, enabling the transcription of a fusion protein that acts as a dual fluorescence-bioluminescence tracer capable of BRET-mediated fluorochrome excitation. All of these data and the corresponding materials and methods employed have been previously described (Iglesias and Costoya 2009).

Hypoxia as a Tumoural Aggresivity Marker in Cancer

One of the most recognizable features of a tumoural cell is the chaotic growth that is intimately related to tumour aggressiveness and invasiveness. As normal cells do, these tumoural cells secrete angiogenic signals to attract additional blood supplies as a response to hypoxia, which usually ensues as soon as the tumour enlarges beyond a millimetre or two in diameter. As a consequence of the low levels of oxygen (hypoxia), the angiogenic switch of these tumoural cells is activated resulting in secretion of hypoxic transcription factors and the number of blood vessels supporting the tumour rises exponentially to fulfil the exacerbated need of nutrients and oxygen (Alberts et al. 2009). This angiogenic process is tightly regulated and results in the participation of several transcription factors, with HIF-1α

being one of the most important. HIF-1 is a HIF-1α/HIF-1β heterodimer that binds the hypoxia response elements (HREs) of target genes under hypoxic conditions. The HIF-1β subunit is constitutively expressed, while in the case of HIF-1□□subunit its expression and transcriptional activity are precisely regulated by the cellular O_2 concentration (Wang et al. 1995). As shown in Fig. 1.2 , by interacting with the coactivator CBP/p300, HIF-1 activates transcription of target genes involved in glucose transportation and glycolysis, angiogenesis, survival and proliferation, and invasion and metastasis (Bárdos and Ashcroft, 2004). In fact, HIF-1□□is overexpressed in may cancer types and is associated with poor prognosis and its expression correlates with metastatic potential of those tumours (Semenza et al. 2003; Zhong et al. 1999).

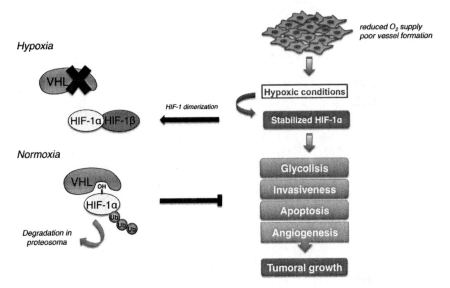

Figure 1.2. In normoxic conditions where oxygen is available the transcription factor HIF-1α becomes hydroxylated and subsequently poly-ubiquitined by the E3 ubiquitin ligase pVHL. On the other hand, in hypoxic conditions such as those within tumoural masses, the formation of neovessels and therefore oxygen supply is deficient and HIF-1α is stabilized and dimerizes with HIF-1β translocating to the nucleus and exerting its transcriptional activity on several essential processes for tumour development.

Design and Characterization of the Biosensor

Figure 1.3 shows the scheme of the biosensor. The HIF-1 sensor is formed by a novel chimeric enhancer able to bind the HIF-1α transcription factor more efficiently than the canonical hypoxia response elements (HRE). This chimeric enhancer that comprises a (Egr-1)-binding site (EBS) from the Egr-1 gene, a metal-response element (MRE) from the metallothionein

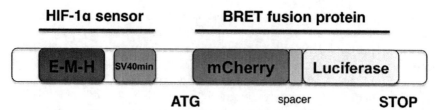

Figure 1.3. Schematic outline of genetically encoded biosensor, the E-M-H enhancer (EGR/ MGR/3xHRE) and the SV40 minimal promoter comprise the HIF-1α sensor moiety, while the tracer module is formed by the fusion protein of mCherry and the firefly luciferase (FLuc).

gene, and a triplet of hypoxia-response elements (3xHRE) from the phosphoglycerate kinase 1 gene (Lee et al. 2006). A SV40 minimal promoter is located downstream of the chimeric enhancer E-M-H. The specificity of this biosensor for HIF-1α is of great advantage when compared to other angiogenesis biosensors based on promoter regions of other transcription factors such as VEGF (Salnikow et al. 2002). VEGF regulates and is regulated by numerous physiological and pathological processes, making a high number of cytokines and growth factors signalling pathways that are known to modulate VEGF expression at the transcriptional level. Some examples of this are IL-1β and IL-6 cytokines, PDGF-BB, TGF-β, and transcription factors such as basic fibroblast growth factor, EGF and HGF, which makes this promoter too promiscuous to be taken solely as a reliable marker of hypoxia (Akagi et al. 1998).

On the other hand, the dual tracer moiety is formed by a fusion protein of mCherry and the firefly luciferase (FLuc). Although initially mPlum was tested as a prospective fluorochrome, it was eventually discarded due to its low brightness (data not shown and Shaner et al. 2005). On the other hand, mCherry presents an excitation wavelength of 585 nm, which makes this fluorochrome an ideal acceptor of bioluminescent light (575 nm), as well as its near NIR-emission avoids the autofluorescence phenomena occurring in living tissue.

At first, we wanted to assess the fluorescent and bioluminescent activity of the fusion protein in order to disregard any sequence discrepancy with the previously reported excitation/emission wavelengths. Accordingly, we registered the spectrophotometric profiles of mCherry and the firefly luciferase, observing the same excitation/emission wavelengths reported before (Shaner et al. 2004), indicating that fusing the luciferase and mCherry together did not affect the *in vitro* performance of the fluorescent protein (data not shown). We next corroborated these data by testing the *in vitro* functionality of the cloned fluorescent protein (Fig. 1.4A). We performed several transfections with growing molar ratios of our vector (E-M-H-mCherry-Luc) along with an expression plasmid enconding the HIF-1α transcription factor (pcDNA3-HIF-1α) into the human HEK 293 cell line.

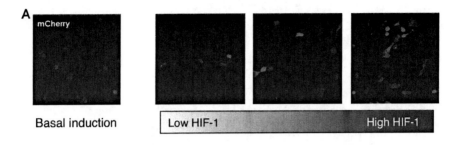

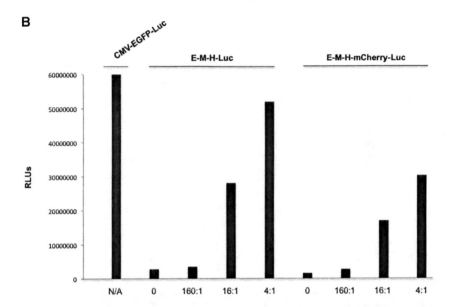

Figure 1.4. (A) *In vitro* fluorescence activity of the biosensor in HEK 293 cells. Basal activity denotes induction due to endogenous HIF-1α levels. Cells were transfected with increasing quantities of a plasmid encoding HIF-1α. **(B)** Luciferase activity of the fusion protein for E-M-H-Luciferase and E-M-H-mCherry-Luciferase.

As expected, the fluorescence signal observed was proportional to the quantity of HIF-1α transfected with the biosensor, indicating that the system is proportionally responsive to the amount of transcription present in each assay.

Next, we tested the luciferase activity and performance of the system *in vitro*. As shown in Fig. 1.4B we observed the same proportionality of the bioluminescent signal in relation with the concentration of the transcription factor HIF-1α. Intriguingly, we observed that one of the control groups where the parental vector E-M-H-Luc was transfected, displayed a similar signal than that of the biosensor with the fusion protein. This discrepancy hinted of a probable energy transfer between FLuc and mCherry that we later confirmed, and to rule out any non-expected hindrance of the luciferase catalytic site caused by mCherry that would result in a weaker FLuc activity. As means of transfection normalization and to rule out discrepancies on transfection efficiency in the different experimental groups, all data were normalized against the β-galactosidase activity of each group.

Subsequently, we wondered if this fluorescent and bioluminescent performance could be translated into an *in vivo* environment. Therefore, we next co-transfected HEK 293 cells with our biosensor and either pcDNA3-HIF-1α, or a transfection control (pcDNA3). Thus, we obtained two groups of cells that contained either the activated biosensor (with artificially high levels of HIF-1α) or non-activated cells that would only display a basal activity due to endogenous HIF-1α. Upon confirming the optical activities of these cells both groups were injected subcutaneously as xenografts in the hindquarters of immunodeficient SCID mice.

Fluorescent signals were measured 24 hr upon injection as shown in Fig. 1.5A. Accordingly, we confirmed that the system remains active in the xenografts formed by HEK 293 cells transfected with the E-M-H-mCherry-Luc (ECL) biosensor, and that their intensity directly correlates to the quantity of the transcription factor HIF-1α present in those cells. Likewise, luciferase activity was also registered *in vivo* (Fig. 1.5B). Upon administration of D-luciferin, we observed a similar output as before with both xenografts, activated with HIF and non-activated, emitted bioluminescent light but with higher intensity in the case of cells with the activated system. Taken

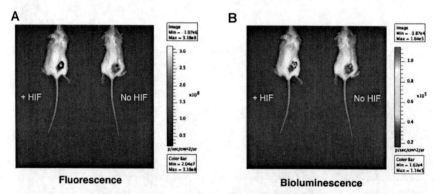

Figure 1.5. (A) *In vivo* mCherry fluorescence in a xenograft implanted subcutaneously in SCID mice. The left mouse carries the "activated biosensor" ('+ HIF'), HEK 293 cells transfected with E-M-H-mCherry-Luciferase and pcDNA3-HIF-1α while the right mouse was injected with the 'non-activated' system ('No HIF') in cells transfected with E-M-H-mCherry-Luciferase and pcDNA3 as a negative control. **(B)** *In vivo* luciferase activity in SCID mice. Left mouse carries the activated biosensor and right mouse the no-activated one.

together, these data demonstrate that our hypoxia biosensor is able to proportionally induce the transcription of the mCherry-luciferase tracer when the concentration of HIF-1α is high enough to bind the response elements located upstream to the fusion protein coding sequence. A similar response was also observed both *in vitro*, in HEK 293 cells transfected with increasing concentrations of HIF-1α, and *in vivo* xenografts of these transfected cells, as shown in Fig. 1.5A and Fig. 1.5B.

As discussed before, we observed a marked decrease when registering the bioluminescent activity of the biosensor and comparing it to that of the parental vector E-M-H-Luc (Fig. 1.4B). We hypothesized that it could be either a consequence of a resonant energy transfer (RET) between FLuc and mCherry, or that by fusing those two proteins together the catalytic site of FLuc resulted in reducing the enzyme's ability to bind to its substrate. Consequently, we first tested whether or not this transference was taking place *in vitro* by comparing the spectrophotometric profiles of whole cell lysates of cells transfected with the parental vector (E-M-H-Luc) or with our biosensor (E-M-H-mCherry-Luc). As shown in Fig. 1.6A, the luciferase alone

A

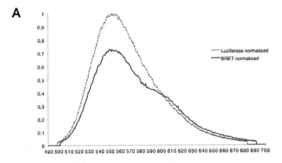

B

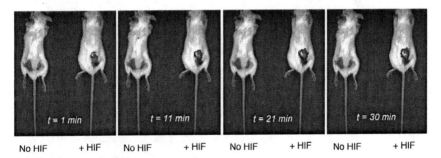

Figure 1.6. (A) *In vitro* BRET performance of the genetically encoded biosensor. Solid line represents luciferase activity of the E-M-H-Luciferase vector; dashed line represents luciferase activity of the E-M-H-mCherry-Luciferase vector. **(B)** *In vivo* BRET performance of the system at various times. Maximum BRET emission was reached 30 min upon injection of D-luciferin (150 mg/kg).

displays a maximum value at the expected wavelength of 575 nm. However, it also displays a lower second peak at a wavelength corresponding to that of mCherry emission maximum wavelength. In addition, a fall of the bioluminescent activity was also observed in this case that would be consistent with the existence of BRET, as the second emission peak suggests. This would imply that part of the bioluminescent light would be absorbed by the fluorochrome rather equalling the difference between both peaks registered by the spectrofluorometer detector.

With this in mind and once we had demonstrated that BRET could be registered *in vitro* in whole cell lysates we wanted to confirm whether or not this phenomenon was also occurring in xenografts in SCID mice. We finally investigated whether or not this BRET phenomenon could be also detected *in vivo*. We consequently registered the fluorescent emission of the activated system while at the same time blocking the excitation filter in order to avoid any excitation source other than the FLuc luciferase. Figure 1.6B shows some of the most representative points of the series including the peak emission of BRET in SCID mice at 30 min upon D-luciferin injection.

CONCLUSION

Fluorescence and bioluminescence imaging are experiencing slow but steady advances to become another tool in clinical environments. These kind of optical methods provide a functional insight that is rarely achieved using other traditional yet spatially powerful techniques such as CT or MRI. As an addition to these optical methods, BRET can be considered an emerging technique that has the best from both fluorescence and bioluminescence. Given that BRET does not depend on an external source of excitation but rather on a chemical reaction it does not present the characteristic tissue autofluorescence that is common in living organisms, and at the same time, the fluorescent light emitted by the fluorochrome is better suited for 3D tomographic reconstructions than bioluminescent light, at the same time allowing its application at deeper locations than fluorescence alone (Dinca et al. 2010). We have described several examples of biosensors used primarily in oncology that not only highlight the tumoural mass but at the same time also inform us on specific biological processes related to tumoural development and maintenance. We have also described the development and characterization of a BRET-based hypoxia biosensor that uses the firefly luciferase (FLuc) as a bioluminescence donor and a NIR fluorochrome, mCherry, as fluorescent acceptor. This genetically encoded biosensor is induced by the hypoxia transcription factor HIF-1α, which acts as key regulator of the angiogenic switch of tumoural cells in response to hypoxic conditions. We have demonstrated that this factor binds the response element located in the regulatory module of the construction efficiently inducing the transcription of the fusion protein, displaying at the same time a proportional response to the concentration of HIF-1α within the cells carrying the biosensor. Although the development of a BRET-based biosensor (So et al. 2006) is not a novelty in the field, combining NIR fluorescence and bioluminescence results in a valuable alternative approach for future inducible biosensors that take advantage of BRET.

KEY FACTS

- The green fluorescent protein (GFP) was first cloned in 1992 from the jellyfish *Aequorea victoria*, by Douglas C. Prasher. This wild-type GFP had lower excitation and emission peaks than their engineered counterparts used currently, mainly EGFP (enhanced green fluorescent protein).
- The sea pansy (*R. reniformis*) luciferase emits light in the blue part of the spectrum at 480 nm when reacts with coelenterazine h, while the *Photynus pyralis* FLuc is a yellow luciferase emitting at 560 nm.
- One of the first applications of BRET was to investigate the dimerization of cyanobacterial circadian clock proteins in bacterial culture. The pair donor-acceptor used back then eventually became one of the most used, *Renilla reniformis* luciferase (RLuc) as donor and GFP as acceptor.
- Optical imaging is already being used as intraoperative aid for surgeons aiming to remove regional lymph nodes or metastasis, both in breast and ovary cancer respectively, improving the clinical management of these tumours and therefore their prognosis.
- Indocyanine green (ICG) is a synthetic dye traditionally used for medical diagnoses because of its ability to penetrate in deeper tissues in angiography studies. Currently, it is being tested for assessing vascular leakage associated with tumour invasion.

DEFINITIONS

- *Bioluminescence*: production of light as a result of a chemical reaction catalysed by a class of enzymes denominated luciferases, found in multiple living organisms.
- *Fluorescence*: physical phenomenon where an external source of light excites a molecule, called fluorochrome, and this emits light at a higher wavelength.
- *BRET*: Bioluminescence resonance energy transfer, a photophysical phenomenon occurring between a donor-acceptor pair where the donor is a light emitting luciferase (RLuc or FLuc) and the acceptor

a fluorochrome excited by the bioluminescent emission of the luciferase.

- *D-luciferin*: (4S)-2-(6-hydroxy-1,3-benzothiazol-2-yl)-4,5-dihydrothiazole-4-ca rboxylic acid. It is the substrate of the firefly luciferase that in the process becomes oxydized (oxyluciferin) and emits the characteristic yellow light.
- *Coelenterazine*: 6-(4-hydroxyphenyl)-2-[(4-hydroxyphenyl)methyl]-8-(phenylmethyl)-7H-imidazo[3,2-a]pyrazin-3-one. It is the substrate of several luciferases found in aquatic microorganisms such as *Renilla reniformis* and *Gaussia princeps*.
- *HIF-1*: the hypoxia inducible factor-1 transcription factor is a heterodimer formed by the alpha and beta subunits. It is part of a family of transcription factors characterized by their basic helix-loop-helix (bHLH) DNA binding domain.
- *VEGF*: the vascular endothelial growth factor is a transcription factor involved in the formation of new vessels primarily during embryo development (*de novo* formation) but also in angiogenesis (from an existing vessel).
- *Quantum dot*: nanocrystal structures with semiconductor properties that can display fluorescent activity with emission peaks in the red-near infrared part of the spectrum.

SUMMARY POINTS

- Fluorescence and bioluminescence imaging are experiencing slow but steady advances to become another tool in clinical environments.
- These imaging techniques provide a functional insight that is not always achieved with other spatially powerful methods such as CT or MRI.
- BRET does not depend on an external source of excitation but rather on a chemical reaction, which facilitates the construction of self-illuminating probes for *in vivo* imaging.
- Functional imaging allows the visualization of biological processes associated with characteristic features of the disease, e.g. metastatic disease.
- We have designed a genetically encoded biosensor that serves as a valuable proof of concept and test benchmark for future hypoxia sensing probes based on small molecules or nanodevices powered by BRET.

ACKNOWLEDGEMENTS

We thank the members of Molecular Oncology Laboratory MOL for helpful discussions. We also thank M.E. Vazquez for useful inputs and assistance with the spectrophotometric analysis. We also thank Prof. R.Y. Tsien and Dr. W.H. Suh for kindly providing us with some of the reagents used in our study. This study was supported by the Spanish Ministry of Education and Science SAF2008-00543 and SAF2009-08629, Xunta de Galicia INCITE08PXIB208091PR (JAC) and by Fundacion de Investigacion Medica Mutua Madrileña (J.A.C., P.I.). Some of the figures were adapted from Biosensors & Biolectronics, 10, Iglesias, P. and Costoya, J.A., a novel BRET-based genetically encoded biosensor for functional imaging of hypoxia, 13126–13130, License number 2599470235384 (2011), with permission from Elsevier.

ABBREVIATIONS

BLI	:	Bioluminescent Light Imaging
BLIT	:	Bioluminescent Light Imaging Tomography
BRET	:	Bioluminescence Resonant Energy Transfer
CT	:	(X-Ray) Computed Tomography
ECL	:	E-M-H-mCherry-Luc
E-M-H	:	EGR-MRE-HRE
EGR	:	Early Growth Response
FLI	:	Fluorescent Light Imaging
FLIT	:	Fluorescent Light Imaging Tomography
FLuc	:	Firefly (*Photynus pyralis*) luciferase
FRET	:	Fluorescence Resonant Energy Transfer
GFP	:	Green Fluorescent Protein
HRE	:	Hypoxia Response Element
HIF-1	:	Hypoxia Inducible Factor-1
ICG	:	Indocyanine Green
MRE	:	Metal Response Element
MRI	:	Magnetic Resonance Imaging
NIR-F	:	Near Infrared Fluorescence
PET	:	Positron Emission Tomography
RLuc	:	Sea pansy (*Renilla reniformis*) luciferase
SPECT	:	Single Photon Emission Computed Tomography
VEGF	:	Vascular Endothelial Growth Factor

REFERENCES

Akagi Y, W Liu, B Zebrowski, K Xie and LM Ellis. 1998. Regulation of vascular endothelial growth factor expression in human colon cancer by insulin-like growth factor-I. Cancer Res 58: 4008–4014.

Alavi A, P Lakhani, A Mavi et al. 2004. PET: a revolution in medical Imaging. Radiol Clin North Am 42: 983–1001.

Alberts B et al. 2008. Molecular biology of the cell. 5th edn. Garland Science, New York.

Bárdos JI and M Ashcroft. 2004. Negative and positive regulation of HIF-1: a complex network. BioEssays 26: 262–269.

Bhang HC, KL Gabrielson, J Laterra, PB Fisher and MG Pomper. 2011. Tumor-specific imaging through progression elevated gene-3 promoter-driven gene expression. Nat Med 17: 123–130.

Brenner DJ et al. 2007. Computed Tomography—An Increasing Source of Radiation Exposure N Engl J Med 357(22): 2277–2284.

Dacres H, J Wang, MM Dumancic and SC Trowell. 2010. Experimental Determination of the Förster Distance for Two Commonly Used Bioluminescent Resonance Energy Transfer Pairs. Anal Chem 82: 432–435.

Dinca EB, RV Voicu and AV Ciurea. 2010. Bioluminescence imaging of invasive intracranial xenografts: implications for translational research and targeted therapeutics of brain tumors Neurosurg Rev 33: 385–394.

Dunn AK, T Bolay, MA Moskowitz and DA Boas. 2001. Dynamic imaging of cerebral blood flow using laser speckle. J Cereb Blood Flow Metab 2: 195–201.

Edinger M, YA Cao, YS Hornig, DE Jenkins, MR Verneris, MH Bachmann, RS Negrin and CH Contag. 2002. Advancing animal models of neoplasia through *in vivo* bioluminescence imaging. European Journal of Cancer 38: 2128–2136.

Hastings JW. 1983. Biological diversity, chemical mechanisms, and the evolutionary origins of bioluminescent systems. J Mol Evol 19: 309–321.

Iglesias P and JA Costoya. 2009. A novel BRET-based genetically encoded biosensor for functional imaging of hypoxia. Biosens Bioelec 10: 3126–3130.

Keereweer S, JD Kerrebijn, PB van Driel, B Xie, EL Kaijzel, TJ Snoeks, I Que, M Hutteman, JR van der Vorst, JS Mieog, AL Vahrmeijer, CJ van de Velde, RJ Baatenburg de Jong and CW Löwik. 2010. Optical Image-guided Surgery—Where Do We Stand? Mol Imaging Biol [Epub ahead of print].

Lee JY, YS Lee, KL Kim et al. 2006. A novel chimeric promoter that is highly responsive to hypoxia and metals. Gene Therapy 13: 857–868.

Mahmood U, and R Weissleder. 2003. Near-Infrared Optical Imaging of Proteases in Cancer Mol Cancer Ther 2: 489–496.

Mankoff DA. 2007. A Definition of Molecular Imaging. The Journal of Nuclear Medicine 48(6): 18N–21N.

Medintz IL, HT Uyeda, ER Goldman and H Mattoussi. 2005. Quantum dot bioconjugates for imaging, labelling and sensing. Nat Mat 4(6): 435–446.

Michelini E, M Mirasoli, M Karp et al. 2004. Development of a Bioluminescence Resonance Energy-Transfer Assay for Estrogen-Like Compound *in vivo* Monitoring. Anal Chem 76: 7069–7076.

Ntziachristos V, C Bremer and R Weissleder. 2003. Fluorescence imaging with near-infrared light: new technological advances that enable *in vivo* molecular imaging. Eur Radiol 13: 195–208.

Pfleger KDG and K Eidne. 2006. Illuminating insights into protein-protein interactions using bioluminescence resonance energy transfer (BRET). Nat Methods 3: 165–173.

Prinz A, M Diskar and FW Herberg. 2006. Application of bioluminescence resonance energy transfer (BRET) for biomolecular interaction studies. Chembiochem 7: 1007–1012.

Salnikow K, T Kluz, M Costa, D Piquemal, ZN Demidenko, K Xie and MV Blagosklonny. 2002. The Regulation of Hypoxic Genes by Calcium Involves c-Jun/AP-1, which Cooperates with Hypoxia-Inducible Factor 1 in Response to Hypoxia 22(6): 1734–1741.

Sampath L, W Wang and EM Sevick-Muraca. 2008. Near infrared fluorescent optical imaging for nodal staging. J Biomed Opt 13: 041312.

Seaman ME, G Contino, N Bardeesy and KA Kelly. 2010. Molecular imaging agents: impact on diagnosis and therapeutics in oncology. Expert Reviews in Molecular Medicine 12: e20.

Semenza, GL. 2003. Targeting HIF-1 for cancer therapy. Nat Rev Cancer 3: 721–732.

Shaner NC, RE Campbell, PA Steinbach et al. 2004. Improved monomeric red, orange and yellow fluorescent proteins derived from *Discosoma* sp. red fluorescent protein. Nat Biotechnol 22: 1567–1572.

Shaner NC, PA Steinbach and RY Tsien. 2005. A guide to choosing fluorescent proteins. Nature 2: 905–909.

So MK, C Xu C and AM Loening. 2006. Self-illuminating quantum dot conjugates for *in vivo* imaging. Nat Biotechnol 24: 339–343.

Soltesz EG, S Kim, SW Kim et al. 2006. Sentinel lymph node mapping of the gastrointestinal tract by using invisible light. Ann Surg Oncol 13: 386–396.

Tanaka E, HS Choi, H Fujii et al. 2006. Image-guided oncologic surgery using invisible light: Completed pre-clinical development for sentinel lymph node mapping. Ann Surg Onc 13: 1671–1681.

Torigian DA, SS Huang and M Houseini. 2007. Functional imaging of cancer with emphasis on molecular techniques. CA Cancer J Clin 57: 206–224.

Uhrbom L, E Nerio and EC Holland. 2004. Dissecting tumor maintenance requirements using bioluminescence imaging of cell proliferation in a mouse glioma model. Nat Med 10: 1257–1260.

Wang GL, BH Jiang, EA Rue and GL Semenza. 1995. Hypoxia-inducible factor 1 is a basic-helix-loop-helix-PAS heterodimer regulated by cellular O2 tension. Proc Natl Acad Sci USA 92: 5510–5514.

Weissleder R and V Ntziachristos. 2003. Shedding light onto live molecular targets. Nat Medicine 9: 123–128.

Wunderbaldinger P, K Turetschek and C Bremer. 2003. Near-infrared fluorescence imaging of lymph nodes using a new enzyme sensing activatable macromolecular optical probe. Eur Radiol 13: 2206–2211.

Zhong H, AM De Marzo, E Laughner et al. 1999. Overexpression of hypoxia-inducible factor 1 alpha in common human cancers and their metas- tases. Cancer Res (1999) 59: 5830–5835.

2

Use of a Surface Plasmon Resonance (SPR) Biosensor to Characterize Zwitterionic Coatings on SiO$_2$ for Cancer Biomarker Detection

Norman D. Brault,[1,a] Shaoyi Jiang[1,b] and Qiuming Yu[1,c,*]

ABSTRACT

The recent push to discover new cancer therapeutics from human matrices, such as serum or plasma, has been limited by the inability to fully verify low concentration biomarkers as being clinically relevant. For biosensing platforms to successfully aid in the development pipeline, they must meet several major design requirements. First, the sensing device must possess high sensitivity with the ability to resolve small changes in analyte binding, preferable in real-time. Second, due to the abundance of irrelevant proteins in serum (or plasma), the platform must effectively reduce non-specific protein adsorption. Finally, in order to possess high sensitivity and specificity, the sensing surface must

[1]Department of Chemical Engineering at the University of Washington, USA.
[a]E-mail: ndb16@u.washington.edu
[b]E-mail: sjiang@u.washington.edu
[c]E-mail: qyu@u.washington.edu
*Corresponding author

List of abbreviations after the text.

also enable the efficient immobilization of biorecognition elements for detecting target analytes with high affinity.

Advances in microelectromechanical system process technologies have led to numerous micro- and nano-scale biosensing platforms based on silicon substrates. Therefore, we briefly review current approaches for creating protein-resistant surface coatings using both "graft-from" and "graft-to" approaches. The recent development of zwitterionic polymer conjugates containing two carboxybetaine methacrylate (CBMA) polymers linked to two 3,4-dihydroxy-L-phenylalanine (DOPA) residues provides a convenient and simple approach for forming protein-resistant coatings on silica substrates as determined with a surface plasmon resonance biosensor. The zwitterionic nature of CBMA polymers significantly reduces protein adsorption while abundant carboxylic acid moieties provide for efficient antibody immobilization using common amino-coupling chemistries. By combining the adhesive properties of DOPA with zwitterionic CBMA, we introduce a new "graft-to" technology for cancer biomarker detection and show its ability to sensitively detect a model protein directly from undiluted human serum.

The transferability of the new "graft-to" technology enabled by zwitterionic polymer conjugates onto the sensing platform of a Si-based biosensor is demonstrated with a suspended micro-channel resonator (SMR). Successful *in situ* polymer attachment and antibody functionalization led to the detection of a cancer biomarker directly from complex media for the first time with a SMR device. The application of this new approach to other areas in the biomedical field, including nanoparticles for theranostic applications, illustrates the great potential for this novel surface coating.

INTRODUCTION

The mantra, "no biomarker, no drug" is frequently heard in a pharmaceutical industry heavily concerned with developing new cancer therapies (de Bono and Ashworth 2010). While some provide a specific target for selective cell cytotoxicity, biomarkers (e.g. proteins, metabolites, DNA, etc.) also play a vital role in early disease diagnostics, monitoring the therapeutic response, and improving patient stratification for treatment. The extreme complexity and heterogeneity of cancer both between patients and between cells within a patient has led to a continued push for discovering more biological indicators. However, the major shortcoming in the development pipeline is the inability of biosensors to fully verify these analytes as reliable targets resulting in few candidates reaching the patient's bedside (Brennan et al. 2010; Kulasingam et al. 2010).

Cancer biomarkers can be identified from several sources including human bodily fluids, tumor tissues, human cancer cell lines, and animal models. Due to the minimally invasive accessibility, abundance, and the ability of the circulatory system to reflect numerous and dynamic pathological states, plasma and serum are the most common choices for analysis. However, the complexity of these media (concentrations that span over 12 orders of magnitude with 22 proteins representing 99% of the total protein mass) has severely hindered the sensitive detection of biomarkers which are typically present at ng/mL to pg/mL quantities. Consequently, this has led to their inability to be verified as clinically relevant (Kulasingam et al. 2010).

These shortcomings have given rise to several major requirements for biosensor design. The low concentration of target analytes in complex media requires that the device possess high sensitivity thereby allowing for the quantification of small changes in response, preferably in real-time. Due to the presence of many irrelevant proteins, the platform must also effectively reduce non-specific protein adsorption (i.e. biofouling) from the plasma (or serum). Last, the biosensing surface must be able to sufficiently immobilize molecular recognition elements (e.g. antibodies) in order to provide highly specific detection (Vaisocherova et al. 2009). The ability to meet these challenges will better enable the verification of cancer biomarkers with high sensitivity and specificity.

In the following, we present a brief overview of current biosensing technology along with several protein-resistant materials frequently used in detection assays. As a result of the numerous advances in microelectromechanical system (MEMS) process technologies, many micro- and nano-scale biosensing devices are based on silicon (Hunt and Armani 2010; Libertino et al. 2009). Therefore, approaches for creating non-fouling surfaces on Si-based platforms are specifically addressed. Recently, the development of zwitterionic polymer conjugates containing the adhesive moiety, 3,4-dihydroxy-L-phenylalanine (DOPA), has enabled a new "graft-to" technology for the convenient attachment of non-fouling materials onto SiO_2 surfaces (Brault et al. 2010). Subsequent immobilization of antibodies onto the adsorbed polymer conjugates lead to the highly sensitive and specific detection of cancer biomarkers directly from undiluted human serum using a surface plasmon resonance (SPR) biosensor. The capability of attaching this material onto the SiO_2 surfaces of other micro/nano-scale platforms, thus indicative of the diagnostic potential for these zwitterionic conjugates, is then demonstrated with a suspended micro-channel resonator (SMR) (von Muhlen et al. 2010). We conclude with the future outlook of this new polymer system for additional applications in the biomedical field.

BIOSENSORS

While key components of biosensors include the microfluidics for sample delivery and the detection assay itself, the primary difference between platforms are the physical properties which are used for monitoring biomolecular interactions. For example, SPR sensors monitor changes in the optical properties of reflected light (Homola 2008). Others can measure changes in mechanical properties, such as the frequency of vibration for the SMR (Burg et al. 2007), or even monitor differences in electrical properties (e.g. conductance) as for field-effect transistors (FETs) (Zheng et al. 2005). Despite the apparent differences between biosensing devices, each technique can provide the high sensitivity necessary for cancer biomarker detection.

SPR Biosensors

SPR biosensing is an affinity-based optical technique that enables label-free and real-time detection of biomolecular interactions. Figure 2.1A shows a SPR platform which adapts the Kretschmann geometry of the attenuated total reflection configuration with wavelength modulation. The sensing chip consists of a glass slide coated with an adhesion-promoting titanium film (~2 nm) followed by a SPR active gold layer (~48 nm). Several materials, such a thin polymer films, are typically attached to the gold surface to provide the antibody immobilization and protein resistant background necessary for detection of analytes. Additionally, the use of a multichannel flow-cell allows several independent measurements to be conducted simultaneously.

The principles of SPR biosensing based on wavelength modulation have been reviewed extensively in the literature (Homola 2008). A polychromatic light beam is first directed through a prism where it contacts the gold surface of the substrate at a fixed angle of incidence. This leads to the coupling of optical energy (i.e. light at a specific wavelength) and the creation of a surface plasmon resonance which propagates along the boundary of the metal-dielectric interface (e.g. gold and water). The specific wavelength of light used to excite the surface plasmon resonance, the resonant wavelength, is highly sensitive to refractive index changes occurring in the dielectric within close proximity to the gold surface (i.e. less than 200–400 nm). The coupling and subsequent dissipation of energy associated with a specific resonant wavelength can be detected as a narrow "dip" in the spectrum of reflected light using a spectrophotometer (Fig. 2.1B). As the refractive index increases, such as for the binding of analytes onto immobilized receptors, the resonant wavelength also increases. Thus, by monitoring changes in the reflected light, highly sensitive label-free detection in real-time is enabled.

A

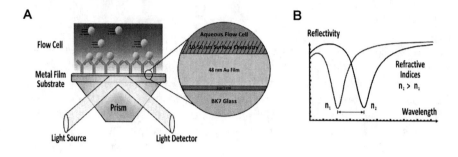

B

C

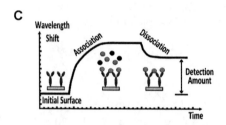

Figure 2.1. A surface plasmon resonance (SPR) biosensor based on wavelength modulation. **(A)** SPR gold substrates are typically modified with surface chemistry to enable probe molecule immobilization and a reduction in non-specific protein binding. Detection of analytes proceeds with a polychromatic light source that gets directed through a prism and strikes the SPR-active gold layer at a fixed angle of incidence; **(B)** The specific wavelength of light which couples to the gold surface plasmon resonance is detected by a spectrophotometer as a "dip" in the reflected spectrum. As the refractive index of the dielectric (i.e. solution side of the chip) increases, the resonant wavelength also increases; **(C)** Monitoring the resonant wavelength shift enables highly sensitive and label-free detection in real-time.

Figure 2.1C depicts a SPR sensor-gram, a plot of the resonant wavelength shift versus time, for the detection of antigens binding to an antibody functionalized sensor surface. After first flowing buffer to establish a stable baseline, a solution of antigens is injected into the device. The binding (association) of analytes to immobilized probe ligands increases the refractive index at the interface which increases the resonant wavelength. Upon flowing buffer, loosely bound analytes are removed (dissociated) from the surface thereby decreasing the resonant wavelength. After a sufficient amount of time the baseline flattens out. The difference between the starting and ending buffer baselines allows the specific amount of bound analyte to be quantified and converted to a surface coverage. These SPR devices have a limit of detection of ~0.1 ng/cm^2 (Homola 2006). Due to their relative ease of use and ability to sensitively monitor biomolecular interactions, these biosensors have been applied in numerous fields including medical diagnostics, food safety, national security, and environmental monitoring.

Silicon-based Micro/Nano-Biosensors

Emerging biosensing configurations have sought to create micro-scale and even nano-scale platforms with the goals of improving the detection sensitivity, decreasing the sample volume, and manufacturing portable devices. These small scale sensors also allow for reduced diffusion path lengths and overall faster kinetics (Libertino et al. 2009). To achieve these outcomes, many researchers have been focusing on Si-compatible systems due to the maturity of silicon technology in the semiconductor industry and the advances in MEMS processing techniques for this material. A variety of micro- and nano-scale biosensors have been developed based on different transducing mechanisms utilizing silicon. Several examples include the SMR, single silicon nanowire arrays, and micro-ring resonators, which are based on mechanical vibrations, electronic FETs, and photonic resonance, respectively (Burg et al. 2007; Ramachandran et al. 2008; Zheng et al. 2005).

SMR biosensors are composed of a small microfluidic channel which passes through a resonating cantilever vibrating in a vacuum. The adsorption of biomolecules onto the sensor surface decreases the resonating frequency thereby enabling label-free detection of analytes with sub-femtogram resolution. The dimensions of the micro-cantilever are $200 \times 33 \times 7 \ \mu m^3$ (length x width x thickness) with channels containing a cross-sectional area of $3 \times 8 \ \mu m^2$ (Burg et al. 2007). Silicon nanowire-based FET biosensors use a single Si-nanowire as a gate between the source and drain on SiO_2 on Si substrates. Charged proteins that adsorb onto the functionalized silicon nanowire induce a change in the source-drain conductivity at a fixed gate voltage thereby enabling detection with picogram sensitivity (Zheng et al. 2005). However, both of these examples represent a common disconnect within the biosensing field; an increase in sensor sensitivity does not necessarily translate to an increase in assay sensitivity. The inability to effectively reduce non-specific protein adsorption from undiluted human plasma (or serum) onto sensing surfaces has severely limited the full exploitation of these devices. Due to the presence of a native oxide layer on silicon surfaces upon exposure to air, it is desirable to develop convenient and effective surface coatings for SiO_2 in order to provide the non-fouling background necessary for highly sensitive and specific detection from complex media.

NON-FOULING SURFACE COATINGS

Non-specific protein adsorption onto surfaces (i.e. biofouling, Fig. 2.2A) primarily occurs via hydrophobic or electrostatic interactions (Ostuni et al. 2001). For biosensing, this can lead to an overwhelming background noise

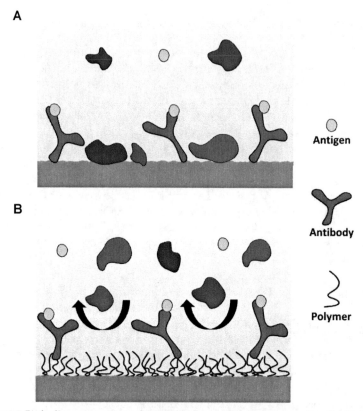

Figure 2.2. Biofouling on sensing surfaces. **(A)** Non-specific protein adsorption (i.e. biofouling) onto a sensing surface occurs primarily via hydrophobic or electrostatic interactions. For biosensing, this generates a large background noise and results in reduced detection limits and false-positives. **(B)** Protein resistant surface coatings reduce non-specific adsorption due to the presence of a hydration layer (i.e. a strongly structured layer of water) and thereby improve the signal-to-noise ratio necessary for highly sensitive and specific detection.

which decreases the detection sensitivity of low concentration biomarkers and increases false-positives. Protein-resistant surface coatings (Fig. 2.2B) can significantly reduce non-specific adsorption due to the presence of a hydration layer (i.e. a strongly structured water interface) thereby improving the signal-to-noise ratio and increasing the detection sensitivity and specificity (Chen et al. 2005). Several methods for reducing protein adsorption on biosensing platforms have been implemented.

Material Selection

Blocking agents (e.g. BSA, fish gelatin, etc.) and surface coatings are commonly employed in biosensors in order to reduce or eliminate fouling from complex media. The use of blocking agents suffer from several limitations including cross-reactivity with assay components and only a minor reduction in non-specific binding. This has given rise to surface coatings which have been found to be both more effective and robust. Ethylene glycol (EG) and its derivatives, such as poly(ethylene glycol) (PEG) or oligo-ethylene glycol (OEG) are the most commonly used materials for preventing protein adsorption. An example of an EG-based material is shown in Fig. 2.3A. Experimental evidence indicates that a combination of tightly bound hydrogen bonding-induced hydration layers, which generate a large repulsive force, in addition to steric effects of longer PEG chains are responsible for the non-fouling properties of this material (Jiang and Cao 2010). However, while these properties enable EG to resist fouling from diluted protein solutions (e.g. plasma diluted with PBS), it is only partially effective against 100% human serum (or plasma) (Ladd et al. 2008).

Despite its benefits, the use of EG for detection of cancer biomarkers underscores a vital criterion for biosensing; in order to obtain highly sensitive detection, the immobilization of molecular recognition elements (e.g. antibodies) must be both efficient and occur without negatively affecting the protein resistance of the surface coating. Relatively complex

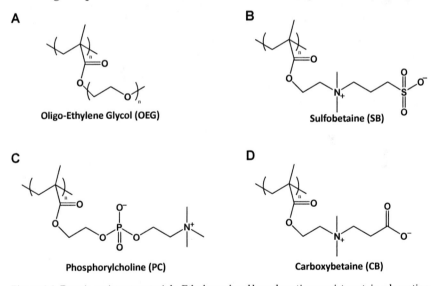

A

Oligo-Ethylene Glycol (OEG)

B

Sulfobetaine (SB)

C

Phosphorylcholine (PC)

D

Carboxybetaine (CB)

Figure 2.3. Protein resistant materials. Ethylene glycol based coatings resist protein adsorption by forming a tightly bound hydrogen-bonding induced hydration layer that provides a repulsive force against non-specific binding. **(A)** Zwitterionic materials such as sulfobetaine **(B)**, phosphorylcholine **(C)**, and carboxybetaine **(D)** offer improved protein resistance by achieving much stronger hydration via electrostatic interactions. (Adapted from Jiang and Cao. Copyright 2010 Wiley-VCH Verlag GmbH & Co. KGaA. Reproduced with permission.)

chemical reaction steps are necessary to functionalized EG-based materials. Furthermore, the use of blocking agents to pacify unreacted activated groups is also necessary. Both of these requirements typically result in worsening the non-fouling properties and thereby limit the overall effectiveness of this material for biosensing applications (Hucknall et al. 2009).

Recently, zwitterionic polymers have been shown to offer improved protein resistance from complex media compared to that of EG. These materials, such as sulfobetaine (SB), phosphorylcholine (PC), and carboxybetaine (CB) as shown in Fig. 2.3B-D, achieve much stronger hydration via electrostatic interactions, which provides the primary physical mechanism for improved non-fouling properties (Chen et al. 2005). It has been demonstrated that highly dense zwitterionic polymer films with controlled lengths exhibited undetectable adsorption to both single protein solutions and undiluted human serum and plasma using a SPR biosensor (Yang et al. 2009). Furthermore, the presence of a carboxylate group in each monomer of CB polymers enables the convenient attachment of antibodies via common N-ethyl-N'-(3-dimethylaminopropyl) carbodiimide /N-hydroxysuccinimide (EDC/NHS) amino-coupling chemistry. The hydrolysis of unreacted NHS-esters simply converts the activated groups back into the original non-fouling zwitterionic background without the use of blocking agents. This has been shown to result in highly sensitive cancer biomarker detection (~10 ng/mL) directly from undiluted human plasma using thin films of CB polymers formed via surface initiated-atom transfer radical polymerization (SI-ATRP) (Vaisocherova et al. 2008).

Protein Resistant Coatings for Oxide Surfaces

The nearly continuous design and manufacture of novel Si-based sensor platforms with unprecedented sensitivity have made non-fouling surface coatings for SiO_2 surfaces highly desirable. In order to coat silica surfaces with thin films of protein-resistant zwitterionic polymers, two methods can be adopted, "graft-from" and "graft-to", as shown in Fig. 2.4 (Currie et al. 2003). For the "graft-from" approach (Fig. 2.4A), the original silica substrate is first modified with a monolayer of silane initiators to introduce the reactive group (e.g. bromine) necessary for subsequent polymerization (Zhang et al. 2006). After adding the appropriate monomer and catalysts, the polymerization reaction proceeds allowing for the formation of dense films over a wide range of controlled thicknesses (Yang et al. 2009). Zwitterionic polymers "grafted-from" glass substrates via SI-ATRP have been previously shown to be highly resistant to protein adsorption (Zhang et al. 2006).

The "graft-to" approach (Fig. 2.4B) enables the convenient attachment of protein resistant surface coatings by exposing the substrate to pre-synthesized polymer conjugates composed of a non-fouling polymer

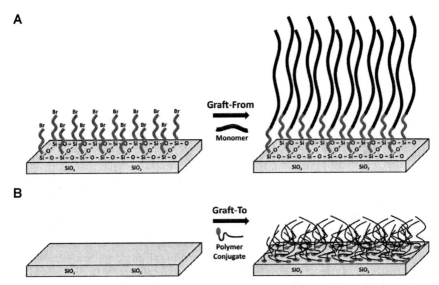

Figure 2.4. Two approaches to form protein resistant surfaces on silica substrates. **(A)** The "graft-from" technique first modifies the original substrate with a monolayer of silane polymerization initiators. Upon the addition of the monomer and catalysts, the reaction proceeds and can result in the formation of dense films with controlled thicknesses. **(B)** The "graft-to" approach can be much more convenient for the smaller geometries of micro/nano-scale biosensors. This method enables the attachment of protein resistant surface coatings by exposing the substrate to pre-synthesized conjugates a non-fouling polymer covalently linked to an adhesive moiety.

covalently linked to an adhesive moiety (Gao et al. 2010). The adhesive group can be a single molecule, such as DOPA, or a polymer, such as poly-L-lysine. DOPA is a molecule found in mussel adhesive proteins and has been shown to strongly adhere to numerous types of substrates including noble metals, native oxides, and ceramics (Lee et al. 2007).

While there are advantages and disadvantages of each method, the adoption of either the "graft-from" or "graft-to" approach will depend upon the particular application. The "graft-from" approach offers the ability to obtain high surface densities of non-fouling groups with finely controlled polymer lengths, both of which have been found to be very important for preventing protein adsorption (Yang et al. 2009). On the other hand, this technique is relatively time consuming and is difficult to implement directly onto devices *in situ* or in the small and confined geometries of the microfluidic systems being designed into novel biosensor platforms (Currie et al. 2003, Gao et al. 2010). The major advantage of the "graft-to" method is that it provides simple and convenient attachment of polymers directly onto device sensing components even within nano-scale geometries. However, the lack of film thickness control and limited surface coverage are the major concerns for this approach (Dalsin et al. 2005).

Advances in "Graft-to" Technology

The ability of DOPA to strongly adhere to numerous substrates has made it highly attractive as an adhesive moiety for new "graft-to" technologies. Previous reports have shown the ability of DOPA-PEG conjugates to form protein resistant coatings on oxide substrates. Furthermore, the surface coverage of these polymer conjugates could then be increased by increasing the number of anchor residues (i.e. one, two, or three DOPA groups per polymer chain) (Dalsin et al. 2005). Conjugates composed of zwitterionic poly(sulfobetaine methacrylate) (pSBMA) and a single DOPA residue have been successfully synthesized and "grafted-to" gold surfaces containing methyl-, hydroxyl-, and amino-terminated self-assembled monolayers. While a significant reduction in protein adsorption was obtained from complex media, the lack of available functional groups for ligand immobilization in pSBMA limited its future use for biosensing applications (Li et al. 2008).

In order to maximize the surface density of non-fouling groups and provide for functionalization capabilities, zwitterionic poly(carboxybetaine methacrylate) (pCBMA) polymers were combined with DOPA residues to create a novel "graft-to" technology. Here, two DOPA-pCBMA polymer conjugates were linked together to create DOPA$_2$-pCBMA$_2$ (Fig. 2.5). The di-DOPA anchor combined with two pCBMA chains was successfully

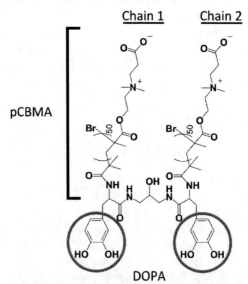

Figure 2.5. The DOPA$_2$-pCBMA$_2$ chemical structure. These polymer conjugates are formed by chemically linking two carboxybetaine methacrylate (CBMA) polymer chains to two 3,4-dihydroxy-L-phenylalanine (DOPA) residues thereby maximizing the surface density of non-fouling and functionalizable groups "grafted-to" a substrate.

attached to gold substrates. Following antibody immobilization, the excellent non-fouling background enabled a target protein to be detected directly from undiluted human plasma using a SPR biosensor (Gao et al. 2010). This demonstrated the importance of developing protein resistant surface coatings which could be conveniently attached to a sensing surface all while obtaining the immobilization capabilities and the post-functionalization non-fouling properties necessary for highly sensitive detection from complex media.

ZWITTERIONIC COATINGS FOR SILICA SUBSTRATES ANALYZED WITH A SPR BIOSENSOR

The presence of SiO_2 in many novel and highly sensitive biosensors has created the need to develop a convenient approach to form non-fouling and functionalizable surface coatings for this material. The sensitivity offered by SPR devices combined with their versatility make them appropriate tools for evaluating new surface chemistries developed for other sensing platforms. Figure 2.6 shows the key procedures for using SPR biosensors to evaluate the performance of a new "graft-to" technology using zwitterionic polymer conjugates developed for silica surfaces (Brault et al. 2010). After

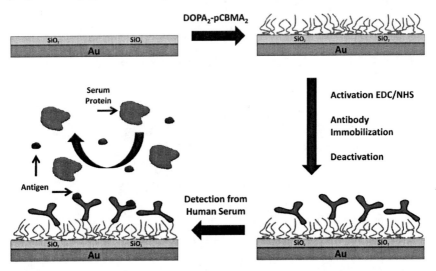

Figure 2.6. The key steps of using SPR biosensors for evaluating the performance of a new zwitterionic "graft-to" technology on silica. After the formation of stable SiO_2 substrates, the polymer conjugate is conveniently grafted *in situ* by flowing the solution through the SPR biosensor. Following antibody immobilization and deactivation of residual activated groups by converting them back into the non-fouling zwitterionic background, the functionalized surface can be used for cancer biomarker detection directly from complex media. (Adapted with permission from Brault et al. Copyright 2010 Elsevier.)

the formation of stable SiO_2 substrates, the polymer attachment, non-fouling properties, immobilization of probe molecules, and subsequent detection of a target analyte directly from undiluted human serum can all be studied in real-time using a SPR biosensor.

The protein, activate leukocyte cell adhesion molecule (ALCAM) was used as a model cancer biomarker. ALCAM is a 105 kDa protein with a normal presence in human blood with evidence for being linked to multiple carcinomas (Ofori-Acquah and King 2008). Thus, a monoclonal antibody to ALCAM (anti-ALCAM) was used to determine the detection sensitivity and specificity of functionalized $DOPA_2$-$pCBMA_2$ coated silica surfaces for detection from complex media.

SiO$_2$ Thin Film Coated SPR Chips

In order for the SiO_2 thin film coated onto the SPR chips to serve as a model system for other biosensor platforms, it must be compatible to a variety of conditions and maintain its stability during detections. Therefore, SiO_2 coated chips were tested under a variety of pH values (1–10), solutions/ organic solvents (e.g. 3M NaCl in PBS, DMF/water, THF, ethanol, and acetone), and temperatures (25°C–40°C). Highly stable silica substrates (Fig. 2.7) were obtained by coating an additional titanium layer (1 nm) on top of a standard gold chip (Fig. 2.1A) followed by depositing SiO_2 (20 nm) via plasma enhanced chemical vapor deposition.

Since SPR sensitivity depends upon the distance of the binding event from the active layer (i.e. gold) (Homola 2008), the change in the sensor response due to the additional titanium and silica layers has to be calibrated.

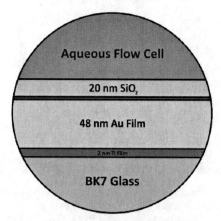

Figure 2.7. Silica substrates for SPR biosensing. Stable silica films are formed by coating an additional adhesion promoting layer of titanium (1 nm) on top of the original gold chips, followed by a thin film of silica (20 nm).

The calibration can be completed using either an experimental approach or via theoretical simulations. The average value of the calibration factor is 1.37 for this system, using both methods. This means that a 1 nm shift in the resonant wavelength for the silica substrates corresponds to a ~1.4 nm shift on standard gold chips (or a protein surface coverage of ~23 ng/cm²). The SPR sensitivity is slightly decreased to 0.14 ng/cm² from 0.1 ng/cm² due to the existence of the additional titanium and silica. These thin layers also have a negligible effect on the plasmonic properties of the gold layer as a deep, narrow SPR "dip" can be obtained. Hence, these stable SiO_2 films enable the use of SPR biosensors for studying the "graft-to" attachment of the polymer conjugates, subsequent antibody immobilization, and cancer biomarker detection from complex media.

Attachment of Polymer Conjugates

The convenient attachment of $DOPA_2$-$pCBMA_2$ onto silica substrates can be easily monitored with a SPR biosensor. As shown in Fig. 2.8, the grafting of the polymer conjugates to the SiO_2 results in an increase in the resonant wavelength. The total surface coverage of bound $DOPA_2$-$pCBMA_2$ can then be easily calculated as the difference between the water baselines. Furthermore, the minor decrease as a result of flowing PBS indicates that the adsorbed material is firmly attached and cannot easily be removed. In

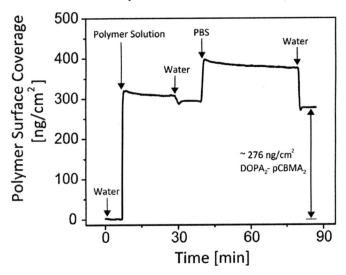

Figure 2.8. The convenient attachment of $DOPA_2$-$pCBMA_2$ onto silica substrates as monitored with a SPR biosensor. The difference between the starting and ending baselines in the sensorgram quantifies the total amount of absorbed polymer. (Adapted with permission from Brault et al. Copyright 2010 Elsevier.)

order to increase the amount of polymer conjugates "grafted-to" the surface and subsequently optimize the non-fouling and protein immobilization properties, a variety of experimental grafting conditions have been tested including pH (3–10), temperature (25°C–40°C), and ionic strength (10 mM to 1 M). The optimal condition for a 20 min *in situ* attachment protocol is pH 8.5 Tris buffer (10 mM) at room temperature. Decreasing pH and increasing the ionic strength decreases the net polymer adsorption thereby providing the ability to control the final film thickness. Temperature has a negligible effect over the range tested.

For DOPA$_2$-pCBMA$_2$ to achieve highly sensitive detection and serve as a reliable material for biosensing applications, the non-fouling properties of the surface coating have to be determined. The SPR sensor-grams for undiluted human plasma and serum being flowed over the DOPA$_2$-pCBMA$_2$ coated silica surface are shown in Fig. 2.9. The results indicate that challenging the surface to complex media does not reduce the non-fouling properties of the DOPA$_2$-pCBMA$_2$ coated silica thereby enabling it to be used for ligand immobilization and subsequent cancer biomarker detection.

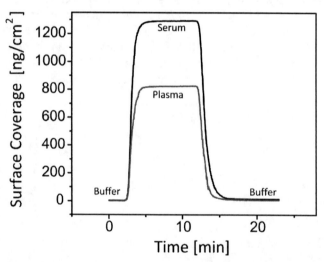

Figure 2.9. The non-fouling properties of the DOPA$_2$-pCBMA$_2$ coated silica substrates to undiluted human serum and plasma as measured with a SPR biosensor. The small difference between the starting and ending PBS buffer baselines indicate that challenging the surface to complex media does not reduce the protein resistant properties of the zwitterionic polymer conjugates. (Adapted with permission from Brault et al. Copyright 2010 Elsevier.)

Immobilization of Antibodies

Material properties that enable non-fouling and efficient immobilization of molecular recognition elements are two vital characteristics of surface coatings for biosensing applications. Following the successful attachment of $DOPA_2$-$pCBMA_2$ onto the silica substrates, anti-ALCAM antibodies are covalently immobilized to the sensing surface via commonly used EDC/NHS amino-coupling chemistry. A simple deactivation step hydrolyzes the remaining NHS-activated esters back into the original low-fouling zwitterionic background without the use of blocking agents.

In order to increase the immobilization efficiency, a slightly basic buffer solution that provides a pH greater than the isoelectric-point of the antibody must be used. This is because of the slight positive charge created near the interface of the zwitterionic CB surface and the buffer solution due to the consumption of the carboxylic groups during EDC/NHS activation. The attractive electrostatic interactions drive the antibodies to the surface leading to higher levels of immobilization. The same strategy was also applied to the immobilization of antibodies onto zwitterionic CB polymer surfaces made via SI-ATRP (Vaisocherova et al. 2008; Vaisocherova et al. 2009; Yang et al. 2009). In addition to EDC/NHS chemistry, other methods can also be used to immobilize antibodies to surfaces, such as physical adsorption (e.g. with hydrophobic coatings) and affinity-based immobilization (e.g. avidin-biotin linkages). Specifically oriented antibodies can also be achieved under certain conditions but the increase in sensitivity which accompanies proper orientation does not often justify the added assay complexity (Rusmini et al. 2007). Regardless, the ability to successfully immobilize anti-ALCAM using EDC/NHS chemistry combined with a simple deactivation step enables the functionalized "graft-to" surface coating to be used for cancer biomarker detection.

Detection of Cancer Biomarkers

The cancer biomarker, ALCAM, has been used to investigate the sensitivity of the anti-ALCAM functionalized $DOPA_2$-$pCBMA_2$ coated silica surface for detection directly from undiluted complex media. Figure 2.10 shows the binding specificity achieved for this system. Here, anti-ALCAM is immobilized on two SPR channels using identical procedures. After establishing a stable buffer baseline, undiluted human serum is flowed through one channel while serum spiked with a known concentration of ALCAM is flowed through the second channel. The larger detection for the spiked sample is due to the additional specific binding of the desired antigen/antibody interaction. Repeating this experiment using spiked concentrations ranging from 25 ng/mL to 1 µg/mL results in a standard curve with a limit of detection of ~64 ng/mL as shown in Fig. 2.11.

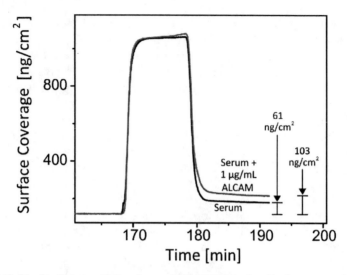

Figure 2.10. The binding specificity of an anti-ALCAM functionalized sensor surface. An antibody to the cancer biomarker ALCAM (anti-ALCAM) is immobilized on two SPR channels using identical procedures. After establishing a stable baseline with PBS buffer, undiluted human serum and serum spiked with a known concentration of ALCAM are flowed through channels 1 and 2, respectively. The larger detection for the spiked sample is due to the additional specific binding of the desired antigen/antibody interaction. (Adapted with permission from Brault et al. Copyright 2010 Elsevier.)

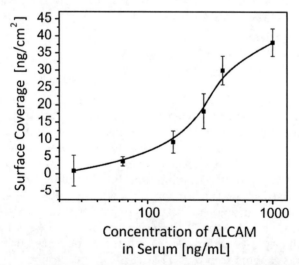

Figure 2.11. The standard detection curve for an anti-ALCAM functionalized $DOPA_2$-$pCBMA_2$ coated surface on silica substrates using a SPR biosensor. The limit of detection from undiluted human serum using an antibody to the cancer biomarker ALCAM (anti-ALCAM) is ~64 ng/ mL. The plot shows the mean plus one standard deviation (n = 3). (Adapted with permission from Brault et al. Copyright 2010 Elsevier.)

APPLYING DOPA$_2$-pCBMA$_2$ TO THE SMR BIOSENSOR PLATFORM

The convenient and robust "graft-to" technology for coating DOPA$_2$-pCBMA$_2$ polymer conjugates onto silica surfaces has been transferred to other Si-based biosensing platforms for the detection of cancer biomarkers from complex media. The grafting of these conjugates onto the highly sensitive Si-based SMR device has been achieved using the simple *in situ* attachment protocol developed with SPR biosensors. The resulting non-fouling properties outperformed PEG based materials. Furthermore, successful antibody functionalization yielded highly sensitive detection from undiluted complex media for the first time using a SMR biosensor (von Muhlen et al. 2010). Figure 2.12 shows the sensor response curves for the direct detection of ALCAM spiked into undiluted fetal bovine serum. The limit of detection from the serum was found to be ~10 ng/mL.

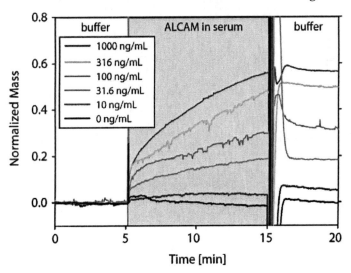

Figure 2.12. The sensor response curves for the direct detection of the cancer biomarker, ALCAM, spiked into undiluted serum using a suspended micro-channel resonator biosensor. The *in situ* attachment of DOPA$_2$-pCBMA$_2$ followed by antibody immobilization enables the detection of the target analyte down to 10 ng/mL. (Adapted with permission from von Mulen et al. Copyright 2010 American Chemical Society.)

APPLICATIONS TO OTHER AREAS OF HEALTH AND DISEASE

The ability to sensitively detect ALCAM directly from complex media using the SMR device indicates the great potential of the DOPA$_2$-pCBMA$_2$

surface coating approach. This material also holds promise for many other Si-based platforms such as Si nanowire arrays and micro-ring resonators. Additionally, nanoparticle-based systems also suffer from instability and aggregation due to non-specific protein binding which can lead to reduced blood circulation half-lives for *in vivo* applications. Therefore, the use of the "graft-to" technology developed here can also be applied to these systems for improving drug targeting, gene delivery, and *in vivo* imaging. For example, magnetic iron oxide nanoparticles coated with DOPA-pCBMA polymer conjugates exhibit excellent stability in serum. Sufficient peptide immobilization significantly improved cell targeting efficiency thereby offering great promise for *in vivo* theranostics using magnetic resonance imaging (Zhang et al. 2010). Other potential areas such as separation and isolation of circulating cancer cells from blood and medical implants are just a few of the numerous applications where the simple and convenient attachment of non-fouling and functionalizable surface coatings can be applied.

KEY FACTS OF SURFACE PLASMON RESONANCE (SPR) BIOSENSORS

- SPR biosensors are affinity-based optical devices which enable label-free and real-time measurements of biomolecular interactions with high sensitivity. They have been applied in numerous applications ranging from medical diagnostics to environmental monitoring.
- As molecules bind to immobilized receptors on SPR substrates they increase the refractive index near the interface which results in a change in the SPR characteristic detected in the reflected light.
- SPR biosensors can monitor changes in refractive index on the order of 10^{-7} refractive index units and within a distance of ~200–400 nm from a SPR-active gold surface.
- Direct detection, sandwich, and inhibition assays are the three primary detection formats used with SPR biosensors.
- SPR biosensing technology has two major limitations. First, the specificity of detection is solely based on the affinity of the molecular recognition element used. Secondly, these sensors suffer from interfering effects, such as non-specific protein binding, thus requiring methods for reducing unwanted interactions near the surface.

DEFINITIONS

- *Surface Plasmon Resonance*: Surface plasmon resonance is an electromagnetic wave that propagates along the interface between a metal film (e.g. gold) and a dielectric (e.g. water). Surface plasmon resonance is characterized by a propagation constant and an electromagnetic field distribution which decays exponentially into the dielectric. Changes in refractive index that occur within the probe range of the electromagnetic field result in changes in the propagation constant which can be accurately measured via optical techniques.

- *Resonant Wavelength*: For SPR sensors based on wavelength modulation with prism coupling, the specific wavelength of light which can excite a surface plasmon resonance is called the resonant wavelength. The resonant wavelength is then absent in the reflected light, creating a dip in the spectrum, and used to quantify biomolecular interactions.

- *"Graft-from"*: A surface polymerization technique in which the substrate is first modified with a monolayer of a chemical initiator containing a specific reactive group (e.g. bromine). Addition of monomer and catalysts allow polymers to be grown from the surface.

- *"Graft-to"*: A surface coating technique in which pre-synthesized polymer conjugates containing a polymer chemically linked to an adhesive group are used to adhere to various substrates. The adhesive group can either be a single compound or another polymer.

- *Zwitterionic Polymers*: Zwitterionic polymers contain both cationic and anionic (i.e. positive and negative) charges within each monomer.

- *EDC/NHS Chemistry*: A reaction chemistry which couples carboxylic acid groups to primary amines using zero-length cross-linking reagents. The EDC first reacts with the carboxylic acid moiety which subsequently reacts with NHS to create a relatively stable intermediate. Upon the introduction of primary amine containing molecules, the NHS-intermediate reacts to form a peptide bond. Un-reacted NHS groups can be hydrolyzed using slightly basic aqueous conditions thereby reforming the original carboxylic group.

SUMMARY POINTS

- For biosensors to aid in cancer biomarker discovery and achieve highly sensitive and specific detection directly from complex media they must meet three major requirements: possess high sensitivity, reduce non-specific protein adsorption, and enable efficient immobilization of molecular recognition elements.

- Advances in processing technologies have given rise to many micro- and nano-scale biosensing devices based on silicon. The recent development of polymer conjugates containing the adhesive moiety, 3,4-dihydroxy-L-phenylalanine, and zwitterionic carboxybetaine methacrylate provides a novel "graft-to" approach for the convenient attachment of a non-fouling and functionalizable material onto SiO_2.

- Using a surface plasmon resonance biosensor, the successful *in situ* grafting of the zwitterionic polymer conjugates to silica substrates enables sensitive cancer biomarker detection directly from undiluted human serum.
- The convenience and robustness of this new technology has been applied to a Si-based biosensor platform, the suspended microchannel resonator. Successful *in situ* attachment of the zwitterionic polymer conjugates and subsequent antibody immobilization enabled highly sensitive detection of cancer biomarkers from complex media for the first time with this device.
- Other potential areas such as coatings for nanoparticles, separation and isolation of circulating cancer cells from blood, and medical implants are just a few of the numerous applications where this new approach can be applied.

ABBREVIATIONS

ALCAM	:	Activated Leukocyte Cell Adhesion Molecule
Anti-ALCAM	:	Antibody to ALCAM
BSA	:	Bovine Serum Albumin
CB	:	Carboxybetaine
CBMA	:	Carboxybetaine Methacrylate
DMF	:	Dimethylformamide
DOPA	:	3,4-dihydroxy-L-phenylalanine
EDC	:	N-ethyl-N'-(3-dimethylaminopropyl) Carbodiimide
EG	:	Ethylene Glycol
FET	:	Field-effect Transistors
MEMS	:	Microelectromechanical System
NHS	:	N-hydroxysuccinimide
OEG	:	Oligo Ethylene Glycol
PBS	:	Phosphate Buffered Saline
PC	:	Phosphorylcholine
pCBMA	:	Poly(Carboxybetaine Methacrylate)
PEG	:	Poly(Ethylene Glycol)
pSBMA	:	Poly(Sulfobetaine Methacrylate)
SB	:	Sulfobetaine
SBMA	:	Sulfobetaine Methacrylate
Si	:	Silicon

SI-ATRP	:	Surface Initiated-Atom Transfer Radical Polymerization
SMR	:	Suspended Micro-channel Resonator
SPR	:	Surface Plasmon Resonance
THF	:	Tetrahydrofuran

REFERENCES

Brault ND, CL Gao, H Xue, M Piliarik, J Homola, SY Jiang and QM Yu. 2010. Ultra-low fouling and functionalizable zwitterionic coatings grafted onto SiO2 via a biomimetic adhesive group for sensing and detection in complex media. Biosens Bioelectron 25: 2276–2282.

Brennan DJ, DP O'Connor, E Rexhepaj, F Ponten and WM Gallagher. 2010. Antibody-based proteomics: fast-tracking molecular diagnostics in oncology. Nat Rev Cancer 10: 605–617.

Burg TP, M Godin, SM Knudsen, W Shen, G Carlson, JS Foster, K Babcock and SR Manalis. 2007. Weighing of biomolecules, single cells and single nanoparticles in fluid. Nature 446: 1066–1069.

Chen SF, J Zheng, LY Li and SY Jiang. 2005. Strong resistance of phosphorylcholine self-assembled monolayers to protein adsorption: Insights into nonfouling properties of zwitterionic materials. J Am Chem Soc 127: 14473–14478.

Currie EPK, W Norde and MAC Stuart. 2003. Tethered polymer chains: Surface chemistry and their impact on colloidal and surface properties. Advances in Colloid and Interface Science 100: 205–265.

Dalsin JL, LJ Lin, S Tosatti, J Voros, M Textor and PB Messersmith. 2005. Protein resistance of titanium oxide surfaces modified by biologically inspired mPEG-DOPA. Langmuir 21: 640–646.

de Bono JS and A Ashworth. 2010. Translating cancer research into targeted therapeutics. Nature 467: 543–549.

Gao CL, GZ Li, H Xue, W Yang, FB Zhang and S.Y. Jiang. 2010. Functionalizable and ultra-low fouling zwitterionic surfaces via adhesive mussel mimetic linkages. Biomaterials 31: 1486–1492.

Homola J. 2006. Surface plasmon resonance based sensors. Springer, Berlin, New York.

Homola J. 2008. Surface plasmon resonance sensors for detection of chemical and biological species. Chemical Reviews 108: 462–493.

Hucknall A, S Rangarajan and A Chilkoti. 2009. In Pursuit of Zero: Polymer Brushes that Resist the Adsorption of Proteins. Advanced Materials 21: 2441–2446.

Hunt HK and AM Armani. 2010. Label-free biological and chemical sensors. Nanoscale 2: 1544–1559.

Jiang SY and ZQ Cao. 2010. Ultralow-Fouling, Functionalizable, and Hydrolyzable Zwitterionic Materials and Their Derivatives for Biological Applications. Advanced Materials 22: 920–932.

Kulasingam V, MP Pavlou and EP Diamandis. 2010. Integrating high-throughput technologies in the quest for effective biomarkers for ovarian cancer. Nat Rev Cancer 10: 371–378.

Ladd J, Z Zhang, S Chen, JC Hower and S Jiang. 2008. Zwitterionic polymers exhibiting high resistance to nonspecific protein adsorption from human serum and plasma. Biomacromolecules 9: 1357–1361.

Lee H, SM Dellatore, WM Miller and PB Messersmith. 2007. Mussel-inspired surface chemistry for multifunctional coatings. Science 318: 426–430.

Li GZ, G Cheng, H Xue, SF Chen, FB Zhang and SY Jiang. 2008. Ultra low fouling zwitterionic polymers with a biomimetic adhesive group. Biomaterials 29: 4592–4597.

Libertino S, V Aiello, A Scandurra, M Renis, F Sinatra and S Lombardo. 2009. Feasibility Studies on Si-Based Biosensors. Sensors 9: 3469–3490.

Ofori-Acquah SF and JA King. 2008. Activated leukocyte cell adhesion molecule: a new paradox in cancer. Translational Research 151: 122–128.

Ostuni E, RG Chapman, RE Holmlin, S Takayama and GM Whitesides. 2001. A survey of structure-property relationships of surfaces that resist the adsorption of protein. Langmuir 17: 5605–5620.

Ramachandran A, S Wang, J Clarke, SJ Ja, D Goad, L Wald, EM Flood, E Knobbe, JV Hryniewicz, ST Chu, D Gill, W Chen, O King and BE Little. 2008. A universal biosensing platform based on optical micro-ring resonators. Biosens Bioelectron 23: 939–944.

Rusmini F, ZY Zhong and J Feijen. 2007. Protein immobilization strategies for protein biochips. Biomacromolecules 8: 1775–1789.

Vaisocherova H, W Yang, Z Zhang, ZQ Cao, G Cheng, M Piliarik, J Homola and SY Jiang. 2008. Ultralow fouling and functionalizable surface chemistry based on a zwitterionic polymer enabling sensitive and specific protein detection in undiluted blood plasma. Anal Chem 80: 7894–7901.

Vaisocherova H, Z Zhang, W Yang, ZQ Cao, G Cheng, AD Taylor, M Piliarik, J Homola and SY Jiang. 2009. Functionalizable surface platform with reduced nonspecific protein adsorption from full blood plasma-Material selection and protein immobilization optimization. Biosens Bioelectron 24: 1924–1930.

von Muhlen MG, ND Brault, SM Knudsen, SY Jiang and SR Manalis. 2010. Label-Free Biomarker Sensing in Undiluted Serum with Suspended Microchannel Resonators. Anal Chem 82: 1905–1910.

Yang W, H Xue, W Li, JL Zhang and SY Jiang. 2009. Pursuing "Zero" Protein Adsorption of Poly(carboxybetaine) from Undiluted Blood Serum and Plasma. Langmuir 25: 11911–11916.

Zhang L, H Xue, CL Gao, L Carr, JN Wang, B Chu and SY Jiang. 2010. Imaging and cell targeting characteristics of magnetic nanoparticles modified by a functionalizable zwitterionic polymer with adhesive 3,4-dihydroxyphenyl-L-alanine linkages. Biomaterials 31: 6582–6588.

Zhang Z, T Chao, SF Chen and SY Jiang. 2006. Superlow fouling sulfobetaine and carboxybetaine polymers on glass slides. Langmuir 22: 10072–10077.

Zheng GF, F Patolsky, Y Cui, WU Wang and CM Lieber. 2005. Multiplexed electrical detection of cancer markers with nanowire sensor arrays. Nat Biotechnol 23: 1294–1301.

3

Microcantilever-based Biosensor Array for Tumor Angiogenic Marker Detection

Riccardo Castagna[1] and Carlo Ricciardi[1,a,*]

ABSTRACT

The development of cantilever-based biosensors for molecular recognition is a recent advance in life science and biochemistry that has generated great expectations in the scientific community for its fundamental and technological perspectives. Cantilever-based sensors are ultrasensitive label-free detectors that have been successfully applied to the identification of nucleic acids and disease proteins, as well as single viruses and bacteria. As for most of immunoassays and biosensors, cantilever surface needs to be functionalized with a proper probe to selectively bind the target molecule.

In the following chapter, we provide the basic knowledge concerning cantilever working principles and detection methods, while focussing mainly on recent developments concerning the application of microcantilever biosensor array to tumour angiogenic marker detection. Microcantilever biosensors are able to detect minimum masses of angiogenic growth factors as Angiopoietin-1 with very high precision (few hundreds of picograms with less than 0.5% of relative uncertainty).

[1]Politecnico di Torino, Applied Science and Technology Department, Corso Duca degli Abruzzi 24, 10129 Torino, Italy.
[a]E-mail: carlo.ricciardi@polito.it
*Corresponding author

List of abbreviations after the text.

Specificity tests performed with different angiogenic growth factors such as Angiopoietin-1 and Vascular Endothelial Growth Factor A_{165} show that contributions coming from non-specific biomolecular interactions are nearly two orders of magnitude lower than typical signals due to specific recognition.

Microcantilever biosensors can also be integrated on microfluidic platforms to develop a Lab-On-Chip able to real-time monitor the kinetics of antibody-antigen complex formation. Such a device is a good candidate for a sensitive and specific, as well as rapid, cheap and portable instrument for next generation diagnostic tools that will be employed at or near the site of patient care (Point-Of-Care testing).

INTRODUCTION

Angiogenesis is the process that leads to the formation of new blood vessel growth from existing ones and plays an essential role in the development of tissues in the vertebrate embryo (Carmeliet 2000). It is also involved in a wide variety of physiological and pathological conditions in adults, including wound repair, metabolic diseases, inflammation, cardiovascular disorders, and tumour progression.

Tumour angiogenesis is a complex dynamic process consisting of extracellular matrix re-modelling, endothelial cell proliferation and capillary differentiation, coordinated by several classes of growth factors (GFs) acting through cognate tyrosine kinase receptors (TKRs) (Steeg 2006). Foremost among GFs and TKRs is the vascular endothelial growth factor (VEGF) family and VEGFRs (VEGF receptors), protagonists of several studies delineating the signal transduction pathways distal to activation of VEGFRs (Cébe-Suarez et al. 2006). Beside the vascular endothelial growth factor (VEGF), most wide studies concern the Angiopoietin family of molecules, Angiopoietin-1 (Ang-1) and Angiopoietin-2 (Ang-2), and their receptor Tie-2 (Brindle et al. 2006). It is well established that the Ang-Tie-2 pathway is involved in tumour angiogenesis, even if the exact roles of angiopoietins on tumour angiogenesis are still under debate (Metheny-Barlow and Li 2003). Nevertheless, experimental and clinical studies have demonstrated that increased expression of Ang-1 and -2 promotes or inhibits tumour angiogenesis, and correlates with a reduced or extended survival time of patients, and with a declined or improved clinical outcome. In general, these studies suggest that Ang-1 is a pro-angiogenic factor that promotes endothelial cell survival and tumour angiogenesis, especially in the presence of vascular endothelial growth factor.

Thus, even if it is clear that a dynamic network, spatially oriented among biomolecules, mediates the mechanism through which cells process extracellular signals from membrane receptors by consequent transduction of biological responses, a major problem is to understand how a receptor generates a specific signal. For instance, in the same cell type the same receptor induces different responses. To explain this phenomenon one hypothesis is based on quantitative differences in protein recruited downstream the receptor, in the number of receptors activated, in the amount of ligands and in the time frame of the stimulus. The low concentration markers released during such kind of phenomena are not detectable with conventional biological analysis techniques. Therefore, to achieve new and relevant insight in system biology it is necessary to develop new tools for fine and precise quantitative measurements (Kelly et al. 2008).

For this purpose, microcantilever (MC) biosensors have shown the potentiality to relevantly improve these kind of measurements. In fact the opportunity to operate with very small quantities of material and to skip fluorescent labelling, are generally the striking advantages of micro- and nano-cantilever biosensors.

To date, cantilevers have been successfully used to detect viable cells, virus particles, pathogens, proteins, toxins, DNA molecules, and other chemicals at various concentrations in and out of liquid systems (Lavrik et al. 2004; Ziegler 2004). Several studies focused on the quantification of cancer markers (Ricciardi et al. 2010b; Wu et al. 2001), highlighting the opportunity to understand the molecular mechanism involved in tumour development.

A quantitative evaluation of molecules involved in the receptor-ligand binding interaction can provide important information for a deeper understanding of the problem, helping to obtain a most reliable model for signal molecular pathways. Moreover, one of the most important challenges in the fight against cancer is the ability to detect cancer cells early in the disease (Hayes et al. 2000). This goal is centred to reduce most cancer-associated deaths as the available cancer drugs and treatment procedures can lengthen the lifespan of most cancer patients if the disease is detected in early stage of development (Smith et al. 2000).

In the end, MC-based biosensors could lead to the understanding of angiogenesis processes, opening new ways in the field of cancer care and the possibility to design new anti-angiogenic drugs acting during the first steps of tumour development.

WORKING PRINCIPLE

As with most of immunoassays and biosensors, cantilever surface needs to be functionalized with a proper probe to selectively bind the target molecule (typical examples of probe-target complexes are antibodies and proteins or complementary DNA strands). The interactions between the binding sites of probe and target change the mechanical response of the system. Such variation due to the recognition event (and thus linkable to analyte concentration) can be monitored by two different transduction methods: first, measuring the bending of the cantilever due to the surface stress generated by the changes in Gibbs free energy upon chemical species interaction (static mode); second, measuring the resonant frequency shift due to the oscillator mass increment (dynamic mode).

Recent works have suggested that the resonance operation method seems to be the most successful application of MC-based biosensor, being less affected by the thermal drift of beam deflection and stabilization problems with respect to the static approach (Lochon et al. 2006, Shen et al. 2006).

In the dynamic operation mode the MC is externally excited (see below for typical actuation mechanisms) in correspondence with one of its resonance modes. If damping is neglected, a rectangular cantilever beam (i.e. satisfying the geometrical condition *length >> width >> thickness*) can be treated as a simple harmonic oscillator, whose resonance frequency f_0 is simply given by the following expression:

$$f_0 = \frac{1}{2\pi} \sqrt{\frac{k}{m*}}$$

(1)

where k is the spring constant and $m*$ the effective mass.

If the analyte mass adsorbed on the cantilever surface Δm is such that $\Delta m << m*$ and the stiffness of the beam k do not change substantially since the bioassay, the consequent variation of resonant frequency Δf can be directly correlated to the added mass Δm as:

$$\Delta m = -2 \frac{m*}{f_0} \Delta f$$

(2)

This simple relationship is commonly applied for MC-based protein biosensing in vacuum environment, when the mass contribution from non-specific bindings is negligible (Ricciardi et al. 2010b; Waggoner and Craighead 2007).

METHODS

Fabrication

A cantilever-based sensor is commonly fabricated by batch silicon micromachining techniques based on optical lithography and typical of integrated circuit (IC) process technology (Fig. 3.1, inset). Thanks to such technology, it is possible to massively produce micrometrical devices comprising large MC arrays (Fig. 3.1) and thus allow for high-throughput screening tools at reasonable costs.

A complete description of micro and nano cantilever fabrication techniques is out of the scope of this book: for a comprehensive review, please refer to (Lavrik et al. 2004).

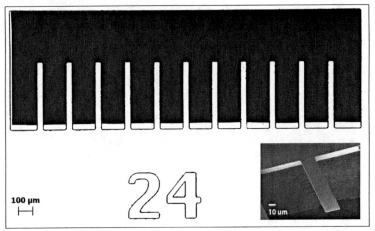

Figure 3.1. Optical micrograph of a microcantilever array. Standard silicon microcantilever array composed of 11 microcantilevers. A Scanning Electron Microscopy (SEM) magnification of a single cantilever is shown as inset.

Actuation and Detection Mechanism

As described above, functionality of MC biosensors is based on the detection of mechanical movements and deformations of their micromachined components. In fact, the general idea behind MC sensors is that physical, chemical, or biological stimuli can affect mechanical characteristics of the micromechanical transducer in such a way that the resulting change can be measured using electronic, optical, or other means. The variety of transduction modes stems from the fact that a stimulus of each type may affect the mechanical state of the transducer directly or may undergo one or several transformations before the measured mechanical parameter of the transducer is affected.

Cantilever vibration can be induced and detected with several techniques (Lavrik et al. 2004), here we focus on the most common actuation-reading scheme, which couples the piezoelectric actuation with the optical read-out (Fig. 3.2). The cantilever actuation using an external piezoelectric crystal is a method derived from the experience of non-contact measurements in

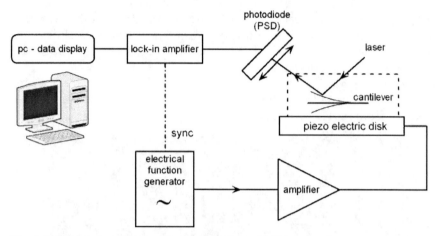

Figure 3.2. Experimental Set-up. Scheme of read-out and data processing system.

AFM systems (Bonnell 2001). A piezoelectric crystal can be driven by an alternated signal at variable frequency and the vibration of the crystal is obtained. The amplitude of the vibration can be modulated by varying the DC component of the applied voltage. If a cantilever is mounted on the piezoactuator, the vibration is transferred to it so that, with a frequency sweep, it is possible to seek the various resonance frequencies of the beam. The piezoactuator method is quite simple to set up and can be controlled electronically through a feedback system (Fadel et al. 2004). Signal output can be used to change the input parameters for a better control of the phenomena. Moreover, no particular cantilever characteristics are required to implement this actuation method (for instance, no conductive layers have to be deposited on the beam), even if a correct clamping between the actuator and the structure to be sensed should be realized for a reliable measurement. It is worth noting that the piezoactuator is able to shake both the device to be measured and its closer environment. This could be a problem for measurements in liquids where standing waves are generated through the acoustic stimulation of the medium.

The optical lever method (or optical beam reflection technique) is the read out scheme commonly used in most commercially-available AFM instruments. The optical lever method appears to be the simplest, even if equally sensitive, among more complex interferometric schemes. This particular optical detection scheme is applicable both on static and dynamic measurements and allows to discern extremely small changes in the cantilever bending and vibration. A laser light is focused on the cantilever (usually in correspondence of its free end) and is reflected off towards a position sensitive photodetector (PSD), a quadrant photodiode whose output voltages depend linearly on the vertical displacement of the light spot projected by the cantilever. The absence of electrical connections with the cantilever, linearity of the response, simplicity, reliability, cost-effectiveness and high level of parallelization are the important advantages that induce most of research groups working on MC biosensors to use the optical lever method. The main drawbacks are the limitation in PSD bandwidth (which is typically on the order of several hundreds kHz) and the need for sufficiently wide reflecting surfaces: which is why such a method does not represent the best choice for nanometer-scale oscillators.

Surface Functionalization

The molecular recognition via cantilever-based biosensors is deeply related with the activation processes of the surface of a MC, the ability of the sensing molecule to recognize its specific target and the evaluation of the frequency shift due to the mass loaded on the MC. Therefore, MC functionalization is a crucial step which determines the successfulness and performances of the measurement. Various biomolecules were immobilized on the MC surface as biochemical probe, among which antibodies were preferred because of their specificity against the complementary antigens and because the general antibody-antigen interactions have been thoroughly studied in the area of biochemistry and biosensing. Thus, in modern diagnostics, antibodies (Abs) have become key sensing molecules, even though they can be produced against almost any component, from small drug molecules to intact cells.

Surface immobilization of Abs is crucial for MC-based biosensor sensitivity and specificity. The most important aspect is the identification of a surface chemistry that allows optimal orientation (antigen-binding regions dangling out of the surface) and a good degree of freedom for the Ab (Skottrup et al. 2008). Generally, sensor surfaces consist of inorganic material (semiconductor, glass, metals, etc.). Since most of literature works are based on silicon MCs, we focus here on the functionalization procedure of silicon surfaces.

Surface functionalization is commonly performed with two strategies: (i) direct physical adsorption and (ii) covalent attachment. Direct physical adsorption is easy to perform but is an uncontrolled process that can lead to protein denaturation when hydrophobic surfaces are used (Skottrup et al. 2008). Moreover, the need for extensive washing in affinity biosensors may lead to ligand leaching from the surface, thereby decreasing the surface bioactivity (Cass 1998). Covalent protein attachment presents many advantages compared to direct adsorption, as ligands are more prone to maintain their conformational stability and do not leach from the surface (Cass 1998). Several strategies exist for the covalent coupling of antibodies to MC surfaces. Two-dimensional surfaces that have proved useful include organosilanes, self-assembled monolayers (SAMs), dendrimers and polyethylene glycol (PEG) brushes (Rusmini et al. 2007).

The orientation and freedom-of-movement of immobilized Abs is important to obtain a maximal functional sensor surface. To reach this goal several studies have shown that the use of linkers (carboxylic groups of BSA or through linear PEG) can considerably enhance the binding efficiency of MC biosensors. In fact, the use of linkers to attached proteins onto the MC surface increases the freedom of Abs to interact with the analyte. Furthermore, there are several methods that focus on the Abs orientation, so that the antigen-binding sites are freely available for analyte interaction. These include a base-layer of proteins, such as protein A or G or Fc-specific antibodies, or a nickel surface that binds histidine-tags in the Fc-region (Skottrup et al. 2008).

Measurement Procedure

An MC-based protein detection is typically composed of the following steps (Ricciardi et al. 2010b; Ricciardi et al. 2010c): (i) thermal oxidation to guarantee numerous hydroxyl (–OH) groups at the silicon surface; (ii) surface amination thanks to a silanization agent that produces a SAM through a simple wet process such as 3-amino-propyl-tri-ethoxy-silane (APTES); (iii) exposition of aldehyde (–CHO) groups by reaction with a linker such as glutaraldehyde (GA); (iv) immobilization of Protein G (PtG) as base-layer; (v) immobilization of specific Ab; (vi) incubation with the target analyte.

After every functionalization and binding step, the resonance curves of the cantilevers are monitored to evaluate the frequency shift and thus, from Eq. 2, quantify the immobilized target mass. From such data, it is also possible to calculate a very interesting variable such as the protein surface density (number of molecules per cm^2), a parameter to quantitatively investigate the stoichiometry of protein-protein interaction and the multimeric state of a target molecule (Ricciardi et al. 2010b). Figure 3.3 reports the first (left) and second (right) mode of vibration of a MC biosensor before and after the aforementioned functionalization and biomolecule binding steps.

MEASUREMENT SENSITIVITY, PRECISION AND SPECIFICITY

A first indication of cantilever mass sensitivity can be deduced directly from the ratio f_0/m in equation 2. If we consider a standard silicon MC with dimensions 400x50x10 μm^3, the mass m is of the order of 10^{-7} grams, the fundamental resonance frequency f_0 is around 10^5 Hz and the cantilever mass

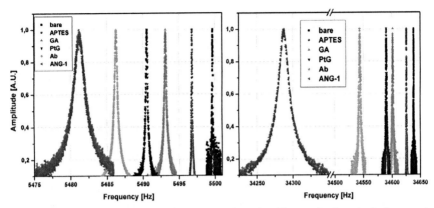

Figure 3.3. Experimental data for Angiopoietin-1 detection. The graphs show typical resonant curves before and after functionalization and protein binding steps: first mode (left panel) and second mode (right panel).

sensitivity parameter f_0/m is therefore roughly 10^{-12} Hz/g. From equation 2, this means that a measured frequency shift Δf of 1 Hz (fairly measurable with standard techniques described above) is ascribed to an immobilized mass of just 1 picogram, i.e. a single bacterium. While nanocantilevers clearly have an intrinsic superior mass sensitivity (Ilic et al. 2004), recent works have shown that microcantilevers can be preferable for biosensing applications because of their faster response (Nair and Alarm 2006) and limited statistical variability (Gupta et al. 2006).

From a diagnostic point of view, measurement precision (i.e. the variability of a measurement around its average value) is as important as limit of detection (LOD). For example, the use of modes of vibration higher than the fundamental one can drastically increase the mass sensitivity (Lochon et al. 2006; Waggoner and Craighead 2007), but commonly this effect is also associated with a detriment of measurement repeatability and reproducibility (Ricciardi et al. 2010b). One possible solution lies in combining the results coming from different modes, for example calculating the arithmetic mean of relative frequency deviation $\Delta f/f$. In such a way, it is possible to give an intrinsic uncertainty (standard deviation of the modes) to each measurement of each MC in the array and use the "weighted average" method to have the best estimation of the true value of the whole array. It has been shown that Ang-1 masses as low as few hundreds of picograms can be detected with less than 0.5% of relative uncertainty using such an approach (Ricciardi et al. 2010b).

Non-specific binding is commonly addressed as an intrinsic drawback and the principal limit of extremely high sensitive label-free technology as microcantilevers (Waggoner and Craighead 2007). Therefore, a lot of work should be done in optimizing the chemical and biological protocols and monitoring MC-based biosensor array not only in response of the targeted antigen, but also in response of other similar biomarkers. MCs have always slightly different geometrical dimensions due to inherent tolerances in the fabrication process; therefore, comparing the experiments in terms of relative frequency deviation $\Delta f/f$ rather than absolute frequency shift is preferable. Ang-1 and VEGF-A$_{165}$ are angiogenic factors, whose expression levels were demonstrated to be crucial in angiogenesis and tumour progression. Ricciardi and co-authors (Ricciardi et al. 2010b) compared the results coming from Ab-immobilized (anti-Ang-1) arrays dipped in PBS solutions containing the "true" antigen, Ang-1, and the "false" antigen VEGF-A$_{165}$ at the same concentration (25 μg/mL). Figure 3.4 displays a histogram, summarizing their results: as it can be clearly seen, the average relative frequency shift induced by incubation with VEGF-A$_{165}$ resulted in nearly two orders of magnitude lower than typical shifts due to specific recognition of Ang-1 (please, note that Fig. 3.4 has a logarithmic y-scale).

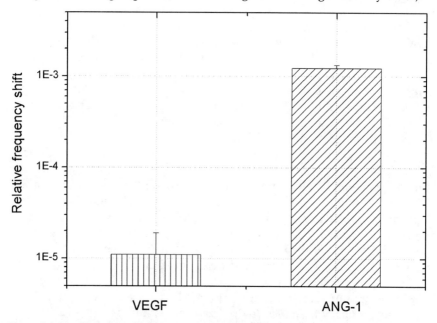

Figure 3.4. Specificity Tests. The histograms show the relative frequency shifts obtained with growth factors specificity test (data from Ricciardi et al. 2010b).

MC-BASED POINT-OF-CARE DEVICE AND REAL-TIME MONITORING OF BIOMOLECULAR INTERACTIONS

The aforementioned measurements (as well as most of literature results on MC biosensors) were performed in air or a vacuum environment, i.e. the

MC arrays were dipped in the solution for the biomolecules incubation (typically for 1–2 hr), washed, dried and placed in a vacuum chamber. Otherwise, the vibration of MC directly in liquid solution would maximize the viscous effects of the environment, causing the cantilever to resonate at lower frequencies, exhibiting extremely noisy curves. Figure 3.5 reports an example of the degradation of MC resonant curve when the vibrating sensor is moving from vacuum to air and liquid environment: it is clear that such a degradation drastically decreases the bioassay LOD. As will be discussed below, the Aspect ratio (AR) i.e. the ratio between length and width of the vibrating structure, can play a very important role in optimizing MC vibration in liquid environment.

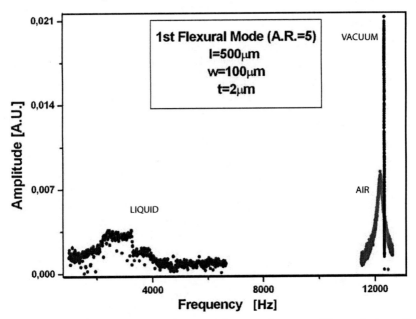

Figure 3.5. Microcantilever resonance curve in different environments. The graph shows the differences between resonant curves obtained in different environments: vacuum, air and liquid.

Despite the intrinsic limitation in sensitivity, operation in liquid would be highly desirable for different reasons (Ricciardi et al. 2010c): first, to exploit real-time measurement and observation of binding and unbinding kinetics; second, to retain biomolecule physiological structure and function; third, to reduce the risk of breaking the MCs in transporting them between different environments as well as during the drying procedure; fourth, to limit residual salt precipitation from the buffer solution when drying the arrays.

Despite using static fluid conditions and large fluid cells, the integration of MC detection in a microfluidic circuit appears a highly performing technological solution to limit sample handling and promote portability and automation of routine diagnostic tests (Point-Of-Care devices). An MC-based Lab-On-Chip (LOC) would guarantee *in situ* and real-time automatic measurements in an actively controlled environment, while reducing reagents volume and assay time. A three level MC-based LOC in which low AR vibrating structures such as microplates are embedded between glass microfluidic channels and a PDMS layer for liquid inlet and outlet was very recently proposed (Fig. 3.6). Thanks to such an optimized design, results in terms of mass sensitivity and assay specificity are not too far from those taken with MC vibrating in air (Ricciardi et al. 2010c).

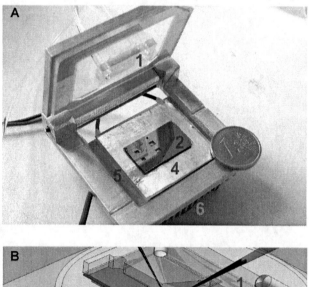

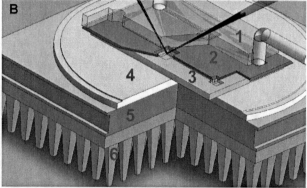

Figure 3.6. Microcantilever-based LOC. The image shows the details of a microcantilever-based LOC: **(A)** picture and **(B)** 3D sketch. Most important parts of the device are labelled as: 1. PDMS interconnections; 2. Cantilever chip; 3. Microfluidic platform (Pirex, SU-8 or PDMS); 4. Piezo Disk; 5. Peltier cell; 6 Heat sink (adapted from (Ricciardi et al. 2010c) with permission).

Figure 3.7 reports the use of such a device for real-time monitoring of resonance frequency of two MCs directly vibrating in PBS solution without (negative control) and with targetted angiogenic factor Ang-1 (at 25 µg/mL). While the first remains substantially unperturbed, the second exponentially decreases and quickly (few minutes) reaches saturation, exhibiting a Langmuir-like kinetics, typical of protein-protein interaction.

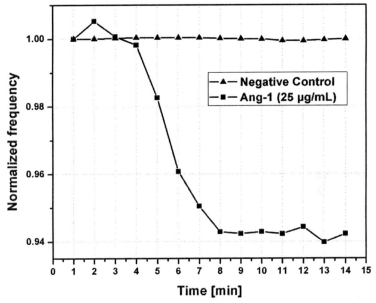

Figure 3.7. Real-time monitoring of antigen-antibody hybridization. The graph shows real-time monitoring of antigen-antibody hybridization compared to negative control experiment (PBS on Ab-coated MC) (adapted from (Ricciardi et al. 2010c) with permission).

These very recent results strongly suggest that MC-based biosensors can be used to monitor the kinetics of biomolecular interactions, and thus are extremely useful in the comprehension of molecular mechanisms involved in tumour development. Furthermore, such a device is a good candidate as a sensitive and specific, as well as rapid, cheap and portable instrument for next generation POC tools.

APPLICATIONS TO OTHER AREAS OF HEALTH AND DISEASE

Recently, MC-based biosensors have been successfully used in the medical field, detecting marker of diseases such as cancer (Ricciardi et al. 2010b; Wu et al. 2001), coronary heart disease (Moulin et al. 2000) and myoglobin (Kang et al. 2006) as well as making significant contributions to genomics and DNA analysis and blood glucose (Pei et al. 2003). Moreover, their high sensitivity and specificity has given interesting results in other areas of human health. In particular, MCs have been used for the detection of pathogen bacteria (Ricciardi et al. 2010a), pathogen spores (Campbell et al. 2007) or the presence of pesticides, such as DDT (Alvarez et al. 2003). These results demonstrate the great potential of MC biosensors for monitoring of human health, environment quality and food safety, facing the big challenges of the next generation of highly sensitive sensors.

KEY FACTS

- Angiogenesis—the process that leads to the formation of new blood vessel growth from existing ones—plays an essential role in the development of tissues in the vertebrate embryo and is involved in a wide variety of physiological and pathological conditions in adults, including wound repair, metabolic diseases, inflammation, cardiovascular disorders, and tumour progression.
- New analytical tools for fine and precise quantitative measurements of multiple biomolecules are needed for early-stage diagnostics and for an indepth comprehension of complex dynamic processes such as cancer progression.
- Cantilever-based microbalances are ultrasensitive label-free detectors that have been successfully applied to the identification of nucleic acids and disease proteins in low concentrations, as well as single viruses and bacteria.
- Thanks to the integrated circuit (IC) process technology, MC sensors are currently fabricated in large arrays that allow for low-cost and high-throughput molecular diagnostics.
- A MC-based biosensor array is integrable on a microfluidic platform to develop a Lab-On-Chip able to real-time monitor the kinetics of antibody-antigen complex formation, and thus is extremely useful in the comprehension of molecular mechanisms involved in tumour development.
- MC-based Lab-On-Chip (LOC) is a good candidate as a sensitive and specific, as well as rapid, cheap and portable instrument for next generation diagnostic tools that will be employed at or near the site of patient care (Point-Of-Care testing).

DEFINITIONS

- *Angiogenesis*: the formation of new blood vessels from the sprouting of existing ones. Physiological angiogenesis occurs during fetal development to create the circulatory system, and in the uterus during the menstrual cycle, as well as occuring around a wound or cut to help with healing. Tumour angiogenesis is the formation of new blood vessels that grow into the tumour, giving it nutrients and oxygen to assist in its growth.

- *Biosensor*: a sensing tool composed of three parts: a biological probe (or bioreceptor), which recognizes and binds the target analyte (DNA, RNA, proteins, cells, etc.); a transducer (mechanical, optical, thermal, piezoelectric, etc.), which converts the perturbation into an electronic signal; and a read out system (computer, digital interface, data logger, etc.). Thus biosensors are detectors that conjugate the sensitivity of transducers with the specificity of biomolecules recognition.

- *Cancer markers*: molecular products metabolized and secreted by neoplastic tissue and biochemically characterized in cells or body fluids. They can indicate the tumour stage and grade as well as give useful evidence for monitoring responses to treatment and predicting recurrence. Cancer markers are represented by many chemical groups, including antigens, hormones, amino and nucleic acids, enzymes, polyamines, and specific cell membrane proteins and lipids.

- *Functionalization*: the modification of a surface to insert chemical functional groups (amine, aldehyde, hydroxyl, etc...) to tune surface chemical and physical properties.

- *Lab-On-Chip (LOC)*: a device that integrates on a single chip multiple laboratory functions such as sample preparation and purification, biochemical reactions, and analyte detection. The dimensions of LOCs can vary from millimetres to a few square centimetres in size and are characterized by the capability of handling extremely small fluid volumes, down to less than picolitres.

- *Limit Of Detection (LOD)*: minimum concentration of detectable analyte. In analytical chemistry it is often estimated as three times noise level.

- *Precision*: in metrology, the variability of a measurement process around its average value.

- *Point Of Care (POC)*: diagnostic testing performed at or near the site of patient care. It includes the entire analytical patient testing activities performed outside the physical facilities of the clinical laboratories. It does not require permanent dedicated space, and can include kits and instruments, which are either hand carried or transported near the patient for immediate testing at that site.

- *Sensitivity*: in metrology, the rate at which the average measurement changes to differences in the true value.

- *Specificity*: in medical sciences, the proportion of negatives that are correctly identified.

SUMMARY POINTS

- New analytical tools for fine and precise quantitative measurements of vascular endothelial growth factors are needed for a deep comprehension of a complex dynamic process such as tumour angiogenesis.
- Microcantilever (MC) biosensors have been successfully applied to detect viable cells, virus particles, pathogens, disease proteins (cancer markers), toxins, nucleic acids, and other chemicals at extremely low concentrations.
- As with most immunoassays and biosensors, cantilever surface needs to be functionalized with a proper probe (typically an antibody) to selectively bind the target molecule: the interactions between the binding sites of probe and target change the mechanical response of the system.
- Resonance operation method (i.e. measuring the resonant frequency shift due to the oscillator mass increment) is suggested to be the most successful application of MC-based biosensors.
- Thanks to the integrated circuit (IC) process technology, MC sensors are currently fabricated in large arrays that allow for low-cost and high-throughput molecular diagnostics.
- After every functionalization and protein binding step, the resonance curves of the cantilevers are monitored to evaluate the frequency shift and thus, from a simple equation, quantify the immobilized target mass. From such data, it is also possible to investigate the stoichiometry of protein-protein interaction, as well as the multimeric state of a target molecule.
- MC-based biosensor arrays are able to detect minimum masses of angiogenic growth factors such as Angiopoietin-1 with very high precision (few hundreds of picograms with less than 0.5% of relative uncertainty) thanks to a combination of results coming from different vibration modes monitoring.
- Specificity tests performed with different angiogenic growth factors such as Angiopoietin-1 and Vascular Endothelial Growth Factor A_{165} show that contributions coming from non-specific biomolecular interactions are nearly two orders of magnitude lower than typical signals due to specific antigen recognition.
- MC biosensor is integrated on a microfluidic platform to develop a Lab-On-Chip (LOC) able to real-time monitor the kinetics of antibody-antigen complex formation, and thus being extremely useful in the comprehension of molecular mechanisms involved in tumour development.

- MC-based LOC is a good candidate as sensitive and specific, as well as rapid, cheap and portable instrument for next generation Point-Of-Care (POC) tools.

ABBREVIATIONS

Ab	:	Antibody
AFM	:	Atomic Force Microscopy
Ag	:	Antigen
Ang-1	:	Angiopoietin-1
APTES	:	Amino-Propyl-Tri-Ethoxy-Silane
AR	:	Aspect Ratio
GA	:	GlutarAldehyde
GF	:	Growth Factor
IC	:	Integrated Circuit
LOC	:	Lab On Chip
LOD	:	Limit Of Detection
MC	:	MicroCantilever
POC	:	Point Of Care
PBS	:	Phosphate-Buffered Saline
PtG	:	Protein G
PSD	:	Position Sensitive photoDetector
SAM	:	Self-Assembled Monolayer
TKRs	:	Tyrosine Kinase Receptors
VEGF	:	Vascular Endothelial Growth Factor

REFERENCES

Alvarez M, A Calle, J Tamayo, LM Lechuga, A Abad and A Montoya. 2003. Development of nanomechanical biosensors for detection of the pesticide DDT. Biosensors and Bioelectronics 18: 649–653.

Bonnell D. 2001. Scanning Probe Microscopy and Spectroscopy: Theory, Techniques, and Applications Wiley-VCH, New York.

Brindle NPJ, P Saharinen and K Alitalo. 2006. Signaling and Functions of Angiopoietin-1 in Vascular Protection. Circ Res 98: 1014–1023.

Campbell GA, D deLesdernier and R Mutharasan. 2007. Detection of airborne Bacillus anthracis spores by an integrated system of an air sampler and a cantilever immunosensor. Sensors and Actuators B: Chemical 127: 376–382.

Carmeliet P. 2000. Mechanisms of angiogenesis and arteriogenesis. Nat Med 6: 389–395.

Cass TAFSL. 1998. Immobilized Biomolecules in Analysis: A Practical Approach. Bioseparation 9: 117–118.

Cébe-Suarez S, A Zehnder-Fjällman and K Ballmer-Hofer. 2006. The role of VEGF receptors in angiogenesis; complex partnerships. Cellular and Molecular Life Sciences 63: 601–615.

Fadel L, I Dufour, F Lochon and O Francais. 2004. Signal-to-noise ratio of resonant microcantilever type chemical sensors as a function of resonant frequency and quality factor. Sensors and Actuators B: Chemical 102: 73–77.

Gupta AK, PR Nair, D Akin, MR Ladisch, S Broyles, MA Alam and R Bashir. 2006. Anomalous resonance in a nanomechanical biosensor. Proceedings of the National Academy of Sciences of the United States of America 103: 13362–13367.

Hayes AJ, WQ Huang, J Yu, PC Maisonpierre, A Liu, FG Kern, ME Lippman, SW McLeskey and LY Li. 2000. Expression and function of angiopoietin-1 in breast cancer. Br J Cancer 83: 1154–1160.

Ilic B. 2004. Attogram detection using nanoelectromechanical oscillators. J. Appl. Phys. 95: 3694–3703.

Kang GY, GY Han, JY Kang, I-H Cho, H-H Park, S-H Paek and TS Kim. 2006. Label-free protein assay with site-directly immobilized antibody using self-actuating PZT cantilever. Sensors and Actuators B: Chemical 117: 332–338.

Kelly KA, SR Setlur, R Ross, R Anbazhagan, P Waterman, MA Rubin and R Weissleder. 2008. Detection of Early Prostate Cancer Using a Hepsin-Targeted Imaging Agent. Cancer Research 68: 2286–2291.

Kyo Seon Hwang JHL, J Park, DS Yoon, JH Park and TS Kim. 2004. *In situ* quantitative analysis of a prostate-specific antigen (PSA) using a nanomechanical PZT cantilever. Lab on a chip 4: 547–552.

Lavrik NV, MJ Sepaniak and PG Datskos. 2004. Cantilever transducers as a platform for chemical and biological sensors. Rev Sci Instrum 75: 2229–2253.

Lochon F, I Dufour and D Rebiere. 2006. A microcantilever chemical sensors optimization by taking into account losses. Sensors and Actuators B: Chemical 118: 292–296.

Metheny-Barlow LJ and LY Li. 2003. The enigmatic role of angiopoietin-1 in tumor angiogenesis. Cell Res 13: 309–317.

Moulin AM, SJ O'Shea and ME Welland. 2000. Microcantilever-based biosensors. Ultramicroscopy 82: 23–31.

Nair PR and MA Alarm. 2006. Performance limits of nanobiosensors. Applied Physics Letters 88: 233120–03.

Pei J, F Tian and T Thundat. 2003. Glucose Biosensor Based on the Microcantilever. Analytical Chemistry 76: 292–297.

Ricciardi C, G Canavese, R Castagna, G Digregorio, I Ferrante, S Marasso, A Ricci, V Alessandria, K Rantsiou and L Cocolin. 2010a. Online Portable Microcantilever Biosensors for Salmonella enterica Serotype Enteritidis Detection. Food and Bioprocess Technology 3: 956–960.

Ricciardi C, S Fiorilli, S Bianco, G Canavese, R Castagna, I Ferrante, G Digregorio, SL Marasso, L Napione and F Bussolino. 2010b. Development of microcantilever-based biosensor array to detect Angiopoietin-1, a marker of tumor angiogenesis. Biosensors and Bioelectronics 25: 1193–1198.

Ricciardi C, G Canavese, R Castagna, I Ferrante, A Ricci, SL Marasso, L Napione and F Bussolino. 2010c. Integration of microfluidic and cantilever technology for biosensing application in liquid environment. Biosens. Bioelect 26: 1565–1570.

Rusmini F, Z Zhong and J Feijen. 2007. Protein immobilization strategies for protein biochips. Biomacromolecules 8: 1775–1789.

Shen Z, WY Shih and W-H Shih. 2006. Self-exciting, self-sensing $PbZr_{0.53}Ti_{0.47}O_3SiO_2$ piezoelectric microcantilevers with femtogram/Hertz sensitivity. Applied Physics Letters 89: 023506-3.

Skottrup PD, M Nicolaisen and AF Justesen. 2008. Towards on-site pathogen detection using antibody-based sensors. Biosensors and Bioelectronics 24: 339–348.

Smith RA, CJ Mettlin, KJ Davis and H Eyre. 2000. American Cancer Society guidelines for the early detection of cancer. CA Cancer J Clin 50: 34–49.

Steeg PS. 2006. Tumor metastasis: mechanistic insights and clinical challenges. Nat Med 12: 895–904.

Waggoner PS and HG Craighead. 2007. Micro- and nanomechanical sensors for environmental, chemical, and biological detection. Lab on a Chip 7: 1238–1255.

Wu G, RH Datar, KM Hansen, T Thundat, RJ Cote and A Majumdar. 2001. Bioassay of prostate-specific antigen (PSA) using microcantilevers. Nat Biotech 19: 856–860.

Ziegler C. 2004. Cantilever-based biosensors. Analytical and Bioanalytical Chemistry 379: 946–959.

4

Electrochemical DNA Biosensors at the Nanoscale

Rosa Letizia Zaffino,[1,3] Wilmer Alfonso Pardo,[1,3] Mònica Mir[1,2,a,*] and Josep Samitier[1,2,3]

ABSTRACT

Electrochemical DNA biosensors at the nanometric scale have gained increasing attention in the last years. The high sensitivity, low cost and easy miniaturization of the electronic detection taken in conjunction with the wide range of applications that offers the detection of DNA, have made these devices a perfect analytical tool in different fields, such as diagnosis of genetic diseases, detection of infectious agents, study of genetic predisposition, development of personalized medicine, detection of differential genetic expression, forensic science, drug screening, food safety and environmental monitoring.

Nanofabrication technologies have brought even more advantages to these kind of devices. The miniaturization of these biosensors contributes towards lesser time on diagnosis and reagents, as well as the reduction of costly preparation and analysis methods, which is of primary relevance in the case of the genosensor. It is expected that the use of nanotechnologies will end the still common preliminary step in most

[1] Nanobioengineering Laboratory, Institute for Bioengineering of Catalonia (IBEC), Barcelona Science Park, Baldiri i Reixac, 10, 08028, Barcelona, Spain.
[2] Centro de Investigación Biomédica en Red de Bioingeniería, Biomateriales y Nanomedicina (CIBER-BBN), Spain.
[a] E-mail: mmir@ibec.pcb.ub.es
[3] Department of Electronics, Barcelona University (UB), Spain.
*Corresponding author

List of abbreviations after the text.

of the existing platforms, the long and expensive DNA amplification with PCR. But the main feature which makes nanobiotechnologies so attractive is the possibility of exploiting the ability of nanomaterials and nanopatterned devices to directly interact with biomolecules and to produce, in the ideal case, a direct readable signal of the interaction event.

INTRODUCTION

The "Human Genome Project", which has recently gained significant achievements, has witnessed the general interests in genomic research programs. The importance in genomic applications have been increased by the high potential benefits that the DNA biosensors are expected to bring to clinical, civil defense and societal settings. The latter range from pharmacogenomic applications, to the diagnosis of disease and forensic purposes. In the field of medical diagnosis, increasing innovations and novel configurations have been developed in order to detect diseases such as cancer in its early stages. Early cancer detection helps in avoiding loss of life and also the high cost of treatments for these kinds of diseases, becoming indirectly in one solution of greater problems public health issues at medium and long term: the cost overruns (Yang et al. 1999).

According to the IUPAC definition (Theavenot et al. 1999); "*A chemical sensor is a device that transforms chemical information, ranging from the concentration of a specific sample component to total composition analysis, into an analytically useful signal. Chemical sensors usually contain two basic components connected in series: a chemical (molecular) recognition system (receptor) and a physicochemical transducer. Biosensors are chemical sensors in which the recognition system utilises a biochemical mechanism.*"

The classification of these devices can be given from either of its two main elements: the biological system of recognition and the transduction element that will eventually lead to a signal detector.

The DNA sensory industry has been, until now, dominated by optical (direct or indirect) read out methods. Optical biosensors based on fluorescence with dyes have been shown to be extraordinarily sensitive, while piezoelectric and surface plasmon resonance methods cannot offer such low detection limits, but inform about the attachment kinetics and the surface coverage. The involved techniques and the relative instrumentations are still costly in view of the massive scale exploitation of these technologies. Indeed, unsolved problems linked with the variability in the rate of fluorophore photobleaching, or the inconsistency between target and labeling, could affect the detection limits and in some cases beyond the minimum required by the clinical protocols. Electrochemical methods appear to be particularly well suited in the general case of biomolecules detection, and especially in the "sample-limited" case of DNA analysis. The simple scalability, without affecting the sensitivity and selectivity, is an attractive principle posed by electrochemical detection methods. Although, there still exist intrinsic difficulties in the manipulation and the measurement of nanosystems, research is still ongoing. (Rogers 1995; Chambers et al. 2009).

The other essential component of a biosensor is the recognition element, which has a biological nature and the remarkable biochemical activity for selective interaction with its counter molecule, generating an output signal of high fidelity and easy detection (Willner et al. 2008). The most frequent reactions between biological components are biocatalysis and bioaffinity. In both cases, the correct formation of the resulting biocomplex will determine the quality of the original signal (Gorodetsky et al. 2009).

Enzymes are the main type of biomolecules that use biocatalysis in biosensor applications. The main property of allosteric enzymes, its regulatory nature, is what gives them great potential as recognition elements (Monoda et al. 1963). Another favorable point for its wide acceptance is the large variety of measurable products derived from the different existing catalytic process (Guan et al. 2004). Other biomolecules used for recognition in biocatalysis are whole cells, microscopic organisms, cellular organelles, membranes and tissues parts (Nice et al. 1999).

The bioaffinity interaction between two complementary biomolecules does not produce a third product, as in the case of biocatalytic coupling. In bioaffinity receptors, the interaction itself needs to be detected, in some cases helped by a label, in order to elucidate the existence of the attached analyte. The bioaffinity couple most widely used is based on antibody-antigen interactions (Buhl et al. 2009). These bioreceptors take advantage of the knowledge about the immuno response produced in biological species due to the entrance of antigenic agents, which in these cases would be our analyte (Guo et al. 2009). The possibility of producing and isolating this receptors in a laboratory, against almost any kind of analytes injected into animals, has paved the way for the growth of this technology.

Another type of affinity biosensor booming today is the system based on receptor/antagonist/agonist, using transmembrane enzymes, ion channels and transcription factors like receptors and their corresponding antagonist (molecules that interact with receptors without actually activating them), and agonist (molecules that interact with receptors causing activation) (Mascini et al. 2001; Yongkang et al. 2003). The interaction between these three modules offers a series of electrochemically measurable signals.

Another widespread bioaffinity system employs the hydrogen bonds created between two complementary DNA strands for the detection of a specific oligonucleotide sequence. Due to the inherent capacity of complementarity that brings a strong but reversible interaction with high simplicity and easy synthesis in structural modifications (Domínguez et al. 2004; Wei et al. 2009). Oligonucleotides have led to a number of recognition structures such as:

Peptide Nucleic Acid (PNA)

In the basic structure of an oligonucleotide polymer, its constituent monomers (nucleotides), differs only at the base carrying the ribose residue, sugar associated with these molecules (Fig. 4.1). So, the main axis of a DNA or RNA molecule is supported on a scaffold of ribose-phosphate. Peptide nucleic acids are chemically synthesized molecules based on this structure, but the ribose-phosphate backbone is replaced with units of N-(2-aminoethyl)-glycine, leading to a molecule of similar characteristics to natural oligonucleotides but with a notable feature; there is no charge. For this reason, DNA-PNA coupling is stronger and more durable for the purpose of recognition, since it avoided the charge repulsion between strands (Brandt et al. 2004; Jayasena et al. 1999).

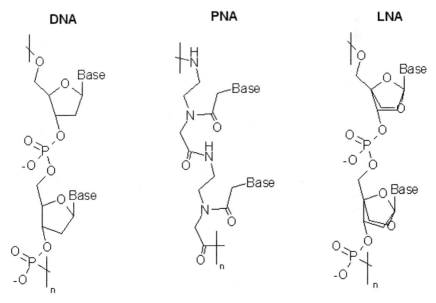

Figure 4.1. Comparison of the chemical structure of DNA, PNA and LNA.

Locked Nucleic Acid (LNA)

LNA is a nucleic acid analogue containing one or more LNA nucleotide monomers with a bicyclic furanose unit locked in an RNA mimicking a sugar conformation (Fig. 4.1). LNA oligonucleotides display unprecedented hybridization affinity toward complementary ss ribonucleic acid (RNA) and complementary ss or ds DNA.

Both modified nucleic acid probes show great hybridization stability and are not easily recognized by either nucleases or proteases, making them resistant to enzyme degradation and are also stable over a wide pH range and ionic strength.

Aptamers

Aptamers are short single stranded DNA or RNA. This bioreceptor is not used for its typical DNA hybridization, but for its interaction with other type of molecules not based on nucleotides, such as ions (Famulok et al. 2000). This DNA artificial interaction with different kinds of molecules is achieved through its particular three-dimensional folding selective for a specific sequence. These simple strands are obtained from libraries of oligonucleotides for an *in vitro* selection process called systematic evolution of ligands by exponential enrichment (SELEX), for selecting the sequence of the library that is more akin to the target molecule.

Molecular Beacons

The molecular beacons are ssDNA or RNA hairpins structures that have a fluorophore at one end and at the other a quencher that closes the hairpin structure when these elements are closer to each other, thus blinding the fluorescence. When the target sequence binds to the loop, where the recognition sequence is located, the hairpin opens and leads the fluorophore to emits its signal (Wang et al. 2008). This kind of configuration was translated to an electrochemical read out by Plaxco, changing the electrode distance of a ferrocene molecule attached at the end of the loop, instead of the fluorophore-quencher couple.

The immobilization of nucleic acids on electrodes can be performed through various types of forces such as physisorption (adsorption), affinity (avidin-biotin coupling), chemisorption (self assembled monolayers (SAMs)) and covalent interactions (carbodiimide method). Chemisorption is the most common interaction in the immobilization of nucleic acids and is widely represented in the SAMs. These highly ordered and oriented hierarchical structures are formed spontaneously from molecules predesigned with a thiol moiety.

Molecular Imprint

This recognition method consists of selective binding sites patterned in synthetic polymers using natural biomolecules as DNA templates. This system is based on natural enzyme recognition; the active site has a unique geometric structure that is particularly suitable for a specific substrate. This effective strategy recognition is low in cost and therefore its easy accessibility makes this technique a promising field of study

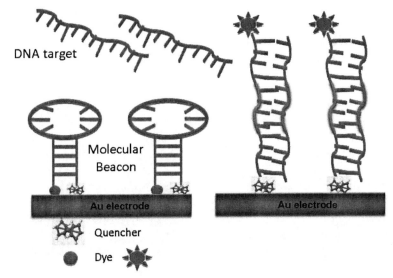

Figure 4.2. Scheme of a fluorescence molecular beacon platform.

NANOSCALE: ADVANTAGES IN ELECTROCHEMICAL DNA BIOSENSORS

Nanobiotechnologies are expected to highly improve the ability of electrochemical DNA biosensors in medical diagnosis in the near future. In the last few years, research has especially focused in the development of devices that make it possible to operate at the point of care, with less time on diagnosis and reagents and avoiding costly preparation and analysis methods. This is of primary relevance in the case of genosensor, where the employment of nanotechnologies is expected to end with long and expensive preparation practices, as the amplification of DNA by PCR, which is still, a common preliminary step in most of the existing platforms. The main feature which makes nanobiotechnologies so attractive is the possibility of exploiting the ability of nanomaterials and nanopatterned devices to directly interact with the biomolecules and to produce, in the ideal case, a direct readable signal of the interaction event.

The diameter of the nanostructures, such as nanowires, is comparable with that of the molecules or chemical species to be detected so that the coupling between biomolecules with nanomaterials can be realized in a highly efficient manner; indeed, one expects that significant changes of the signal are produced following the binding of few molecules.

The efficiency of different nanobiosensing platforms can be described on the basis of a simple diffusion-capture (reaction-diffusion) model, describing the kinetics of absorption of biomolecules on nanosensors, and the Poisson-Boltzmann equation, defining the electrostatic interaction between biomolecules in ionic solutions (solvation effect). This simple theoretical model makes it possible to account for some strikingly reported experimental observations. In general, the detection limits of nanosensors are as high as the greater is the active surface of the device. For example, a typical 3D nanowire sensor has a detection limit of three to four orders of magnitude higher compared to a planar ion selective field effect transistor (ISFET) sensor. Apart from the geometry of the system, the other relevant parameter affecting the efficiency of the detection is the settling time; i. e. the minimum requested time in order to capture a certain number of analyte molecules (Sheehan et al. 2005). A statistical interpretation of the nanoscale biosensors detection limit based on diffusion-limited capture of analyte molecules suggests that femtomolar detection is available.

Based on above considerations, it is easy to figure out why nanosensors based on electrical readout have increasingly gained popularity. Some of these electrochemical nanodevices for DNA detection are introduced below.

DNA NANOWIRE SENSORS

These devices are based on semiconductor nano-objects connected to a metallic source and drain electrodes in a field-effect transistor (FET) geometry. The semiconductor is usually functionalized with a molecular receptor, which selectively binds to the analyte. When the target binds to the bioreceptor, the properties of the superconductor near the surface modifies, so that the conductivity changes and is the same target molecule which acts as an electrical gate for its own detection.

Nanowire Based on Single Walled Carbon Nanotubes (SWCNT)

SWCNT configures as the smallest available nanostructure, with a diameter of the order of 1nm. This size is comparable to the size of the individual biomolecules, and to the range of the electrostatic screening length relevant in the physiological environment. Moreover, the scarce carrier density charge of SWCNT is comparable with that of proteins at the sensor surface, which makes the SWCNT particularly well suited in electrical detection assays. Indeed, they share a set of interesting physical properties that derive from the completely covalent sp^2 bonding that is characteristic of the defect-free grapheme sheet (Saito et al. 1998).

It is well accepted that DNA strongly interacts with the SWCNT, the simulations show that DNA binds to the external surface of uncharged, or

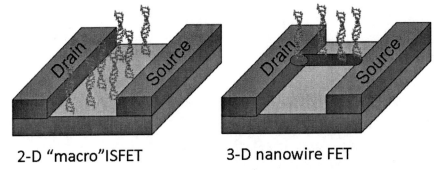

2-D "macro"ISFET   **3-D nanowire FET**

Figure 4.3. Schematic representation of 2-D and 3-D FET based sensors.

positively charged SWCNT on a time scale of a few hundred picoseconds (Zhao et al. 2007), being in some cases an irreversible interaction to the sidewalls of SWCNT (Tang et al. 2006). The binding mode of DNA on uncharged SWCNT is qualitatively different for the case of positively charged SWCNT. Indeed, it is known that adsorption of DNA on the sidewalls of SWCNT does not affect the internal structure of the stacking inside the molecule.

Although numerous studies have focused on the sensing mechanisms of SWCNT, a clear understanding of it is still lacking. The proposed mechanisms range from: the electrostatic gating to the change in the gate coupling, the changes in the carriers mobility and the unconventionally Schottky barrier effect. In order to identify the sensing mechanism experimentally, the source-drain current (I) versus the gate voltage potential (Vg) curves for a SWCNT transistor immersed in an eletrolyte solution were studied by Dekker (Yuan et al. 2008) in the case of ambipolar conduction (i.e. both for hole than electron transport). After being grown by standard chemical vapour deposition (CVD) on a thermally oxidized wafer, SWCNT were deposited between Ag/Cr contacts, on an isolating SiO2 surface, obtained through lithography in a field-effect transistor layout. The I-Vg characteristics were studied for a large number of devices, and for all of them, the electrostatic gating and/or Schottky barrier mechanism, have been individuated as the principle sensing mechanism. Indeed, a better reproducibility of the results is observed for the electrostatic gating mechanism along the bulk of the SWCNT instead of that for the Schottky barrier modulation at the contacts. This shows the importance of the electrode-SWCNT contact in establishing the sensing mechanism with respect to the channel doping.

In order to further elucidate this point, an area-selective photoresist cupping was provided to study the effects of the channel and the junction on the observed change of the drain current. The charge density modification near the electrode results to be the principle factor accounting for almost all the observed changes in I_d (32% vs 6%) compared to the SWCNT channel doping.

A simple protocol for label-free detection of DNA hybridization has been tested (Tang et al. 2006) for two random sequences of 15mer and 30mer respectively. Thiolated DNA is anchored, in this case, to the surface of Au electrodes, by exploiting the well-known affinity between gold atoms and the terminal sulfur groups of the thiol molecule. A network of about 100 SWCNT grown almost parallel between the electrodes, and a platinum wire inserted in the buffer solution, was used as top gate electrode (Fig. 4.4). Electrical detection of DNA hybridization was performed by real time measurement of the source-drain current following the addition of complementary and mismatched ssDNA by means of a semiconductor analyzer. A decrease of about the 25% of the conductance is reported after hybridization with the complementary ssDNA for both sequences, while no differences were observed on the addiction of PBS or the mismatched sequence in the device functionalized with MHC and the capture probe. In order to give further insight into the sensing mechanism, the authors performed a parallel analysis by means of fluorescence measurements, quartz crystal microbalance (QCM) and X-ray photoelectron spectroscopy. On the basis of this study, they concluded that the modulation of the SB at the metal-SWCNT contact, by means of the efficient duplex hybridization that causes the lowering of the work function of gold contacts, is the leading sensing mechanism.

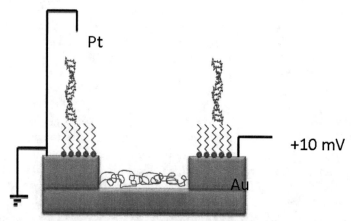

Figure 4.4. Representation of the nanowire device developed by Tang et al. (Tang et al. 2006).

Silicon Nanowire (SiNW)

Semiconductor nanowires based on silicon bridges, as well as SWCNT, enable an efficient charge transfer between the surface-attached DNA and the nanowire. Moreover, SiNW has the interesting advantage that they can be prepared by exploiting either a "bottom-up" or "top-down" approaches. Unlike SWNCT, the electrical performances of SiNW are highly reproducible and tunable during the growth process, which can be well controlled.

Hahm and Lieber (2004) demonstrated the effectiveness of a SiNW based biosensor in the direct electrical ultrasensitive DNA mismatch detection (Fig. 4.5). This SiNW biosensor was functionalized with a PNA as capture probe and it was used for detection of two different mutations of the cystic fibrosis transmembrane receptor, which are a manifestation of the disease. The use of PNA receptor, instead of the correspondent DNA sequence, increases the hybridization efficiency, because of the neutral character of the PNA chain that helps to achieve hybridization at low ionic strength and mismatch discrimination of PNA is more efficient than that of DNA (Ratilanien et al. 2000; Egholm et al. 1993). The problem of maintaining a low ionic strength is crucial in FET because they respond to changes in the surface charge, and increased ionic strength comprises the electrical double layer around the wires (Zhang et al. 2006).

P-type SiNW, synthesized using the gold nanocluster catalyzed chemical vapor deposition (CVD) method (Egholm et al. 1993) were used in this assay. NWs were assembled in a FET configuration sensor and also in this case, the functionalization was achieved by PNA immobilization

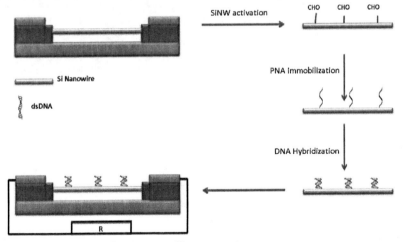

Figure 4.5. DNA functionalization on a silicon nanowire sensor.

of PNA surface. Increase of the conductance is reported following the addiction of femtomolar (fM) concentrations of both wild type DNA, and mutated DNA. The increase in conductance is consistent with the increase in the negative surface charge density subsequent the binding of DNA to the NW. The device is able to detect, in an efficient and specific fashion, concentrations down to 10 fM in a totally label-free and real-time method; this low detection limit is well below the achievable ones with current analysis routines.

The same group was also able to show the label-free real-time multiplexed detection of protein cancer markers with ultrasensitive performances, in the order of fM. But for this purpose antibody molecules were attached on the SiNW sensor (Zheng et al. 2005).

A reliable and scalable fabrication technique for producing uniform and well aligned SiNW, has been shown (Gao et al. 2007) to be efficient and sensitive in the label-free electrical detection of DNA hybridization. The device is fabricated by combining deep ultraviolet lithography and self-limiting oxidization, and allows sensitivity down to fM concentrations. SiNW arrays were obtained on a patterned and etched silicon-on-insulator (SOI) wafer, which was further submitted to oxidation, contact metal deposition and passivation. Microfluidic channels embed on the SiNW arrays and provide isolation of all the electrical contacts from the aqueous solution. The SiNW were functionalized with PNA capture probe via the silane chemistry. The application of the device in the ultrasensitive DNA detection was established by monitoring the resistance after immersion in hybridization buffer with different complementary DNA concentrations. No detectable resistance changes were observed at the control SiNW array, while different changes were reported following the addition of complementary DNA samples at distinct concentrations. A general increase of the resistance follows after exposure of the devices to the complementary strands, with some variations in the settling of the response corresponding to different concentrations.

At low concentrations the resistance shows a linear dependence with the hybridization time. So, at ultralow concentrations, longer hybridization times are required to reach the same sensitivity. Comparing this behavior with that obtained by switching to the neutral buffer solution, the authors concluded that the reported changes in the resistance are a consequence of the DNA hybridization, which induces a decrease in the carrier concentrations on the surface of the n-type SiNW used, giving rise to a field effect on the NWs.

NANOSENSORS BASED ON GOLD NANOPARTICLES (AuNpS)

Gold nanoparticles (AuNps) constitutes a prominent example of such nanoprobes whose properties can now be well controlled during fabrication, in such a way that the shape, size, as well as the chemical-physical properties can be tailored for an efficient coupling with different biomolecules. The target binding event occurring at the nanoparticle surface produces a change, usually in the optical or electrical properties of the nanoprobe that can be usefully exploited for biosensing. Moreover, they enable electron transfer between redox protein and the electrode surface, which allows in performing electrochemical sensing without the need of a transducer element. Indeed, AuNps provide a stable surface for the immobilization of the biomolecules without interfering with their ordinary biological activity due to their high biocompatibility. The well explored conjugation chemistry at the gold surface makes it possible to realize efficient coupling between the biological recognition element and the surface. AuNps does not emit light, as it happens in the case of Quantum Dots which are considered their semiconductor counterpart, but instead absorb and scatter it in the surface plasmon resonance (SPR). As a consequence, they can also be easily detected by exploiting the plasmonic coupling properties, by the fluorescence quenching or by addressing the conductivity changes.

At low concentrations, ranging from high attomolar to mid-picomolar, AuNps are usually subjected to silver-enhancement treatment, whereupon they promote the deposition of silver metal in the presence of silver ion and a revealing agent, the hydraquinone.

Use of a gold nanoparticle based array for biosensing, was shown by Park and colleagues (Park et al. 2002). In this device, a short oligonucleotide capture probe is located between the microelectrodes gap, while a longer target oligonucleotide in solution, is provided with recognition elements complementary to the capture probe and labeled with AuNps. When the binding event is accomplished, the gold nanoparticles fill the micorelectrodes' gap and a silver-enhanced treatment with a photographic developing solution that uses AuNps to promote the reduction of the Ag(I) and hydroquinone, is used here to increase the sensitivity of the device (Fig. 4.6). The microelectrodes, far apart at 20 um, were obtained by standard photolithography on a silicon wafer and the SiO_2 surface was functionalized with SMPB (succinimidyl4-melamidophenil-butyrate), where they were left to react during 24 hr. Once the device is treated with the target and the nanoparticles, it is then submitted to the silver-enhancement procedure with the photographic solution. The detection of the array is then tested by monitoring the gap resistances by increasing the time exposure to the silver-enhancement treatment, with complementary and not complementary

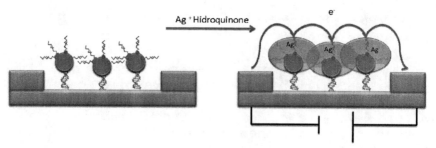

Figure 4.6. Schematic representation of the signal amplification of a nanosensor with AuNP and AgNps.

strands. The deposition of silver is turned on by the nanoparticles and thus by the hybridization event. In the control experiments carried out with denatured strands, no detectable signals were measured.

A similar approach, also involving the use of gold nanoparticles labeling and silver-enhancement treatment, but which exploits a different detection technique, has been shown to be useful for the detection of DNA sequences related to the BRCA1 breast cancer gene. (Wang et al. 2001). Silver-enhancement is here used in order to induce selective and catalytic deposition of silver on the gold labels, and avoiding spontaneous precipitation on other parts of the device. A biotinylated DNA probe is bound to a streptadivin coated magnetic latex sphere. When the hybridization event occurs, it is followed by the formation of the biotin-streptadivin couple and the catalytic silver precipitation on gold labels, which is detected with the potentiometric stripping protocol. The removal of non-hybridized DNA is achieved by means of magnetic separation, which allows an efficient minimization of nonspecific binding. A detection limit of 10 pg for 50 ug/L and hybridization time of 20 min, can be achieved by exploring this technique. Lower detection limits are expected to be found for longer hybridization times.

Two different array formats, which also rely on the use of magnetic beads to trigger the direct electrochemical detection, were explored as biosensing electrochemical genosensor platforms based on gold nanoparticles. The two alternative designs, one in a so-called two strands assay format and the other with a sandwich format, have been proven to be effective in the detection of hybridization, one to the breast cancer gene BRCA1, and the other one to the cystic fibrosis gene. In the former case, the capture probe is immobilized onto biotinylated paramagnetic beads; once this step is accomplished, the hybridizing solution with the target is added and then, submitted to a solution containing streptavidin-coated AuNps.

At this point, the detection is carried out by the direct differential pulse voltametry (DPV) measurement of the AuNps tag in the conjugate.

A similar procedure is involved in the test of the alternative array design. In the sandwich assay format a further hybridization step is necessary to conjugate the target probe attached to paramagnetic beads and second a biotinylated probe for signaling with streptavidin-coated AuNps. In both cases, the devices show great discrimination efficiency when tested with a three base mismatch sequence and a non-complementary strand. Indeed, no current signal is observed in these cases, while a clear current DPV peak is reported for the complementary strands. The two strands assay formats reach sensitivity of 600 nM.

NANOPORE BASED SENSORS

Next generation of DNA sequencing will be fundamentally based on single molecule detection approaches, providing a faster response and making it possible to avoid expensive and time-consuming sample preparation routines. Among the feasible single molecule based detection platforms, an electronic method through which the bases of large DNA molecules can directly be read, without the need of any chemical manipulation or labeling protocol, is still a challenging aim, and could be accessible in the near future by exploiting the properties of the nanopore. These kind of sensors were successfully introduced in an analogy with the ionic nanochannels through which the homeostatic equilibrium of cells is controlled. The detection principle is based, as in ordinary coulter counter, on a particle-size discrimination criterion: when a molecule passes through the nanopore a translocation event signal coinciding with the closure of the nanopore is produced. Nanopores with embedded electrodes to monitor the transverse tunneling current inside them could provide the technology needed to meet this aim. The core of detection is hidden behind the following features of the tunneling current, the exponential sensitivity is directly related with the electrodes separation distance and the atom position between the electrodes. Although, we are still far from sequencing every single base in a DNA sequence, as technical challenges are needed to outfit the nanopores with sufficiently tiny electrodes and a better control of the translocation speed. In fact, in order to use this method for sequencing one has also to consider that the tunneling amplitude is also sensitive to changes in the atomic or molecular positions due to the thermal fluctuations, which can be a problem in the presence of contaminant molecules. As a consequence, it is still not possible to obtain a single base sensitivity found on the reading of the ionic current.

Identification of the four DNA bases by means of tunneling currents has been reported by two groups, based on slightly different protocols; in one case (Chang et al. 2010) functionalized electrodes in nanoscale gap were used, while in the other device (Thundat 2010) nanosized reconfigurable electrodes were exploited. In the former case, electrode functionalization was carried out to increase the order of detection selectivity by using a reagent, which limits the possible orientations of the molecules passing the gap and reducing the gap resistance. Tunneling measurements were accomplished on a scanning probe microscope interfaced to a digital microscope. A low noise signal with a characteristic conductance of 20 pS, was recovered when both the probe and the gold substrate were functionalized with 4-mercaptobenzoic acid. However, the current fell after the solution containing the four nucleosides was placed between the electrodes. Concentrations of the nucleosides were adjusted in such a way to obtain approximately equal spikes inside the tunnel gap. The signals were filtered through a custom program which analyzed the height of the spikes and retained only the responses above the noise of the baseline. For most of the collected spikes, the behavior is characteristic of the binding and unbinding of molecules inside a gap. Measured distributions show dependence from the functionalization of the electrodes. Signals coming from pyrimidine registered were less frequent than from purine. When measurements were repeated with a functionalized substrate and a bare gold probe, the major change observed only pertained to the width of the distribution and the nucleotides peaks were not differentiated. Current peaks in the case of dA and dG result were well distinguishable only when both the probe and the substrate were functionalized. Also, the lifetime duration of current spikes was almost equal when a bare and one functionalized electrode were used. Although , it is not possible to ascertain where the signals really originate, as it is not possible to exclude that the measured currents only come from single nucleotides. Similar results were also found in the case of dC and dT, the main difference was that in this case a shorter gap size was needed, corresponding to a resistivity of 40 pS, as the pyrimidines are smaller molecules than purines.

The other approach exploits the possibility to statistically identify the single nucleotides through electron transmissivity that is related to their HOMO-LUMO gap, and providing in this way the efficiency of this kind of detection protocol. The latter is based on the observation of the temporal changes in a two-probe tunneling current associated with the trapping of nucleotides between the electrode gap. For this purpose, the gap size was adjusted in order to fit the nucleotides length. In this experiment, molecules are weakly connected to the metal electrodes in such a way that a marginal change in the molecular conformation will also result in an appreciable change in the current, due to the modification of the electrode-molecule distance. On the other hand, a narrower gap reflecting a stronger electrode-molecule coupling, will be followed by an increase in the tunneling current. The electron transport features for this system were investigated by studying the bias-voltage dependence of the tunneling current. The nanofabricated electrode provides a direct electrical and label-free nucleosides sequencing method. In order to analyze the I-V characteristics, I pulses were statistically examined. Well defined single peaks appear in the current distributions indicating the preferred conformation of the guanine inside the gap, and which has been interpreted as the alignment of the molecules along the electrostatic potential gradient induced by the applied voltage. It is important to underline that the trapping duration of the nucleotides inside the gap is influenced by the induced electrostatic field. The plots also show a linear increase of the current with the increase of the potential, which is viewed as the signature of a possible electron transport mechanism occurring in the nucleotides. Experiments were repeated by adding the different solutions containing equimolar quantities of the other nucleotides. After the addition of thymine and guanine it was possible to distinguish two single peaks which show that it is able to detect single nucleotides on the basis of two-probe tunneling current detection. When superposing the current histograms of guanine, cytosine and thymine a remarkable overlap is found, indicating that a single shot measurement result is not adequate to identify the nucleotides type. Moreover, the I-V characteristics were still more difficult to interpret in the case of adenine, where a high base level of current and significant noise were present. From the available measurements it is possible to conclude that the adenine shows a relatively high-degree of no-specific binding to gold. This result avoids, for the moment, the possibility of a label free direct electrical detection of single-nucleotide by means of the tunneling current approach described here. Precise control of the DNA dynamics in the proximity of the nanoelectrodes is needed.

Among nanomaterials, graphene is gaining popularity in the scientific community and two physicists who were able to synthesize graphene for the first time were awarded the Nobel Prize this year. The enthusiasm for this discovery is motivated by the versatility and the unique features that exist in graphene . Graphene is a single-atom thick hexagonal lattice (~0.3 nm) that can now be synthesized in different ways. The single atom thickness enables the transverse conductance measurements, and its good electrical properties and the mechanical robustness are highly interesting for biosensing purposes, as they offer the possibility of directly solving the problem of locating an electrode inside the nanometric gap. Graphene nanopores could also be employed both as electrodes and as membrane material. Indeed, electrons in graphene move faster than ions in solid state nanopores, opening sequencing protocols faster. In the case of DNA detection, the proper gap size should be around 1~1.5 nm so that ssDNA can pass without folding. A theoretical study (Nelson et al. 2010) based on ab initio density functional theory, predicts the feasibility of a graphene nanopore based device able to reach single-base detection by measuring the ionic current blockade, which is expected to be different in correspondence of the translocation of the four distinct bases. Indeed, the conductance must be independent from the nucleobases orientations in the gap, as it happens in the case of tunneling-current like devices. Theoretical simulations predict higher measured currents in the case of ionic-current blockade devices, of the order of mA, opposite for tunneling current and ionic current ones for which measured currents only reach values around nA. However it is mandatory to consider the possibility of an overestimation of these values as the calculation excludes different dissipation sources. Also, the theoretical analysis takes into account the current dependence from the gap size, and the results show that for wider gaps the peaks become broader, and the overall current decreases exponentially with the nanogap width. This demonstrates the need for a method that could differentiate the changes in the current due to base variations from those arising for the gap size. The analysis of nonlinear current-voltage characteristics could be used to solve this problem.

The main problem envisaged is the conductance variations introduced by the geometric fluctuations of the nucleobases inside the gap, which could be controlled by stabilizing the nucleotides while passing the gap, by means of a functionalization of the nanogap or by modulation of the bias applied voltages. A graphene nanopore based device for single-nucleotides detection has been proposed and tested by Schneider et al. (2010). The nanopore is a small hole connecting two chambers containing electrolyte solution. As the molecules pass the gap they partially block the ionic flow, so that molecules can be detected as drops in the I-V characteristics. The ionic blockade current signatures observed here, compared favorably with the performance obtained with SiN pore. Indeed, the current signal recorded in bare graphene nanopore is noisier than in the case of SiN. In this assay, a monolayer of graphene is transferred over a substrate of SiN where a 5μm sized hole was produced. Once obtained, the pores were mounted into a microfluidic cell, and the saline solution is added at each side of the nanopore membrane, measurements of the ionic transport through the nanopore were performed. The values of the resistances across nanopores of different size were also measured showing that resistance decreases with the increase of the pore diameter. Indeed, the linear behavior of the current vs the voltage shows that this is generated by the ionic flow through the pore and not by the process occurring at the graphene membrane. Translocation events of the DNA nucleotides through the nanopore were detected as spikes in the conductance profile. Three kinds of events can be individuated: the molecule passes in a linear head-to-tail fashion (not folded), is partially grabbed and then translocates as before (partially folded) and finally the molecule is grabbed in the middle (folded). A part the amplitude of the translocation event has also been analyzed the time duration. The latter result is independent from the membrane thickness with an average value of 2.7 + –0.8 ms, for practical applications it would be highly useful to have shorter times with higher spatial resolution. Further experiments will focus on the exploration of the single strand translocation, and then with the single base detection with the final aim of DNA sequencing.

KEY FACTS

- *Hybridization*: The process of interacting two nucleic acid strands, joining two complementary strands of DNA/DNA, RNA/RNA, DNA/RNA. These reactions can be used to detect and characterize nucleotide sequences using a particular nucleotide sequence as a probe.
- *Biomolecule*: A biomolecule is a chemical compound found in living organisms. These chemicals consist mainly of carbon, hydrogen, oxygen, nitrogen, sulfur and phosphorus. Biomolecules are the building blocks of life.
- *Buffer*: Buffer is a solution whose pH does not change with the addition of an acid or base. It has a mixture of weak acid and its conjugate salt, or mixture of weak salt and its acid conjugate.
- *DNA/RNA:* DNA and RNA are biological macromolecules consisting in an acidic chain to multiply repeat units of phosphoric acid, sugar with purine and pyrimidine bases; they are involved in the preservation, replication and expression of hereditary information in every living cell.
- *Nanotechnology*: Nanotechnology is the study of developing materials or devices on an atomic and molecular scale, structures sized between 1 to 100 nanometer, in at least one dimension.

DEFINITIONS

- *Self assembles monolayer*: A self assembled monolayers (SAMs) is an organized layer of amphiphilic molecules in which one end of the molecule, the "head group" shows a special affinity for a substrate. SAMs also consist of a tail with a functional group at the terminal end.
- *Human Genome Project*: Genome, is the set of genes, where the hereditary material of a living organism lies, encoded in a sequence of four alternating letters, which are the basic constituents of the DNA. The Human Genome Project refers to a set of initiatives aimed at the sequenciation of the human genome and of the other species. The foundation of the Project officially dates back to 1990, at which time it was perceived as the challenging

scientific and technical target of the end of the Millennium, witnessing a unified effort in biological research. In a handwritten note of one the first defining meetings, the aim of the project is "To have all the sequence public and available for both research and development in order to maximize its benefit for society". The goal of the Project was, indeed, to furnish the researchers with tools and strategies to understand at a genetic level the origin and the evolution of the diseases, and the possibility on the other hand to develop new medical protocols based on this specific knowledge. Globally, the methodology adopted was to focus first on the more relevant sequences in the DNA, and then going deeper in the analysis of more specific maps according to the advance in hardware and software solutions needed for the job. The first draft of the human genome, corresponding to about the 90% of the total, was published in Nature in 2001, two years later the full sequence was completed.

- *Electrochemical detection methods*: Electrochemical detection methods are based on the measurement of the current produced by the reduction or the oxidation of a given analyte. Detection is accomplished by means of an electrochemical cell which is obtained by placing two electrodes in an electrolyte solution. Reduction or oxidation of the analyte at the electrode is induced by the application of an external potential. By correctly choosing the applied potential, according to the monitored reduction/oxidation reaction, and the material of the working electrode, rapid response time, a wide dynamic range with sample reduction and low volume dead, can be achieved. Electrochemical methods, accordingly, can offer high selectivity and low detection limits at modest a cost, and have been widely exploited in biosensor applications. Different kinds of electrochemical measurements can be performed giving rise to the principal electroanalitycal methods: potentiometry (measurement of the potential difference at the electrode), coulometry (measurement of the current produced by the total oxidation of the analyte), and voltammetry (measurement of the current in function of a constant o varying potential, as in the case of differential pulse voltammetry DPV).

- *Schottky Barrier*: The formation of the so called Schottky Barrier (SB), at the metal-semiconductor (MS) interface, is the intrinsic feature of the MS junction enabling its operations as a semiconductor device. The SB, in fact, operates as a rectifying barrier for the electrical conduction at this interface, so that it can be employed as a dyode. The origin of the potential barrier is the mismatch between the energy of the carrier of the semiconductor (conduction band minimum energy level for a n-type semiconductor, valence band maximum energy level in p-type semiconductor) and the Fermi energy level at the MS junction. The height of the barrier (SBH) reflects the magnitude of this mismatch. The lower potential which characterizes this junction, compared with a conventional p-n one, improves its switching speed which permits its application to high frequency signals rectification.

- *The Landauer formula*: This formula obtained within the more general theory of the electronic transport developed by Landauer. It is highly useful and widely applied to determine the transport properties in nanoscaled devices. Moreover , the Landauer theory is the standard theoretical framework through which the electron transport in molecular systems is treated. At a practical level, it permits to calculate the conductance of a one dimensional (1D) conductor connected with two metallic reservoirs. At its roots the Landauer formula is based on the concept of the tunneling current, and then in general the phenomenon of tunneling in quantum systems.

SUMMARY POINTS

- Genosensors have a lot of different applications such as diagnosis of genetic diseases, detection of infectious agents, study of genetic predisposition, development of personalized medicine, detection of differential genetic expression, forensic science, drug screening, food safety and environmental monitoring.
- Electrochemistry transduction has the advantages of high sensitivity, short time response, low cost and easy miniaturization.
- Nanofabrication technologies contributes to less time on diagnosis and reagents, as well as the reduction of costly preparation and analysis methods
- Nanowire based sensors have demonstrated to be highly sensitive, achieving detection limit in the order of fM.
- Nanopores sequencing devices need further development for single nucleotide detection. However, these sensors are able to detect the hybridization of DNA sequences.

ACKNOWLEDGEMENTS

This work was financially supported by the ONCOLOGICA Consortium, funded by the Consorcios Estratégicos Nacionales en Investigación Técnica (CENIT) programme of the Centro para el Desarrollo Tecnológico Industrial (CDTI) and financed by the Spanish Ministry of Science and Innovation (MICINN).

The Nanobioengineering group participates in the CIBER-BBN, an initiative funded by the VI National R&D&i Plan *2008–2011, Iniciativa Ingenio 2010, Consolider Program, CIBER Actions* and financed by the Instituto de Salud Carlos III with assistance from the *European Regional Development Fund.*

The Nanobioengineering group has support from the Commission for Universities and Research of the Department of Innovation, Universities, and Enterprise of the Generalitat de Catalunya (2009 SGR 505).

ABBREVIATIONS

APTMS	:	Aldehyde Propyltrimethoxylane
AuNp	:	Gold nanoparticle
BRCA	:	breast cancer gene
CEA	:	carcinoembryonic antigen
CHEMFET	:	Chemical Field Effect Transistor
CVD	:	Chemical Vapour Deposition
DPV	:	Differential Pulse Voltammetry
DNA	:	Deoxyribonucleic acid
dA	:	deoxyadenosine
dC	:	deoxycytosine
dG	:	deoxyguanosine
dsDNA	:	Double Stranded DNA
dT	:	deoxythymidine
FET	:	Field Effect Transistor
HOMO	:	High Occupied Molecular Orbitals
ISFET	:	Ion Sensitive Field Effect Transitor
LNA	:	Locked nucleic acid
LUMO	:	Low Unoccupied Molecular Orbitals
MHC	:	Mercaptohexanol
NW	:	Nanowire
Np	:	Nanoparticle
PBS	:	Phosphate Buffered Saline
PCR	:	Polymerase Chain Reaction
PNA	:	Peptide nucleic acid
PSA	:	Prostatic Specific Antigene
QCM	:	Quarz crystal microbalance
RNA	:	Ribonucleic acid
		Self assembled monolayer
SB	:	Schottky Barrier
SELEX	:	Systematic Evolution of Ligands by Exponential Enrichment
SiNW	:	Silicon Nanowire

SOI	:	silicon-on-insulator
SPM	:	Scanning Probe Microscope
SPR	:	Surface Plasmon Resonance
SWCNT	:	Single Walled nanotube
ssDNA	:	Single Stranded DNA
TEM	:	Transmission Electron Microscopy
Vg	:	Voltage potential
WKB	:	Wentzel–Kramers–Brillouin approximation

REFERENCES

Brandt O and JD Hoheisel. 2004. Peptide nucleic acids on microarrays and other biosensors. Trends Biotechnol 22: 617–622.

Buhl A, S Page, NH Heegaard, PV Landenberg and BL Luppa. 2009. Optical biosensor-based characterization of anti-double-stranded DNA monoclonal antibodies as possible new standards for laboratory tests. Biosensors and Bioelectronics 25(1): 198–203.

Chambers JP, BP Arulanandam, LL Matta, A Weis and JJ Valdes. 2008. Biosensor recognition elements. Curr Issues Mol Biol 10: 1–12.

Chang S, S Huang, J He, F Liang, P Zhang, S Li, X Chen, O Sankey and S Lindsay. 2010. Electronic Signatures of all Four DNA Nucleosides in a Tunneling Gap. Nano Letters 10(3): 1070–1075.

Domínguez E, O Rincón and A Narváez. 2004. Electrochemical DNA sensors based on enzyme dendritic architectures: an approach for enhanced sensitivity. Anal Chem 76: 3132–3138.

Egholm M, O Buchardt, L Christensen, C Behrens, SM Freier, DA Driver, RH Berg, SK Kim, B Nordén and PE Nielsen. 1993. PNA hybridizes to complementary oligonucleotides obeying the Watson-Crick hydrogen-bonding rules. Nature 365: 566–568.

Famulok M., G Mayer and M Blind. 2000. Nucleic Acid Aptamers-From selection *in vitro* to applications *in vivo*. Acc Chem Res 33: 591–599.

Gao Z, A Agarwal, AD Trigg, N Singh, C Fang, CH Tung, Y Fan, KD Buddharaju and J Kong. 2007. Silicon Nanowire Arrays for Label-Free Detection of DNA. Analytical Chemistry 79(9): 3291–3297.

Gorodetsky AA, MB Buzzeo and JK Barton. 2008. DNA-mediated Electrochemistry. Bioconjugate Chem 19(12): 2285–2296.

Guan J, Y Miao and Q Zhang. 2004. Impedimetric biosensors. Journal of Bioscience and Bioengineering 97(4): 219–226.

Guo S and S Dong. 2009. Biomolecule-nanoparticle hybrids for electrochemical biosensors. Trends in Analytical Chemistry 28(1): 96–109.

Hahm J and CM Lieber. 2004. Direct Ultrasensitive Electrical Detection of DNA and DNA Sequence Variations Using Nanowire Nanosensors. Nano Letters 4(1): 51–54.

Jayasena SD. 1999. Aptamers: An emerging class of molecules that rival antibodies in diagnostics. Clinical Chemistry 45: 1628–1650.

Mascini M, I Palchetti and G Marrazza. 2001. DNA electrochemical biosensors. Fresenius J Anal Chem 369(1): 15–22.

Monoda J, JP Changeuxa and F Jacob. 1963. Allosteric proteins and cellular control systems. Journal of Molecular Biology 6(4): 306–329.

Nelson T, B Zhang and OV Prezhdo. 2010. Detection of Nucleic Acids with Graphene Nanopores: Ab Initio Characterization of a Novel Sequencing Device. Nano Letters 10(9): 3237–3242.

Nice EC and B Catimel. 1999. Instrumental biosensors: new perspectives for the analysis of biomolecular interactions. BioEssays 21: 339–352.

Park SJ, TA Taton and CA Mirkin. 2002. Array-Based Electrical Detection of DNA with Nanoparticle Probes Science 295(5559): 1503–1506.

Ratilainen T, A Holmén, E Tuite, PE Nielsen and B Nordén. 2000. Thermodynamics of Sequence-Specific Binding of PNA to DNA. Biochemistry 39(26): 7781–7791.

Rogers KR. 1995. Biosensors for Environmental Applications. Biosensors & Bioelectronics (10): 533–541.

Saito R, MS Dresselhaus and G Dresselhaus. 1998. Physical Properties of Carbon nanotube. Imperial College Press, London.

Schneider GF, SW Kowalczyk, VE Calado, G Pandraud, HW Zandbergen, LMK Vandersypen and C Dekker. 2010. DNA Translocation through Graphene Nanopores. Nano Letters 10(8): 3163–3167.

Sheehan PE and LJ Whitman. 2005. Detection Limits for Nanoscale Biosensors. Nano Letters 5(4): 803–807.

Tang X, S Bansaruntip, N Nakayama, E Yenilmez, Y Chang and Q Wang. 2006. Carbon Nanotube DNA Sensor and Sensing Mechanism. Nano Letters 6(8): 1632–1636.

Theavenot DR, K Toth, RA Durst, and GS Wilson. 1999. Electrochemical biosensors: recommended definitions and classification. Pure Appl Chem 71(12): 2333–2348.

Thundat T. 2010. DNA sequencing: Read with quantum mechanics. Nature Nanotechnology 5: 246–247.

Wang J, R Polsky and D Xu. 2001. Silver-Enhanced Colloidal Gold Electrochemical Stripping Detection of DNA Hybridization. Langmuir 17(19): 5739–5741.

Wang K, Z Tang, C Yang Y Kim, X Fang, W Li, Y Wu, C Medley, Z Cao, J Li, P Colon, H Lin and W Tan. 2008. Molecular Engineering of DNA: Molecular Beacons. Angew. Chem 47: 2–17.

Wei D, MJA Bailey, P Andrew and T Ryhänen. 2009. Electrochemical biosensors at the nanoscale. Lab on a Chip 9: 2123–2131.

Willner I, B Shlyahovsky, M Zayats and B Willner. 2008. DNAzymes for Sensing, Nanobiotechnology and Logic Gate Applications. Chem Soc Rev 37: 1153–1165.

Yang M, KE Sapsford, N Sergeev, S Sun and A Rasooly. 2009. Meeting Current Public Health Needs: Optical Biosensors for Pathogen Detection and Analysis; Proceedings of SPIE-The International Society for Optical Engineering, 7167, 716702.

Yongkang Y and J Huangxian. 2003. DNA electrochemical behaviours, recognition and sensing by combining with PCR technique. Sensors 3: 128–145

Yuan GD ,WJ Zhang, JS Jie, X Fan, JA Zapien, YH Leung, LB Luo, PF Wang, CS Lee and ST Lee. 2008. p-Type ZnO Nanowire Arrays. Nano Letters 8(8): 2591–2597.

Zhang J , HP Lang, F Huber, A Bietsch, W Grange, U Certa, R Mckendry, HJ Güntherodt, M Hegner and CH Gerber. 2006. Rapid and label-free nanomechanical detection of biomarker transcripts in human RNA. Nature Nanotechnology 1: 214–220.

Zhao X and JK Johnson. 2007. Simulation of Adsorption of DNA on Carbon Nanotubes. Journal of the American Chemical Society 129(34): 10438–10445.

Zheng G, F Patolsky, Y Cui, WU Wang and CM Lieber. 2005. Multiplexed electrical detection of cancer markers with nanowire sensor arrays. Nature Biotechnology 23: 1294–1301.

5

Aptamer-based Biosensors for Cancer Studies

Ilaria Palchetti[1,a] and Marco Mascini[1,b,*]

ABSTRACT

In bioassays for cancer diagnosis, prognosis and theragnostic, antibody-based detection methodologies are still considered the standard assays. These assays are well established and have been able to reach the desired sensitivity and selectivity. However, the use of antibodies could lead to some limitations. In order to circumvent some of these drawbacks, other recognition molecules have been explored as alternatives. In the recent years, attention has turned toward reagents, known as nucleic acid aptamers. Aptamers are made from short strands of DNA or RNA that adopt specific three-dimensional conformations allowing biorecognition of specific target proteins or small molecules. Aptamers are generated by the selection of molecules in a process which represents a systematic evolution of the ligand by exponential enrichment (SELEX) and therefore in this iterative process of *in vitro* selection and amplification, large libraries of oligonucleotides are screened. The SELEX process involves a combination of selection of nucleic acid ligands which interact with the target (i.e. a protein) and amplification of those selected nucleic acids. Iterative cycling of the selection/amplification steps allows selection of one or a small number

[1]Dipartimento di Chimica Ugo Schiff, Università degli studi di Firenze, Via della Lastruccia 3, Sesto Fiorentino (Fi), Italia.
[a]E-mail: ilaria.palchetti@unifi.it
[b]E-mail: Marco.mascini@unifi.it
*Corresponding author

List of abbreviations after the text.

of nucleic acids which demonstrate a high affinity against the target. Innovative features of these molecules for clinical applications in cancer research are summarized in this chapter.

INTRODUCTION

One of the major future challenges in oncology will be the early diagnosis and individualized, tailored care of cancer patients. Cancer continues to be the most feared global disease, with prostate, lung, breast, and colon cancer topping the list of cause of mortality in the United State and Canada in 2006 (Tothill 2009; Berrino et al. 2009). Collectively cancer has also been identified as the second largest cause of death in most developing countries (Berrino et al. 2009; De Angelis 2009). Cancer can be caused by a range of factors and these include genetic or environmental factors such as exposure to carcinogenic chemicals, radiation or microbiological causes including: bacterial (e.g. stomach cancer) or viral infections (e.g. cervical cancer). As the causes of cancer are so diverse, clinical testing is also very complex.

In cancer, the disruption of the normal cell signaling pathways leads to the inactivation of the tumor suppressor genes and the activation of oncogenes. These multi-factorial changes (genetic and epigenetic) can cause the onset of the disease and the formation of cancer cells which will exhibit higher growth capability than normal mammalian cells. However, in terms of diagnosis, no single gene is universally altered during this process, and the patterns of change differ in tumors from different locations (organ), as well within tumors from the same location. All these changes which take place can be so variable and overlapping that it is difficult to select a specific change or marker for the diagnosis of specific cancers (Tothill 2009). Thus, it is worth noting that multi-marker profiles (presence and concentration level) can be essential for the diagnosis of early disease onset and for providing information to assist clinicians in making successful treatment decisions and increasing patient survival rate.

A range of biosensor platforms are reported in the literature for cancer disease diagnosis (Tothill 2009). However, most of these papers deal with the use of classical antibody-antigen recognition system (McShane et al. 2005), based on different transduction techniques, from electrochemical to piezoelectric and optical methods.

In this chapter, innovative bioreceptors such as specific nucleic acid aptamers, claimed to overcome problems of stability and synthesis reproducibility encountered with classical antibody (Mascini et al. 2012) will be described. In particular, they will be discussed as bioreceptors in biosensors for multiplexed analysis of biomarkers and in detection of cells that cause metastasis.

APTAMERS A NOVEL CLASS OF BIORECEPTORS

Nucleic acid aptamers are short, single stranded DNA or RNA oligonucleotides, which adopt stable three dimensional sequence-dependent structures. This intrinsic property makes them efficient binding molecules, capable of binding to molecular targets ranging from small ions and organic molecules to large proteins and even cells. They can vary in size between 25 and 90 bases and adopt complex secondary and tertiary structures, which facilitate specific interactions with other molecules; from this their name "aptamer", a word from the Latin expression "aptus" (to fit) and the Greek word "meros" (part) (Ellington and Szostak 1990).

The functionality of aptamers is based on their stable three-dimensional structure, which is dependent on the primary sequence, the length of the nucleic acid molecule and the environmental conditions.

The selection process is called systematic evolution of ligands by exponential enrichment (SELEX), first reported in 1990 (Ellington and Szostak 1990; Tuerk and Gold 1990).

The SELEX process involves iterative cycles of selection and amplification starting from a large library of oligonucleotides with different sequences (generally 10^{15} different structures). After incubation with the specific target and the partitioning of the binding from the non-binding molecules, the oligonucleotides that are selected are amplified to create a new mixture enriched in those nucleic acid molecules having a higher affinity for the target. After several cycles of the selection process, the pool is enriched in the high affinity sequences at the expense of the low affinity binders.

The number of cycles required depends on the stringency conditions, but, once obtained and once the sequence is known, unlimited amounts of the aptamer can be easily achieved by chemical synthesis. In addition to this very important aspect of having an unlimited source of identical affinity recognition molecules available, aptamers can offer advantages over antibodies that make them very promising for analytical applications. The main advantage is overcoming the use of animals or cell lines for the production of the molecules. Antibodies against molecules that are not immunogenic are difficult to generate. On the contrary, aptamers are isolated by *in vitro* methods that are independent of animals: an *in vitro* combinatorial library can be generated against any target. In addition, generation of antibodies *in vivo* means that the animal immune system selects the sites on the target protein to which the antibodies bind. The *in vivo* parameters restrict the identification of antibodies that can recognize targets only under physiological conditions limiting the extension to which the antibodies can be functionalized and applied. Moreover, the aptamer selection process can be manipulated to obtain aptamers that bind a specific region of the target and with specific binding properties in different binding conditions. After selection, aptamers are produced by chemical synthesis and purified to a very high degree by eliminating the batch-to-batch variation found when using antibodies. By chemical synthesis, modifications in the aptamer can be introduced enhancing the stability, affinity and specificity of the molecules. Often the kinetic parameters of aptamer–target complex can be changed for higher affinity or specificity. Another advantage over antibodies can be seen in the higher temperature stability of aptamers and they can recover their native active conformation after denaturation; in fact antibodies are large proteins sensitive to the temperature and they can undergo irreversible denaturation. Moreover aptamers provide significant advantages over antibodies as therapeutics and for *in vivo* sensing, including non-toxicity and lack of immunogenicity, and fast tissue penetration with short blood residence time.

Aptamers with affinity for a large variety of molecules, including virtually any class of proteins (enzymes, membrane proteins, viral proteins, etc.), peptides, drugs, toxins, low-molecular-weight ligands, ions and cells have been isolated. The folding of nucleic acid around the target provides numerous discriminatory intermolecular interactions. These interactions fall in the class of non covalent bonding and are mainly stacking, shape complementarity, electrostatic and hydrogen-bonding interactions. Multiple interactions contribute to the same aptamer-target complexes. The molecular interactions govern the specific recognition of and discrimination between different target classes in aptamer complexes.

The design for aptamer-based biosensor (or aptasensor) largely relies on the inherently different recognition modes of each aptamer-target complex. Aptamers generally incorporate small molecules into their nucleic acid structure, leaving little room for interaction with a second molecule. Generally small molecules are detected by a single-region binding assay. By contrast, protein targets are structurally complicated, allowing the interplay of various discriminatory contacts. As a result, protein can be assayed via both single-region binding and dual region binding assay (sandwich assay).

APTAMER-BASED BIOSENSORS FOR CANCER STUDIES

Several aptamers have already been developed against cancer related proteins (PDGF, VEGF, NFkB, tenascin-C, or PMSA) (Ireson and Kelland 2006; Lupold et al. 2002; Daniels et al. 2003) and have been adapted for numerous biosensing principles mainly in direct and sandwich formats rather than competitive formats.

As an example of a direct assay, Lai et al. 2007, reported on a platelet derived growth factor (PDGF) DNA aptamer modified with methylene blue (MB) and immobilized onto a gold electrode. The capability of the aptamer to fold in its characteristic structure when in contact with the target molecule was studied (Fig. 5.1). In the unfolded structure, hence in the absence of PDGF, the aptamer has only one of the three characteristic stems and MB, fixed at the aptamer end, far from the electrode surface. In the presence PDGF the aptamer adopts the three stems structure and the distance between MB and the electrode decreases, improving the electron-transfer activity, with an increase of current.

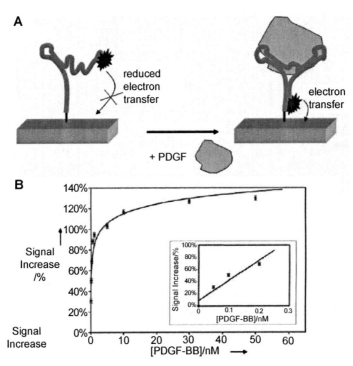

Figure 5.1. Example of a Direct Assay: **(A)** Scheme of the direct aptamer-based electrochemical detection of PDGF. **(B)** Dose–response curve of the sensor for increasing concentrations of PDGF (adapted with permission from Lai et al. 2007).

Regarding sandwich assay, an electrochemical biosensor for PDGF detection via sandwich structure and AuNPs mediated amplification has been reported (Wang et al. 2009). As shown in Fig. 5.2, the aptamer was immobilized on the electrode surface through self-assembly. In the presence of the target PDGF, it can be captured onto the interface through the formation of PDGF-aptamer complex. Then the aptamer modified AuNPs, which are negative charged, recognized the target specifically and bound

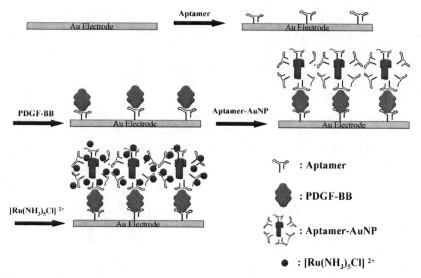

Figure 5.2. Example of a sandwich assay: scheme for the formation of sandwich structure and Au-NPs mediated amplification for PDGF detection (with permission from Wang et al. 2009).

to the electrode surface to form a sandwich structure. Finally, the positive charged $[Ru(NH_3)_5Cl]^{2+}$, used as a probe, was adsorbed to the sandwich structure via electrostatic interaction. The obtained electrochemical signals were directly concerned with the concentration of PDGF.

As already discussed, competitive scheme of assay, is mainly used with small molecules, like drugs such as aminoglycoside antibiotics, even if competitive assay for detection of protein have been reported (Papamichael et al. 2007).

The main differences between the various biosensor formats are the immobilized species (aptamer, antibody or target analyte), the number of experimental steps involved, and in which order the different reagents are exposed to the solid support, when present. The choice of the format depends on the molecular size of the analyte, the availability of reagents and the cost.

Excellent reviews have been recently published, also covering the application of aptamer biosensing in medicine studies (Mascini et al. 2012; Mayer 2009), and readers are referred to these reviews to find more examples of the different sensing procedures, including the coupling with nanomaterials to improve biosensing sensitivity.

This chapter will focus mainly on describing selection procedures that are proposed for multiplexed biomarker analysis or cell detection and applied mainly for cancer studies. Practical examples of aptamers evolved by these procedures and used for biosensing in cancer studies will be also described.

APTAMERS EVOLVED BY PHOTO SELEX IN CANCER BIOSENSING STUDIES

With photochemical SELEX (Photo SELEX), modified ssDNA aptamers capable of photocross-linking the target molecule have been identified (Fig. 5.3). The method is based on the incorporation of a modified nucleotide activated by absorption of light, in place of a native base in either RNA- or

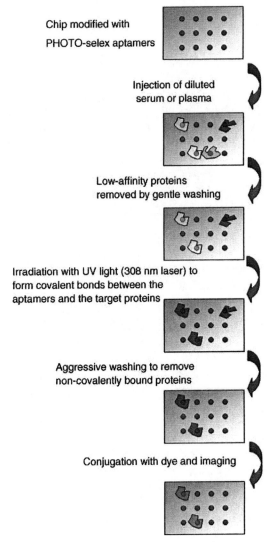

Chip modified with
PHOTO-selex aptamers

Injection of diluted
serum or plasma

Low-affinity proteins
removed by gentle washing

Irradiation with UV light (308 nm laser) to
form covalent bonds between the
aptamers and the target proteins

Aggressive washing to remove
non-covalently bound proteins

Conjugation with dye and imaging

Figure 5.3. The Photo SELEX: Scheme of the photo-aptamer-based assay (with permission from Tombelli et al. 2007).

in ssDNA-randomized oligonucleotide libraries. The aptamers selected with this method have the ability to form a photo-induced covalent bond with the target molecule and have for this reason, greater sensitivity and specificity than those aptamers selected through conventional selection methodologies.

Some interesting approaches such as the possibility of developing a diagnostic system incorporating Photo SELEX evolved aptamers (Golden et al. 2000) capable of simultaneous quantification of a large number of analyte molecules, have been presented (Bock et al. 2004).

The Photo SELEX-evolved aptamers, specific for many different marker proteins, could be fixed to a solid support (chip) and incubated with the sample (e.g. patient serum). After washing, the chip is irradiated with UV light causing a covalent bond formation between the aptamer and target and a universal fluorescent dye is added to conjugate specific amino acids of the covalently bonded proteins, to quantitatively detect the target molecules (Bock et al. 2004). Several advantages of this system, such as minimal sample requirement, quantification of multiple proteins and very high specificity, have been evidenced with respect to single-analyte conventional immunoassays. Moreover, this kind of assay eliminates the need of secondary binding agents such as detection antibodies, still reaching the detection limits necessary for the detection of the targets molecules at their physiological level.

The technology was already applied for multiplexed detection of basic fibroblast growth factor (bFGF), vascular endothelial growth factor (VEGF), and interleukins IL-6, IL-8, IL-12 and IL-16, (Bock et al. 2004).

Aptamers Evolved by Improved SELEX and Photo SELEX Technology in Cancer Biosensing Studies: SOMAmer Approach

SOMAmer (Slow Off-rate Modified Aptamer) are aptamers discovered by SOMAlogic. As mentioned by Brody et al. 2010: *"The idea was to generate novel aptamers that had the low Kds of classic aptamers, and that, in addition, had very slow dissociation rates with their cognate analytes but fast dissociation rates for most other proteins in plasma or serum."*

The authors considered that generally the dissociation rate for most aptamers are fast, and the key fact in this novel technology could have been the selection of slow dissociation rate in the SELEX process itself. Moreover, these novel molecules have functionalities at five-positions on pyrimidines that could provide extra binding interactions.

In two recent papers on PLOS one (Gold et al. 2010; Ostroff et al. 2010) SOMAmers were used for multiplexed proteomic technology for biomarker discovery (Fig. 5.4). In particular (Ostroff et al. 2010), compared the sera of heavy smokers not known to have non-small-cell lung cancer (NSCLC) or known to have benign nodules with the sera of heavy smokers known to have either early-stage or late stage NSCLC. The proposed technology allowed the identification of 44 biomarkers. Analysis of the data suggested that of the 44 biomarkers that indicated NSCLC, many were correlated with each other. The accuracy (expressed as the AUC calculation from the receiver operating characteristic [ROC] curve for a typical classifier using approximately 12 biomarkers) is approximately 90%, and was confirmed on a set of blinded samples held back for that purpose. The data for the entire experiment were collected from serum samples of 1326 patients (with 870 protein measurements per sample) from four independent birepositories. The reported results seem interesting in the view of identification of novel biomarkers.

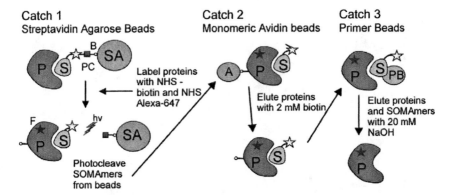

Figure 5.4. Aptamers (SOMAmers) for biomarker discovery. SOMAmers are mixed with the target sample (purified protein or plasma) and incubated to bind to equilibrium. In Catch-1, bound SOMAmer(S)-protein(P) complexes are captured onto streptavidin beads (SA) and the proteins are tagged with biotin (B) (NHSbiotin) and fluorescent label (F) (NHS Alexa 647). Unbound proteins are washed away. Bound complexes are released from the beads by cleaving the photo-cleavable linker (PC) with ultraviolet light. In Catch-2, SOMAmer-protein complexes are captured onto monomeric avidin beads (A), washed, and eluted from the beads with 2 mM biotin. At this stage, SOMAmer-protein complexes are subjected to a kinetic challenge analogous to that used in the proteomics assay. Specific complexes survive the challenge and non-specific complexes dissociate. In the final step, Catch-3, bound complexes are captured onto primer beads (PB) by DNA primer that is complementary to a portion of the SOMAmer and any remaining unbound protein resulting from the kinetic challenge is washed away. Finally, the captured complexes are dissociated with 20 mM NaOH and the target protein is eluted for analysis by PAGE. From Gold et al. 2010 with permission.

APTAMERS EVOLVED BY CELL SELEX IN CANCER BIOSENSING STUDIES

The major cause of mortality in patients with cancer is metastasis, which is caused by tumor cells that escape from the primary tumor into the bloodstream and travel through the circulatory system to distant sites where they develop into secondary tumors. The cells that cause metastasis are called circulating tumor cells (CTCs). Although CTCs are very rare in the early stage of breast cancer patients, for example, they vastly increase in number once the disease develops (Tang et al. 2007; Pu et al. 2010).

Aptamers selected by a process known as Cell SELEX can be created for any type of cancer cell. A typical selection cycle is shown in Fig. 5.5. Briefly, cell concentration and viability need to be determined before selection. The suspension cells are first thoroughly washed to remove serum from culture media, and adherent cells are treated with enzymatic or non-enzymatic dissociation solution to break the adhesion interaction between cells and suspend cells in the media. Secondly, the library is

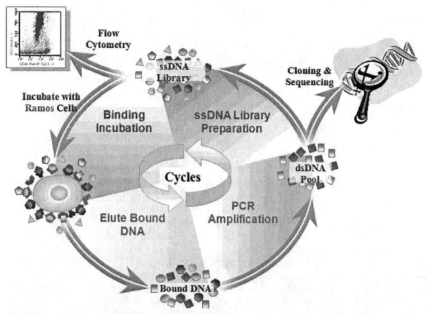

Figure 5.5. The Cell SELEX: Scheme of the cell-SELEX procedure, from Tang et al. 2007 with permission. The ssDNA pool was incubated with target cells (here Ramos cells). After washing, the bound DNAs were eluted by heating to 95°C for 5 min. The eluted DNAs were amplified by PCR. The double-stranded PCR products were separated into ssDNAs, and the sense strand DNAs were collected for the next round selection or tested by flow cytometry to monitor the SELEX progression. When the selected pool was enriched enough, the PCR product of the evolved pool was cloned and sequenced for aptamer identification.

incubated with the target cells for the desired time and temperature. After washing away the unbound DNA, the bound probes are collected by using heat denaturing. Third, the eluent is amplified by PCR or used for counter selection. In counter selection, the negative cells are incubated with eluent, and unbound probes are collected by centrifugation and amplified by PCR. In this way, the nucleic acids that bind to commonly expressed membrane proteins are successfully removed. Fourth, the amplified dsDNA is treated with streptavidin beads. The antisense strand with biotin is retained on the beads, and the sense strand is eluted with sodium hydroxide solution. The eluted ssDNA is considered the enriched pool for the first round and used as library for the next round. In general, the concentration of cells, DNA, ionic strength, incubation time, and temperature can all be varied to provide more stringent conditions favoring the selection of ligands with the highest affinity. To determine if high-affinity ligands are being enriched, it is necessary to monitor the binding of each pool by using flow cytometry or fluorescence microscopy

Using cell-Selex, aptamers able to identify CTCs were reported in literature and used for *in vivo* imaging. Moreover, examples of aptamers evolved by cell-Selex and employed for diagnostic assays were also reported. The group of Tan is particularly active in this field. For example they use aptamer-conjugated gold nanoparticles (AuNPs) for developing a colorimetric assay (Medley et al. 2008). As described by (Medley et al. 2008), aptamer-conjugated AuNPs are targeted to assemble on the surface of a specific type of cancer cell through the recognition of the aptamer to its target on the cell membrane surface. Once AuNPs have assembled on the cell surface, they behave as a larger gold cluster, having, as a consequence of aggregation, sufficient proximity for surface plasmon resonance to overlap. This results in the alteration of light scattering and absorption properties. After optimizing particle size and concentration, 1.0×10^{10} AuNPs were incubated with increasing amounts of target cells and the same amounts of control cells for comparison. The results showed that samples with the target cells present exhibited a distinct color change, while non-target samples did not elicit any change in color (Medley et al. 2008). Even a concentration of cells as low as 1,000 is reported to be readily detected by the naked eye. For more complex samples containing variously colored species to confound the results, this method was still able to rely on spectroscopic detection without any further sample preparation steps. In addition, the assay was able to differentiate between different types of target and control cells based on the aptamer used in the assay.

The same group reported on an aptamer-nanoparticle strip biosensor (ANSB) prepared on a lateral flow device (Liu et al. 2009). A pair of aptamers capable of specifically binding Ramos cells is used to prepare the ANSB. A thiolated aptamer (thiol-TD05) is immobilized on the AuNPs, and a biotinylated aptamer (biotin-TE02) is immobilized on the test zone of the ANSB (Fig. 5.6). Ramos cells interact with aptamer probes of the Au-NP-aptamer conjugates to form the Au-NP-aptamer cell complexes and continue to migrate along the strip. A large number of Au-NPs then accumulate on the test zone and produce a characteristic red band, which can be used for either qualitative, i.e. visual evaluation, or quantitative detection of cells by a portable strip reader. A DNA probe (complementary with the thiol-TD05) is immobilized on the control zone to capture the excess of Au-NP-aptamers, resulting in a second red band. The feasibility of this biosensor is evaluated by detecting Ramos cells spiked in human blood.

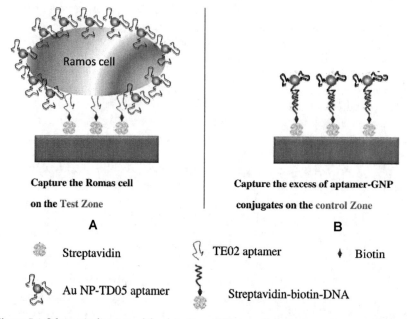

Figure 5.6. Schematic diagram of the detection of Ramos cells on aptamer-nanoparticle strip biosensor (ANSB): **(A)** capturing Au-NP-aptamer-Ramos cells on the test zone of ANSB through specific aptamer-cell interactions and **(B)** capturing the excess of Au-NP-aptamer on the control zone of ANSB through aptamer-DNA hybridization reaction (with permission from Liu et al. 2009).

APPLICATION TO OTHER AREAS OF HEALTH AND DISEASE

This chapter deals with the use of aptamers in biosensing for cancer studies. An overview of innovative technology to develop aptamers with high specificity for cancer studies were described with particular emphasis on multiplexed analysis of cancer biomarkers and on circulating cancer cell detection. These fields in fact seem to be especially benefited by the use of aptamers.

The potential use of aptamers as therapeutics has been already extensively reviewed. Among the other application in medicine, the use of aptamers for cell targeting, such as in flow cytometry, has been extensively examined. As bioreceptors in bioassays, aptamers have been used for many diagnostic applications, from protein analysis to antibiotics investigation.

KEY FACTS

- Nucleic acid aptamers are short, single stranded DNA or RNA oligonucleotides, which adopt stable three dimensional sequence-dependent structures.
- Aptamer are developed using a selection process called SELEX.
- The SELEX process involves iterative cycles of selection and amplification starting from a large library of oligonucleotides with different sequences (generally 10^{15} different structures).
- Several modifications into the SELEX procedure have been introduced recently and in the past in order to improve the aptamer selectivity.
- Several aptamers have already been developed against cancer related proteins and circulating tumor cells.

DEFINITIONS

- *Oncogenes*: gene that can cause cancer.
- *Tumor suppressor gene*: gene that code for proteins which serve as a stop signal.
- *Epigenetic*: study of changes produced in gene expression due to reasons other than in changes in DNA sequence.
- *Metastasis*: spread of cancer to different part of the body.
- *Bioreceptor*: biological or biologically-derived sensing element.
- *Biosensor*: a compact analytical device incorporating a biological or biologically-derived sensing element either integrated within or intimately associated with a physicochemical transducer.
- *Multiplexed analysis*: simultaneous measurement of multiple analites.
- *Proteomic technologies*: Technologies for large scale studies of proteins.

SUMMARY

- Nucleic acid aptamers are gradually entering the arenas of classical antibody applications. This is also underlined by the commercial exploitation of some of these molecules for different applications. Medical therapeutics and diagnostics are still the major areas of interest.
- The advantages of nucleic acid aptamers versus antibodies derive from their synthetic nature and their production by *in vitro* selection process from a combinatorial library.
- Aptamers can vary in size between 25 and 90 bases and adopt complex secondary and tertiary structures, which facilitate specific interactions with other molecules.
- As demonstrated by the high and increasing number of publications on this subject in recent years great progress has been made toward the development of aptamer-based assays.
- Several aptamers have already been developed against cancer related proteins and have been adapted for numerous biosensing principles mainly in direct and sandwich formats.
- Aptamers have been used for multiplexed proteomic technology for biomarker discovery and detection.
- Another field that seems to have been especially benefited by the use of aptamers is the detection of circulating tumor cells.

ABBREVIATIONS

ANSB	:	Aptamer-nanoparticle strip biosensor
AuNP	:	Gold Nanoparticle
bFGF	:	Basic fibroblast growth factor
CTC	:	Circulating tumor cells
DNA	:	DeoxyriboNucleic Acid
HER3	:	Human epidermal growth factor receptor 3
IL	:	Interleukin
MB	:	Methylene Blue
NFkB	:	Nuclear factor kB
NSCLC	:	Non small cell lung cancer
PDGF	:	Platelet-Derived Growth Factor
PMSA	:	Prostate-membrane specific antigen
RNA	:	RiboNucleic Acid
SELEX	:	Systematic Evolution of the Ligand by EXponential enrichment
SPR	:	Surface Plasmon Resonance
VEGF	:	Vascular Endothelial Growth Factor

REFERENCES

Berrino F, A Verdecchia, JM Lutz, C Lombardo, A Micheli and R Capocaccia. 2009. Comparative cancer survival information in Europe. Eur J Cancer 45: 901–908.

Bock C, M Coleman, B Collins, J Davis, G Foulds and L Gold. 2004. Photoaptamer arrays applied to multiplexed proteomic analysis, Proteomics, 4: 609–618.

Brody EN, L Gold, RM Lawn, J Walker and D Zichi. 2010. High-content affinity-based proteomics: unlocking protein biomarker discovery Expert Rev Mol Diagn 10: 1013–1022.

Daniels DA, H Chen, BJ Hicke, KM Swiderek and L Gold. 2003. A tenascin-C aptamer identified by tumor cell SELEX: systematic evolution. Proc Natl Acad Sci USA 100: 15416–15421.

De Angelis R, S Francisci, P Baili, F Marchesi, P Roazzi, A Belot, E Crocetti, P Pury, A Knijn, M Coleman and R Capocaccia. 2009. The EUROCARE-4 database on cancer survival in Europe: Data standardisation, quality control and methods of statistical analysis. Eur J Cancer 45: 909–930.

Ellington AD and JW Szostak. 1990. *In vitro* selection of RNA molecules that bind specific ligands. Nature 346: 818–822.

Gold L, D Ayers, J Bertino et al. 2010. Aptamer-Based Multiplexed Proteomic Technology for Biomarker Discovery. PLoS ONE 5: e15004. doi:10.1371/journal.pone.0015004

Golden MC, BD Collins, MC Illis and TH Koch. 2000. Diagnostic potential of Photo SELEX-evolved ssDNA aptamers J Biotechnol 81: 167–178.

Ireson CR and LR Kelland. 2006. Discovery and development of anticancer aptamers. Mol Cancer Ther 5: 2957–2962.

Lai R, KW Plaxco and AJ Heeger. 2007. Aptamer-Based Electrochemical Detection of Picomolar Platelet-Derived Growth Factor Directly in Blood Serum. Anal Chem 79: 229–233.

Liu G, X Mao, J Phillips, H Xu, W Tan and L Zeng. 2009. Aptamer-Nanoparticle Strip Biosensor for Sensitive Detection of Cancer Cells Anal Chem 81: 10013–10018.

Lupold SE, BJ Hicke, Y Lin and DS Coffey. 2002. Identification and characterization of nuclease-stabilized RNA molecules that bind human prostate cancer cells via the prostate-specific membrane antigen. Cancer Res 62: 4029–4033.

Mascini M, I Palchetti and S Tombelli. 2012. Nucleic Acid and Peptide Aptamers: Fundamentals and Bioanalytical Aspects, ANGEWANDTE CHEMIE-INTERNATIONAL EDITION, 51, 6, 1316–1332.

Mayer G. 2009. The Chemical Biology of Aptamers Angew. Chem Int Ed 48: 2672–2689.

McShane LM, DG Altman, W Sauerbrei, SE Taube, M Gion and GM Clark. 2005. Reporting recommendations for tumour MARKer prognostic studies (REMARK). Eur J Cancer 41: 1690–6.

Medley CD, JE Smith, Z Tang, Y Wu, S Bamrungsap and W Tan. 2008. Gold Nanoparticle Based Colorimetric Assay for the Direct Detection of Cancerous Cells. Anal Chem 80: 1067–1072.

Ostroff R, W Bigbee, W Franklin et al. 2010. Unlocking biomarker discovery: large scale application of aptamer proteomic technology for early detection of lung cancer PloS ONE 5: e15003.

Papamichael KI, M Kreuzer and GG Guilbault. 2007. Viability of allergy (IgE) detection using an alternative aptamer receptor and electrochemical means. Sensors and Actuators B, 121: 178–186.

Pu Y, Z Zhu, H Liu, JI Zhang, J Liu and W Tan. 2010. Using aptamers to visualize and capture cancer cells. Anal Bioanal Chem 397: 3225–3233.

Tang Z, D Shangguan, K Wang, H Shi, K Sefah, P Mallikratchy, HW Chen, Y Li and W Tan. 2007. Anal Chem 79: 4900–4907.

Tombelli S, M Minunni and M Mascini. 2007. Aptamers for diagnostic, environmental and food analysis. Biomolecular Engineering 24: 191–200.

Tothill IE. 2009. Biosensors for cancer markers diagnosis. Seminars in Cell & Developmental Biology 20: 55–62.

Tuerk C and L Gold. 1990. Systematic evolution of ligands by exponential enrichment: RNA ligands to bacteriophage T4 DNA polymerase. Science 249: 505–510.

Wang J, W Meng, X Zheng, S Liu and G Li. 2009. Combination of aptamer with gold nanoparticles for electrochemical signal amplification: application to sensitive detection of platelet-derived growth factor. Biosens. Bioelectron 24: 1598–1602.

6

Fluorescent Biosensors for Cancer Cell Imaging and Diagnostics

May C. Morris

ABSTRACT

Although cancer represents the leading cause of death worldwide, its burden could be largely reduced through implementation of diagnostic approaches for early detection and strategies to monitor disease progression and response to treatment. The development of genetically-encoded autofluorescent proteins, and the design of small synthetic probes with exceptional photophysical properties have catalyzed the development of fluorescent biosensors that can report on the relative abundance and dynamic behaviour of biomolecules. Together with these, major advances in high resolution imaging technologies have provided novel means to image biomolecules in their natural environment in a sensitive yet non-invasive fashion. Molecular imaging with fluorescent biosensors allows the biologist to study dynamic processes in real time in healthy and pathological cells with high spatial and temporal resolution. In addition, this technology has a number of practical applications in analytical chemistry and biotechnology, and is widely applied to several areas of health and

CRBM-CNRS-UMR 5237, University of Montpellier-IFR122, 1919 Route de Mende, 34293 Montpellier, France.
E-mail: may.morris@crbm.cnrs.fr
Corresponding author

List of abbreviations after the text.

disease, including clinical diagnostics and preclinical evaluation of candidate drugs in drug discovery programmes. In particular molecular tracers, targeted probes and "smart probes" which are specifically activated by the tumour environment have been developed for imaging cancer and metastasis, and successfully applied to image-guided surgery. Fluorescent biosensors are expected to improve early cancer detection, and to provide better means of determining cancer origin, stage and grade, thereby paving the way for personalized diagnostics and theranostic applications. This chapter will focus on fluorescent biosensor technology and molecular tracers for imaging biomarkers in cancer and metastasis. Representative examples of molecular tracers, targeted probes and activatable sensors will be presented and future developments for diagnostic and imaging applications will be discussed, in particular strategies aimed at probing intracellular biomarkers that contribute to cancer cell proliferation, multiplexed sensing technologies and potential theranostic applications.

INTRODUCTION

Cancer constitutes a diverse class of diseases which differ widely in their origin and development, but which share the characteristic acquired ability of cells to grow in an uncontrolled fashion, and at a later stage to invade adjacent tissues and spread further throughout the rest of the body through blood and the lymph. According to the World Health Organization, cancer is the leading cause of death worldwide, accounting for 7.9 million deaths in 2007, a figure expected to increase to reach 12 million by 2030. Six major alterations in the physiology of cancer cells, have been recognized to contribute to malignant cell growth. These features are commonly referred to as cancer hallmarks: (1) the acquisition of self-sufficiency in growth signals, (2) the loss of sensitivity to growth inhibitory signals, (3) the loss of ability to undergo apoptosis, (4) the acquisition of limitless replicative potential, i.e. the loss of ability to senescence, thereby allowing for uncontrolled growth and unlimited proliferation (immortality), (5) the development of sustained angiogenesis, and (6) the ability to invade tissues and metastasize at distant sites (Hanahan and Weinberg 2000). In addition, cancer cells present a characteristic lack of surveillance and repair mechanisms, develop means of avoiding the immune system, and display a significantly different metabolic activity from healthy cells (Kroemer and Pouyssegur 2008), as schematized in Fig. 6.1.

Cancer is a multicausal pathology, which is believed to develop following accumulation of inherited and/or acquired mutations in genes encoding proteins whose aberrant behaviour wreaks havoc in the orderly succession of events that lead to cell division. Mutations in well-characterized proto-oncogenes on the one hand, and on tumour suppressor genes,

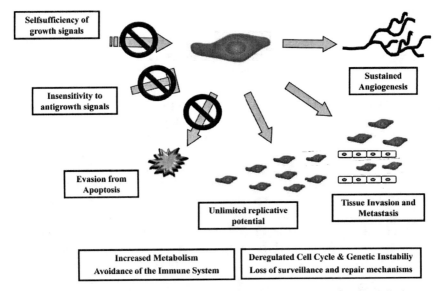

Figure 6.1. Cancer Hallmarks are major alterations in the physiology of cancer cells that are recognized to be characteristic of malignant growth. Together they contribute to deregulated cell cycle and genetic instability due to a characteristic lack of surveillance and repair mechanisms, which are accompanied by increased metabolism and avoidance of the immune system.

checkpoint control genes, and natural inhibitors that normally set brakes on proliferation in healthy cells on the other, are known to be responsible for a loss of coordination between surveillance and repair mechanisms, cell growth and division, thereby leading to uncontrolled cell proliferation and genetic instability (Kastan and Bartek 2004). These mutations are therefore recognized as largely responsible for development of cancer and constitute notorious factors of predisposition. Moreover they are accompanied by a larger set molecular alterations that cooperate in establishing and sustaining cancer cell growth by affecting critical cellular mechanisms that control cell physiology, metabolism and cell cycle progression. In particular, mutations that affect the enzymatic circuitry of cell cycle regulators constitute some of the most frequent alterations in human cancers (for review Kurzawa and Morris 2010, and references therein).

CANCER BIOMARKERS AND DETECTION STRATEGIES

Despite significant advances in our understanding of the molecular traits underlying development of cancer, its inherent complexity makes it very difficult both to diagnose and to target at an early stage, so as to prevent metastasis and progression of the disease to a terminal stage. This being said, it is estimated that one third of cancer cases could be avoided by early detection and treatment, through implementation of screening programmes aimed at identifying biomarkers of this disease. The National Cancer Institute defines a biomarker as "a biological molecule found in blood, other body fluids, or tissues that is a sign of a normal or abnormal condition or disease. A biomarker may be used to see how well the body responds to a treatment for a disease or condition." Biomarkers are typically found in the blood, serum, urine or cerebral spinal fluid, but may also be identified at the surface of cells or within cells. Bona fide cancer biomarkers are invaluable targets for early cancer detection, initial diagnosis, prognosis and staging, and may further be used for monitoring response to therapeutic treatment and/ or disease progression (Ludwig and Weinstein 2005). Disease biomarkers commonly used in clinical settings include seric proteins and cell surface antigens, antibodies and hormones, oncogenes and oncoviral proteins, as well as selected nucleic acid mutations, polymorphisms, amplification or translocation (Fig. 6.2). This being said, the development of genomic, proteomic and bioinformatics-based approaches has yielded a wealth of information as to novel candidate cancer biomarkers with potential clinical value (Ludwig and Weinstein 2005). In particular, gene profiling studies between healthy and cancer cells have led to identification of "proliferation

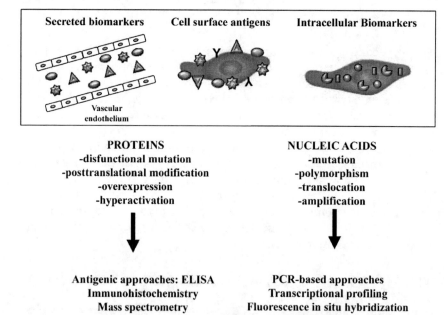

Figure 6.2. **Cancer Biomarkers** are found in bodily fluids, at the surface of cells or within cells and tissues. The molecular nature of biomarkers is variable. Typical examples of protein and nucleic acid biomarkers are listed, together with standard detection approaches.

signatures" which include genes that regulate critical steps of cell cycle progression, DNA synthesis and cell division (Carter et al. 2006; Whitfield et al. 2006). Although these candidate biomarkers constitute attractive targets for development of diagnostic strategies, like many other biomarkers, their relative inaccessibility due to their intracellular localization limits their direct detection *in situ*. As such traditional approaches for detection of biomarkers remains invasive, relying on biopsy followed by fixation and extraction procedures. Commonly implemented screening strategies involve antigenic approaches, such as ELISA or immunohistochemistry, proteomic approaches such as mass spectrometry for identification of protein biomarkers, and PCR-based assays, transcriptional profiling or FISH for probing nucleic acid biomarkers. This overall lack of appropriate methods to probe intracellular biomarkers within their healthy or pathological environment requires novel, sensitive and non-invasive detection strategies. Table 6.1 lists some of the most common biomarkers routinely used for cancer detection, together with potential cancer biomarkers proposed based on gene profiling or proteomics studies.

Table 6.1. Common examples of Cancer Biomarkers for Cancer Detection and Staging.

BIOMARKER FOR DIAGNOSIS	SPECIFIC CANCER TYPE
Secreted Biomarkers (FDA approved)	
CEA (serum)	colon, pancreatic, gastric, liver, lung, breast, ovarian
CA125 (serum)	ovarian, uterus, cervix, breast, etc.
CA15-3 (serum)	breast
alpha-fetoprotein (serum)	testicular, ovarian, liver
beta-human chorionic gonadotropin (serum)	testicular, ovarian, trophoblastic
PSA (serum)	prostate
thyroglobulin (serum)	thyroid
Cell Surface Biomarkers (FDA approved)	
Growth factor receptors :	most solid tumours
EGFR	colon
HER2 / NEU	breast
Oestrogen and progesterone receptors	breast
Intracellular Biomarkers	
Tumour suppressors: -pRB, p53	wide variety of cancers
-BRCA1, BRCA2	breast
Checkpoint proteins: Chk1, Chk2	wide variety of cancers
Cell cycle regulators:	wide variety of cancers
- Kinases: CDK/cyclins, Plk1, Aurora	
- Phosphatases: Cdc25	
Chromosomal abnormalities	
Polymorphisms, translocations	leukaemia

FLUORESCENT BIOSENSORS

One of the major challenges of modern biology and medicine is to visualize and probe biomolecules in their natural environment in a non-invasive yet dynamic fashion, so as to gain insight into their behaviour in both physiological and in pathological conditions, and monitor changes in their spatio-temporal localization patterns, their relative abundance, biological activity or function in response to specific stimuli or to treatment with drugs. The development of fluorescent biosensor technologies, associated with the development of genetically-encoded autofluorescent proteins, and of synthetic fluorescent probes with exceptional photophysical properties, and the concomitant development of high resolution fluorescence imaging technologies have allowed to meet this challenge, thereby providing highly sensitive means of studying biomolecular processes in real time, and a new generation of tools for biomedical imaging and diagnostic applications. Fluorescent biosensors are analytical devices that bear a fluorescent probe, which is genetically, chemically or enzymatically coupled to a sensing moiety responsible for recognition of a biomarker/target, whose spectral properties undergo variations directly related to target binding, thereby yielding an optical signal which is generally proportional to target concentration or activity (for review Morris 2010; Wang et al. 2009). Fluorescence variations can be monitored by one of several approaches depending on the nature of the bioprobe, as well as on the information sought for with respect to the biomarker (activity, abundance, conformation, subcellular localization). Changes in the spectral properties of the fluorescent probe are most often monitored by measuring variations in fluorescence intensity or shifts in fluorescence emission wavelength (associated with ratiometric quantification strategies), through FRET or FLIM approaches when a biosensor bears several probes whose proximity is modulated by the target, or yet by monitoring changes in subcellular localization and/or molecular mobility monitored by FCS and FCCS.

Fluorescent biosensors constitute an extremely diverse class of molecules, ranging from genetic fusions of autofluorescent proteins to synthetic peptides or macromolecular receptors such as proteins or protein fragments which can be site-specifically labelled, at an appropriate position, with a synthetic probe. They may be distinguished as activity or ligand-based biosensors, based on the sequence they present for recognition of their target. Activity biosensors consist of a short sequence that is recognized as a substrate and consequently modified by the target enzyme (e.g. proteolytic cleavage, phosphorylation, acetylation, etc.). Ligand biosensors comprise a domain that binds a characteristic complementary region on the target, through recognition of a specific epitope or conformation. Fluorescent biosensors are also distinguished by the mechanism through which they transduce their encounter with the target. FRET-biosensors bear two fluorescent probes whose proximity is directly affected by target binding, which induces a conformational change. In contrast, environmentally-sensitive or solvatochromic probes are directly involved in target sensing, binding of which modifies the polarity of the solvent in the immediate vicinity of the probe. Positional biosensors report on target activity through changes in their subcellular localization (Fig. 6.3).

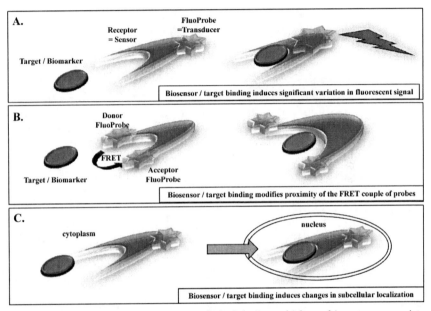

Figure 6.3. Fluorescent Biosensors are analytical devices which combine a sensor moiety involved in recognition of a specific analyte or target, with a physiochemical transducer, a fluorescent probe that emits a detectable and measurable signal upon binding to the target. A. Environmentally-sensitive biosensors B. FRET biosensors C. Positional biosensors.

The specificity and sensitivity of biosensors are critical features to enhance their response and reduce noise and artefacts, and more so for biomolecular imaging and clinical diagnostics. Although these parameters are directly related to the biomarker traits recognized by the biosensor, they can most often be fine-tuned when engineering the biosensor, so as to optimize selectivity and increase sensitivity. A good fluorescent biosensor should recognize and bind its target with respectable affinity, so as to ensure selectivity, and exhibit a change in fluorescence which reflects the presence or activity of the target in a highly sensitive fashion, with a high signal-to-noise ratio. In living cells and *in vivo*, however, fluorescent signals are often flawed by different parameters including autofluorescence which contributes to noise, and absorption of light by tissues at lower wavelengths of the visible spectrum, changes in cell morphology or in local intracellular pH. Therefore, careful consideration should be given in the choice of the most appropriate fluorescent probe for each biosensor application, as well as in standardization aspects.

Genetically-encoded AutoFluorescent Protein Biosensors. The discovery of the Green Fluorescent Protein, its genetic engineering and application to generate genetically-encoded fusion proteins, truly revolutionized fluorescence imaging approaches by providing novel means to engineer cell lines reporting on gene expression and study the spatio-temporal localization of ectopically expressed proteins (Tsien 2005; Zhang et al. 2002). GFP was further engineered to develop a broad range of autofluorescent protein derivatives with different spectral properties, and enhanced photophysical stability, including more recent NIRF probes for *in vivo* applications (Chudakov et al. 2010 and references therein). This palette of AFPs offers a wealth of options as well as means to perform multispectral imaging of cells expressing several genetic constructs simultaneously. In the late 90s, this technology was applied to the development of the first genetically-encoded biosensor, a FRET biosensor dubbed cameleon, designed for intracellular Ca2+ sensing, derived from the calcium-binding protein calmodulin (Miyawaki et al. 1997). Genetically-encoded protein fusions of autofluorescent proteins constitute an important class of biosensors for fundamental research and have been used successfully in cellulo and *in vivo*. The larger parts of these biosensors are single-chain FRET sensors, or positional biosensors, that are applied to monitor changes in enzymatic activities (Fig. 6.4). However these biosensors rely on ectopic expression of fusion proteins, which is rather lengthy and heterogeneous and therefore less adapted for diagnostic screens which require a rapid and standardized response.

Fluorescent Biosensor Proteins and Peptides. Besides the development of AFPs, major advances in fluorescence chemistry have yielded an extraordinary diversity of fluorescent dyes, small synthetic fluorophores with exceptional photophysical properties for biosensor applications and fluorescence imaging. Of particular interest are dyes that respond with extreme sensitivity to changes in their environment, dyes which can be quenched in the absence of the target, and near-infrared dyes which are particularly well suited for *in vivo* applications (Frangioni 2003; Lavis and Raines 2008; Loving et al. 2010). This prompted the development of Fluorescent Biosensor Proteins and Peptides, a class of biosensors directly derived from a polypeptide substrate or a protein binding domain, which is covalently modified with one (or more) synthetic fluorophores (Fig. 6.4). The versatility of FBPs is far greater than that of genetically-encoded biosensors, both in terms of design and engineering, with respect to the choice of the

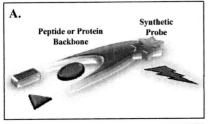
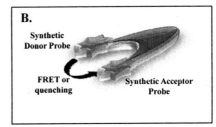
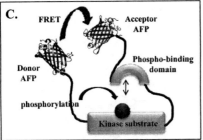
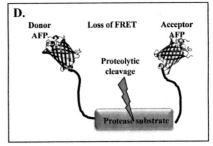

Figure 6.4. Genetically-encoded versus protein/peptide biosensors. Protein/peptide biosensors are derived from protein domains or peptide sequences that are site-specifically labelled with a synthetic probe A. A ligand-protein biosensor may report on the relative abundance and conformation of a specific target B. An activity-protein biosensor may report on enzymatic activity through conformationally-induced FRET, quenching or activation of a pair of synthetic probes. Genetically-encoded biosensors are genetic fusions of autofluorescent proteins. C. A single-chain FRET biosensor reports on phosphorylation through conformational-induced FRET between a donor and acceptor pair of AFPs upon recognition of a phosphorylated kinase substrate sequence by a phosphobinding domain. D. A single-chain FRET biosensor reports on proteolytic activity through loss of FRET between a donor and acceptor pair of AFPs upon cleavage of an intervening protease substrate sequence.

fluorescent label and its position within the biosensor scaffold. Moreover protein and peptide biosensors are easy to synthesize and handle *in vitro*, and provide an important degree of control which allows to circumvent issues associated with ectopic expression of genetically-encoded biosensors. However most FBPs cannot cross cell membranes alone, and therefore require facilitated delivery strategies to penetrate into cells and probe the relative abundance or activity of their intracellular target. Modular FBPs designed in a rational fashion so as to recognize specific protein interfaces, and that incorporate chemical fluorescent probes at strategic positions constitute a promising class of biosensors, and offer a wealth of perspectives for applications in cell biology, tumour profiling and cancer diagnostics.

APPLICATIONS OF FLUORESCENT BIOSENSORS

Fluorescence is particularly well suited to probe dynamic processes due to its intrinsic sensitivity and selectivity. As such fluorescent biosensors provide an extremely sensitive means of detecting analytes, ions, metabolites and biomarkers *in vitro* in complex environments including serum, cell extracts, living cells and *in vivo* for real-time imaging of dynamic processes. Fluorescent biosensors have been designed to report on the relative abundance, on a specific conformation or on overall activity of a given target, as well as to monitor changes in target concentration, conformational changes, variations in enzymatic activity, protein/protein interactions, cofactor and substrate binding and activation steps (Wang et al. 2009; Morris 2010). Importantly, fluorescence lends itself to non-destructive imaging, thereby preserving the sample and the molecules of interest within, and further allowing for multiple acquisitions over regular time intervals, as well as multiplexed acquisitions if several probes are used in combination. Fluorescence imaging also provides a high degree of spatial and temporal resolution at the cellular and subcellular levels. Fluorescent biosensors therefore allow studying the biological behaviour of molecules in their natural environment in a non-invasive fashion, to monitor dynamic changes in their subcellular localization, and to undertake studies of molecular mobility and molecular tracking. As such, fluorescent biosensors are useful tools for a wide variety of applications *in vitro*, in cellulo and *in vivo*, provided they can be introduced into cells and animals efficiently and non-invasively.

To name but a few, fluorescent biosensors have been designed for fundamental studies of cytoskeletal proteins, microtubules, and intermediate filaments, ions, second messengers and metabolites, motor proteins and enzymatic activities, to characterize signal transduction pathways and biomolecular networks in a wide variety of fields, ranging from cell cycle progression to neuroscience. These tools are also quite widely employed in analytical chemistry and biotechnology to monitor production and fermentation processes. Moreover, fluorescent biosensors have become central to drug discovery programmes at different stages of drug identification, characterization and validation (Lang et al. 2006; Giuliano et al. 2007; Willmann et al. 2008). First, they constitute sensitive and selective tools for high throughput screening of complex libraries in multi-well formats or in cell-based screens to identify potential therapeutic candidates that may affect target function, expression or subcellular localization. Once hits are identified, fluorescent biosensors are further employed to validate their therapeutic potential and characterize their mechanism of action *in vitro* and in cellulo. Finally they provide a means of assessing the preclinical relevance of candidate drugs *in vivo*, by characterizing their biodistribution, pharmacokinetics, and therapeutic potential. Last but not least, fluorescent biosensors play a major role in biomedical imaging, and are currently applied to monitor disease progression and assess response to therapeutic intervention. They are further expected to have a significant impact in clinical diagnostics, thereby responding to an urgent demand for sensitive technologies for early detection of cancer (for review Weissleder and Pittet 2008). Table 6.2 provides an overview of the different fields of application of fluorescent biosensors.

Table 6.2. Fluorescent Biosensors Applications.

Fundamental Studies in Life Sciences
Gene expression and subcellular localization
Relative abundance, conformation and activity
Intramolecular and intermolecular dynamics
Protein/protein interactions : substrate, cofactor, partner binding
Signal transduction, transcription, replication, cell growth and division, apoptosis ...

Applied Sciences
Biotechnology : fermentation processes
Analytical chemistry : analyte production
Lab-on-a-chip devices for electrolyte measurements
Fluorescence-based arrays

Drug Discovery Programmes
HTS to identify drug candidates
Cell-based screens to validate drug candidates
Preclinical evaluation: therapeutic potential, biodistribution, pharmacokinetics

Biomedical Applications
Molecular profiling
Clinical diagnostics
Monitoring disease progression and response to treatment
Endoscopy, laparascopy, intravital imaging, whole-body imaging
Image-guided surgery

MOLECULAR TRACERS AND FLUORESCENT BIOSENSORS FOR IMAGING CANCER

Over the past decade, several imaging modalities have been established for imaging cancer, including microcomputed tomography (CT) and magnetic resonance imaging (MRI), which provide high anatomical resolution yet low contrast sensitivity, single-photon emission computed tomography (SPECT), positron emission tomography (PET), and optical imaging technologies such as bioluminescence and fluorescence imaging, which are best suited for monitoring tumour cell biology, cancer progression and metastasis (Massoud and Gambhir 2003; Kaijzel et al. 2007; Dufort et al. 2010). SPECT and PET rely on the injection of radiolabelled tracers and are therefore somewhat hazardous for the patient, despite their reliability and sensitivity; moreover the short half-life of the radionuclides significantly limits longitudinal studies, and microscopic cellular imaging is essentially impracticable. In contrast, fluorescence imaging strategies rely on fluorescent probes which are minimally invasive for the patient, and which can provide high resolution cellular information with respect to molecular targets. As such, fluorescent probes have been developed for imaging cancer and metastasis and applied to animal models for intravital imaging, endoscopy or laparoscopic detection of cancer lesions (Hoffmann 2005; Kaijzel et al. 2007; Sahai 2007; Weissleder and Pittet 2008). More recently, fluorescent tracers have been successfully applied to image-guided surgery, with far more sensitivity and resolution of tumour resection than standard surgery based on tumour detection thanks to human vision and palpation (Dufort et al. 2010).

Optical imaging of tumour genesis, development and metastasis has made considerable progress thanks to the development of new generations of molecular tracers, optical contrast agents and fluorescent probes which specifically light up cancer cells and tumours thanks to one of several ingenious strategies (Pierce et al. 2008). In this respect cancer-specific receptors, as well as physiological properties that characterize cancer cells, such as high metabolic activity, acidic environment and increased angiogenesis, constitute targets for design of specific uptake, targeting or activation strategies (Keereweer et al. 2010). So far, essentially three strategies have been applied to design molecular probes for *in vivo* imaging of cancer: (1) non-targeted molecular contrast agents which accumulate in the vicinity of the tumour naturally; (2) targeted molecular tracers, which are coupled to ligands that direct the probe to cancer-specific receptors; and (3) activatable probes, also known as smart probes, that are specifically activated by the tumour environment. An alternative approach consists in developing probes that report on intracellular biomarkers which are specifically overexpressed/hyperactivated in cancer cells. Figure 6.5 provides a overview of the molecular tracers and biosensors developed to image cancer and metastasis.

Non-targeted molecular contrast agents accumulate naturally and passively into cancer structures, thanks to the angiogenic vasculature and intrinsic properties of tumours, including increased vascular permeability, high pressure and increased metabolic activity. Near-infrared fluorescent (NIRF) probes (emitting between 650 and 900nm) have become a sine qua none for *in vivo* imaging, as this window of light affords minimal absorption by tissues, minimal autofluorescence and light scattering, allowing photons to reach deep tissues and organs (Frangioni 2003). One of the first molecular

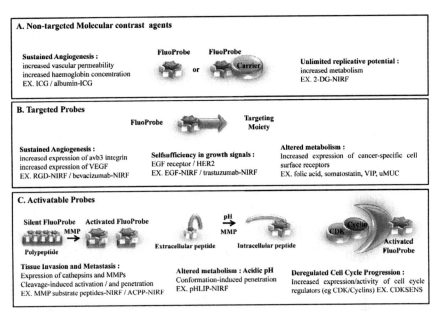

Figure 6.5. **Fluorescent Biosensors and Molecular Tracers for Imaging Cancer.** Three types of molecular tracers have been developed A. Non-targeted molecular tracers. B. Targeted probes that are selectively directed to cancer cells expressing specific cell surface receptors. C. Activatable probes that are activated by proteases and acidic pH in the tumour environment, or sensitive to changes in specific intracellular biomarkers.

tracers developed for *in vivo* imaging of cancer is indocyanine green (ICG), a NIRF probe with a peak of spectral absorption at 790nm, used in the clinic for retinal angiography (Slakter et al. 1995). In fact the majority of NIRF dyes used in optical imaging are carbocyanine dyes, which present particularly well suited spectral properties and high biocompatibility. Some commonly used dyes for near-infrared imaging, including Cy 5.5, Alexa Fluor 680 and 750, IRDye 680 and 800CW. The use of NIRF dyes for optical imaging of animal models is now well established, and these probes have been used to label small ligands, metabolic substrates and drugs, polymeric scaffolds and grafts, antibody fragments and inorganic molecules (Tung 2004; Pierce et al. 2008, Weissleder and Pittet 2008; Keereweer et al. 2010). Noteworthy examples include labelling of human serum albumin with tetra-sulphonated heptamethine indocyanines applied for mapping of sentinel lymph nodes (Ohnishi et al. 2005), and coupling of 2-deoxyglucose (2-DG), a derivative of the glucose analog FDG routinely used in PET imaging, to IRDye 800CW, applied to tumour imaging in xenografted mouse models (Kovar et al. 2009).

Tumour cell targeted probes. Selective targeting strategies are increasingly employed to enhance uptake of fluorescent probes by tumour cells, through covalent attachment of ligands or antibodies, which are specifically recognized by cell-surface tumour associated antigens or cancer-cell specific receptors (Allen 2002; Schrama et al. 2006). Some of the most common moieties for targeting cell surface receptors that are overexpressed on cancer cells include somatostatin analogs and vasoactive intestinal peptide for gastroenteropancreatic tumours (Becker et al. 2001), folic acid derivatives for ovarian and lung cancers overexpressing the folate-receptor, peptides targeting the underglycosylated MUC-1 tumour antigen overexpressed in adenocarcinomas, practically all breast cancers and several hematological malignancies (Moore et al. 2004), and glucose derivatives for targeting GLUT receptors (Kovar et al. 2009). In addition several strategies have been designed to target the angiogenic vasculature such as coupling RGD (Arginine-Glycine-Aspartic Acid) peptide sequences which target $\alpha v \beta 3$-integrin expressed at the surface of both tumour blood vessels and cancer cells (Chen et al. 2009), and anti-tumour monoclonal antibodies such as bevacizumab for targeting VEGF receptors, cetuximab or trastuzumab for targeting EGFR/HER2 (for review Schrama et al. 2006; Keereweer et al. 2010).

Activatable probes. New generations of "smart sensors" have been designed which are not directed to cancer-specific receptors, but instead specifically activated by the tumour environment, that is by cancer-specific proteases, and local acidic pH. In particular, the group of R.Weissleder has developed a wide variety of protease-sensitive probes, which are quenched due to the proximity of coupled NIRF probes, until activated by cancer-specific matrix metalloproteinases (MMP2, 9, 13) or cathepsins (B and D), which cleave the intervening peptide sequence, thereby releasing the fluorescent probes (Weissleder et al. 1999). A different strategy was employed by R. Tsien, who developed an activatable cell-penetrating polyarginine peptide, ACPP-NIRF probe, whose selective cellular penetration was conditioned by extracellular MMPs, whose activity enabled cleavage of a sequence masking the CPP (Jiang et al. 2004). A different strategy was devised by Urano and colleagues, which consisted of conjugating a pH-activatable fluorescent probe to a cancer-targeted monoclonal antibody, whose fluorescence was enhanced upon lysosomal acidification following internalization into viable cancer cells (Urano et al. 2009). More recently peptides whose cellular internalization is pH-sensitive, pHLIP peptides coupled to fluorescent probes, have been applied to tumour imaging. (Reshetnyak et al. 2010).

Fluorescent Biosensors of intracellular cancer biomarkers: probing CDK/ Cyclins. Rather than taking advantage of overexpressed cell surface receptors for targeting purposes, an alternative strategy consists in designing probes that report on the relative abundance or activity of intracellular biomarkers which are specifically overexpressed or hyperactivated in cancer cells. In this respect, cell cycle regulators whose expression or activity is altered in cancer cells constitute relevant biomarkers and pharmacological targets. In particular cyclin-dependent kinases (CDK/Cyclins), heterodimeric kinases, considered as the engines that coordinate timely cell cycle progression, play a key role in sustaining proliferation in cancer cells. Mutations that affect CDK/Cyclin activity confer a selective growth advantage, and overexpression or exacerbated CDK/cyclin activity has been documented in a broad range of cancers and associated with poor prognosis in patients (Malumbres and Barbacid 2001; 2009). As such, CDK/cyclins constitute attractive pharmacological targets for the development of anticancer drugs (Lapenna and Giordano 2009), and alterations in their levels or activities can be considered as valuable biomarkers of cell proliferation. Our group has recently developed a class of fluorescent peptide biosensors to probe CDK/Cyclin kinases, which can be introduced into living cells and animal models for fluorescence imaging thanks to cell-penetrating peptides. CDKSENS biosensors bear an environmentally-sensitive probe whose fluorescence increases significantly upon recognition of CDK/Cyclin complexes. Furthermore CDKSENS can be coupled to NIRF probes, and used for live-cell imaging of CDK/Cyclins and ratiometric quantification of their relative abundance between healthy and cancer cells. This technology allows to measure subtle differences in CDK/cyclin levels and provides a means of identifying cells in which overexpression of these kinases is truly relevant for therapeutic intervention (Kurzawa et al. 2011).

APPLICATIONS TO OTHER AREAS OF HEALTH AND DISEASE

Aside from cancer-related processes, fluorescent biosensors and imaging technologies have been applied to characterize a wide variety of pathological conditions, including inflammatory diseases such as arthritis, cardiovascular and neurodegenerative diseases and viral infection. Although genetically-encoded reporters and fluorescently-labelled protein biosensors or polymeric scaffolds have been developed to probe activities associated with specific pathological conditions, peptide-based probes are undoubtedly the most widely developed for molecular imaging of disease (Tung 2004; Law and Tung 2009; Morris 2010). Peptides offer low antigenicity compared to antibodies, and are rapidly eliminated by the circulation, thereby decreasing their toxicity. Moreover peptides can easily be coupled to fluorescent probes, as well as to ligands or targeting sequences. Peptide-based NIR imaging probes based on proteolytic activation have been developed to probe HIV and HSV. Protease probes have been developed to visualize

Table 6.3. Biosensor Applications in Health and Disease.

DISEASE CATEGORY	BIOSENSOR / TRACER
Cancer and Metastasis	
Passive accumulation in tumours and lymph nodes	ICG, NIRF-labelled albumin
Increased Metabolism	2-deoxyglucose-NIRF
Integrin expression	RGD-based NIRF probes
VEGF expression	bevacizumab-NIRF probes
MMP 2, 9, 13 and cathepsins B and D	-peptide-based protease-sensitive and ACPP probes
Local acidification	-pH-sensitive probes (pHLIP)
Cancer-specific surface receptors	
-somatostatin, vasointestinal peptide, uMUC1	peptide-based receptor-targeted probes
-EGFR, HER2	antibody-based receptor targeted probes
-folate receptor	folic acid analogs
Inflammatory diseases	
Arthritis : MMP and cathepsin expression	protease biosensors
Cardiovascular diseases	
Thrombosis, Atherosclerosis	thrombin biosensors, cathepsin B biosensors
Neurodegenerative diseases	
Apoptosis	caspase biosensors
	annexin-based polarity biosensor
Viral Infection	
HSV, HIV, HCV	Viral protease biosensors
HCV	Fluorescent cell-reporter assay

proteolytic activity of cells infected with Cytomegalovirus (CMV), Human Immunodeficiency virus (HIV) and Herpes Simplex virus (HSV) (for review Tung 2004). Enzyme-activatable peptide probes that are subject to proteolytic cleavage by cathepsins have been developed for detection of arthritis. Along the same lines, peptide-based NIR imaging probes have been developed for cardiovascular diseases, including thrombosis, and atherosclerosis (for review Tung 2004). Common to all of these biosensors, a substrate-based strategy has been employed to monitor proteolytic activities specific to disease (Law and Tung 2009). Notwithstanding, environmentally-sensitive biosensors are being developed to probe molecular features devoid of enzymatic activity, which characterize a pathological condition equally well, as exemplified by the polarity-sensitive annexin-based biosensor developed to detect apoptosis and applied to study neurodegeneration in rat neurons (Kim et al. 2010a). More recently, real-time imaging of hepatitis C virus infection thanks to a fluorescent cell-based reporter system has been described (Jones et al. 2010).

CONCLUDING REMARKS AND PERSPECTIVES

Fluorescent biosensors undoubtedly constitute some of the most promising tools for the detection of biomolecules *in vitro*, in cellulo and *in vivo*, and for monitoring dynamic molecular events in real time in a sensitive yet non-invasive fashion. Proteomic and genomic profiling have yielded a wealth of information concerning biomarkers which can be exploited to develop sensitive detection assays. Moreover, developments in the chemistry of fluorescent probes and in the design of cancer-specific targeting and activation strategies have yielded new tools for imaging cancer which have been successfully applied to mouse models of cancer, and which offer high expectations for biomedical applications. Despite these breakthroughs, one of the major challenges yet to be overcome concerns the sensitivity of biomarker detection at the earliest stages of cancer, such that small primary tumours and metastases will be detectable with sufficient sensitivity and reliability by optical imaging. Further, the multiplexed application of an array of fluorescent biosensors to probe several cancer biomarkers simultaneously would provide significant means of improving cancer characterization and staging, whilst paving the way for personalized diagnostics. Multi-analyte detection could be developed thanks to lab-on-a-chip devices, branched polymer or nanoparticle-based systems. Multiplexed detection strategies would then allow for therapeutic intervention with appropriately selected inhibitor cocktails. Finally, beyond their diagnostic function, fluorescent biosensors can be expected to contribute to cancer theranostics. The combination of specific targeting strategies with optical imaging approaches would provide a means of coupling biomarker detection with tailored therapeutic intervention, the efficiency of which could in turn be determined by monitoring response to treatment (Fig. 6.6). In this respect, multifunctional nanoparticles hold great promise for simultaneous target detection and drug delivery (Kim et al. 2010b). Optical imaging of cancer with fluorescent biosensors is still in its infancy, but clearly has exceptional potential, and future developments in nanotechnology will undoubtedly unleash powerful strategies for cancer diagnostics and personalized medicine that will allow to circumvent the current requirement for biopsies.

KEY FACTS

- Cancer is the leading cause of death worldwide, with a rising incidence estimated to reach 12 million deaths by 2030. Cancer is a multicausal pathology caused by genetic alterations which may be inherited and/or caused by environmental hazards such as chemical carcinogens, radiation, or infectious agents.

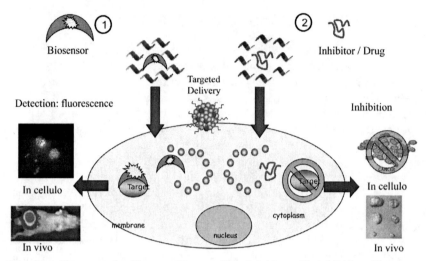

Figure 6.6. Biosensors for Theranostics: coupling detection with inhibition. Fluorescent biosensors can be expected to become useful tools for theranostics, providing a means to detect the target biomarker, and couple tailored therapeutic intervention. Multifunctional nanoparticles hold great promise for targeted delivery of fluorescent biosensors and drugs, for combined optical imaging and treatment of disease.

- Screening approaches implemented for early detection, monitoring disease progression and response to treatment are essential to reduce the cancer burden. Traditional methods to identify cancer cells rely on microscopic analysis, cell fixation and staining following biopsy or other indirect techniques, including antigenic detection of biomarkers, RT-PCR or proteomic approaches.
- Fluorescent biosensors constitute highly sensitive tools for probing molecular targets in their natural environment and offer a means of reporting on their relative abundance, biological activity, subcellular localization and molecular dynamics in real-time with high spatial and temporal resolution in a non-invasive fashion.
- Fluorescent biosensors are employed for a wide variety of applications *in vitro*, in cellulo and *in vivo*, including fundamental studies of gene expression, protein behaviour and dynamics, monitoring industrial production processes in analytical chemistry and biotechnology, high throughput screening assays and preclinical evaluation in drug discovery programmes, and biomedical applications in clinical settings.
- Fluorescent biosensors are particularly well suited to molecular imaging of cancer biomarkers, and are expected to provide significant advances in clinical diagnostics, for early detection and staging, imaging disease progression and response to treatment, as well as for image-guided surgery.

DEFINITIONS

- **Cancer Biomarkers** are biological molecules found in blood, serum, urine or cerebral spinal fluid, tissues or cells, indicative of alterations related to a physiopathological disorder or disease. Common biomarkers, include mutations, amplification or translocation of DNA, hormonal imbalance, high levels of specific antibodies, expression of oncogenes, cell surface receptors, alteres expression or mutations of tumour suppressors.
- **Cancer Hallmarks** are major alterations in the physiology of cancer cells that are recognized to be characteristic of malignant growth (1) self-sufficiency in growth signals, (2) resistance to antigrowth signals, (3) evasion of apoptosis, (4) limitless replicative potential, (5) sustained angiogenesis (6) tissue invasion and metastasis. These are accompanied by an increased metabolism, a characteristic lack of surveillance and repair mechanisms, and avoidance of the immune system.
- **Fluorescent biosensors** are analytical devices constituted of a target recognition sequence or domain (most often a protein domain or peptide sequence) onto which is coupled a fluorescent probe (autofluorescent protein or synthetic fluorophore) whose spectral properties undergo measurable variations upon target/biomarker recognition, thereby allowing to probe the relative abundance, activity, and dynamics of a target/biomarker.
- **Molecular Imaging** consists in imaging a specific molecular target or process thanks to molecular probes or tracers in living cells and organisms without perturbing their function. This technology is typically applied in fundamental studies, to characterize the behaviour of molecules in their physiological environment, to probe disease biomarkers in diagnostic applications, such as cancer, neurological disorders, and cardiovascular diseases, and is used in drug discovery programmes for preclinical and clinical validation of candidate drugs.
- **Theranostics** concerns the coupled application of diagnostics and therapeutics to probe disease biomarkers and monitor disease progression and response whilst simultaneously implementing therapeutic intervention, through a selective targeting approach.

SUMMARY POINTS

- **Cancer** is a multicausal pathology consisting in aberrant and unrestricted growth of cells, which constitutes the leading cause of death worldwide. Traditional approaches for detection of cancer biomarkers remain invasive and indirect, dependent on biopsy, cell fixation and extraction, followed by antigenic approaches (ELISA, immunohistochemistry), RT-PCR or proteomic approaches. Alternatively, the morphological characteristics of cancer cells cultured from a biopsy, can be examined by optical microscopy to assess the origin, stage and grade of the tumour. Implementation of screening programmes for early detection of cancer is necessary to reduce cancer burden, thereby calling for development of non-invasive detection strategies with high sensitivity, resolution and selectivity.

- **The development of fluorescent biosensors** that report on biological targets through changes in their spectral properties, together with major advances in high resolution imaging technologies have provided novel means of imaging biomolecules in their natural environment and dynamic processes in a non-invasive fashion. Genetically-encoded biosensors express one or more autofluorescent proteins in fusion with a target-specific recognition sequence, and can be ectopically expressed in living cells. Fluorescent biosensor proteins and peptides constitute are derived from protein or peptide domains that bind the target, onto which one or several small synthetic probes may be coupled.

- **Applications:** Fluorescent biosensors constitute a sensitive means of probing specific analytes, ions, metabolites, and biomarkers and can provide target information in complex solutions: serum, cell extracts, living cells. Fluorescence biosensors have been designed to report on relative abundance, activity, function, subcellular localization of biomolecules and are well suited to real-time studies of dynamic processes. They constitute sensitive tools for a wide variety of applications *in vitro*, in cellulo and *in vivo*, from fundamental studies of gene expression, protein behaviour and dynamics to more practical problems in analytical chemistry and biotechnology, and biomedical applications, including clinical diagnostics, intraoperative imaging, and drug discovery programmes.

- **Applications to areas of health and disease:** Fluorescent biosensors are widely used for molecular imaging of different aspects of health and disease, in a variety of pathologies, including arthritis and inflammatory diseases, cardiovascular and neurodegenerative diseases, viral infection, cancer and metastasis. They are also widely used in drug discovery programmes for identification of candidate drugs by high throughput screening approaches and for preclinical evaluation of the therapeutic potential, biodistribution and pharmacokinetics of candidate drugs.

- **Imaging cancer and metastasis:** Growth and metabolism of malignant tumour cells are not dictated by the same rules as healthy cells. Cancer hallmarks constitute targets for development of optical imaging strategies. Fluorescent contrast agents, receptor-targeted probes, and "smart probes" which are selectively activated by the tumour environment have been developed for intravital and whole-animal imaging. Further strategies include the development of probes that report on intracellular biomarkers that are specifically overexpressed/hyperactivated in cancer cells, multiplexed sensing platforms or lab-on-a-chip devices, and the design of multifunctional nanoparticles for theranostic applications.

ACKNOWLEDGMENTS

Research in M.C. Morris group is supported by the CNRS (Centre National de la Recherche Scientifique) and grants from the Association de Recherche contre le Cancer (ARC), the Region Languedoc-Roussillon (Subvention "Chercheuse d'Avenir") and Institut National du Cancer (INCA). This chapter is dedicated to my mother and her fight against cancer.

ABBREVIATIONS

ACPP	:	activatable cell-penetrating peptide
AFP	:	autofluorescent protein
CDK	:	cyclin-dependent kinase
CPP	:	Cell penetrating peptide
CT	:	microcomputed tomography
2-DG	:	2-deoxyglucose
EGF	:	Epidermal Growth Factor
FBP	:	fluorescent biosensor protein
FCCS	:	fluorescence corss-correlation spectroscopy
FCS	:	fluorescence correlation spectroscopy
FDG	:	18F-fluoro-deoxyglucose
FISH	:	fluorescence *in situ* hybridization
FLIM	:	fluorescence life-time imaging
FP	:	fluorescent protein
FRET	:	fluorescence resonance energy transfer
GFP	:	Green fluorescent protein
HTS	:	high throughput screening
ICG	:	indocyanine green
MMP	:	matrix metalloproteinase
MRI	:	magnetic resonance imaging

NIRF   :   Near-InfraRed Fluorescence
PET   :   Micropositron emission tomography
SPECT   :   single-photon emission computed tomography
VEGF   :   Vascular Endothelium Growth Factor
VIP   :   vasoactive intestinal peptide

REFERENCES

Allen T. 2002. Ligand-targeted therapeutics in anticancer therapy. Nat Rev Cancer 2: 750–761.

Becker A, C Hessenius, K Licha, B Ebert, U Sukowski, W Semmler, B Wiedenmann and C Grötzinger. 2001. Receptor-targeted optical imaging of tumors with near-infrared fluorescent ligands. Nat Biotechnol 19: 327–31.

Carter SL, AC Eklund, IS Kohane, LN Harris and Z Szallasi. 2006. A signature of chromosomal instability inferred from gene expression profiles predicts clinical outcome in multiple human cancers. Nat Genet 38: 1043–48.

Chen K, J Xie and X Chen. 2009. RGD-human serum albumin conjugates as efficient tumor targeting probes. Mol Imaging 8(2): 65–73.

Chudakov DM, MV Matz, S Lukyanov and KA Lukyanov. 2010. Fluorescent proteins and their applications in imaging living cells and tissues. Physiol Rev 90(3): 1103–63.

Dufort S, L Sancey, C Wenk, V Josserand and JL Coll. 2010. Optical small animal imaging in the drug discovery process. Biochim Biophys Acta 1798(12): 2266–73.

Frangioni JV. 2003. *In vivo* near-infrared fluorescence imaging. Curr Opin Chem Biol 7: 626– 634.

Giuliano KA, DL Taylor and AS Waggoner. 2007. Reagents to measure and manipulate cell functions. Methods Mol Biol 356: 141–63.

Hanahan D and RA Weinberg. 2000. The hallmarks of cancer. Cell 100: 57–70.

Hoffmann RM. 2005. The multiple uses of fluorescent proteins to visualize cancer *in vivo*. Nat Rev Cancer 5: 796–806

Jiang T, ES Olson, QT Nguyen, M Roy, PA Jennings and RY Tsien. 2004. Tumor imaging by means of proteolytic activation of cell-penetrating peptides. Proc Natl Acad Sci USA 101: 17867–17872.

Jones CT, MT Catanese, LM Law, SR Khetani, AJ Syder, A Ploss, TS Oh, JW Schoggins, MR MacDonald, SN Bhatia and CM Rice. 2010. Real-time imaging of hepatitis C virus infection using a fluorescent cell-based reporter system. Nat Biotechnol 28(2): 167–71.

Kaijzel EL, G van der Pluijm and CW Löwik. 2007. Whole-body optical imaging in animal models to assess cancer development and progression. Clin Cancer Res 13(12): 3490–7.

Kastan MB and J Bartek J. 2004. Cell Cycle Checkpoints and cancer. Nature 432: 316–323.

Keereweer S, JD Kerrebijn, PB van Driel, B Xie, EL Kaijzel, TJ Snoeks, I Que, M Hutteman, JR van der Vorst, JS Mieog, AL Vahrmeijer, CJ van de Velde, RJ Baatenburg de Jong and CW Löwik. 2010. Optical Image-guided Surgery-Where Do We Stand? Mol Imaging Biol [Epub ahead of print]

Kim YE, J Chen, JR Chan and R Langen. 2010a. Engineering a polarity-sensitive biosensor for time-lapse imaging of apoptotic processes and degeneration. Nat Methods 7: 67–73.

Kim K, JH Kim, H Park, YS Kim, K Park, H Nam, S Lee, JH Park, RW Park, IS Kim, K Choi, SY Kim, K Park and IC Kwon. 2010b. Tumor-homing multifunctional nanoparticles for cancer theragnosis: Simultaneous diagnosis, drug delivery, and therapeutic monitoring. J Control Release 146(2): 219–27.

Kovar JL, W Volcheck, E Sevick-Muraca, MA Simpson and DM Olive. 2009. Characterization and performance of a near-infrared 2-deoxyglucose optical imaging agent for mouse cancer models. Anal Biochem 384(2): 254–62.

Kroemer G and J Pouyssegur. 2008. Tumor cell metabolism: cancer's Achilles' heel. Cancer Cell 13(6): 472–82.

Kurzawa L and MC Morris. 2010. Cell Cycle Markers and Biosensors, Chem Bio Chem 11(8): 1037–47.

Kurzawa L, M Pellerano, JB Coppolani and MC Morris. 2011. Fluorescent peptide biosensor for probing the relative abundance of cyclin-dependent kinases in living cells. PloS One, 6(10): e26555.

Lapenna S and A Giordano. 2009. Cell cycle kinases as therapeutic targets for cancer. Nat Rev Drug Discov 8(7): 547–66.

Lang P, K Yeow, A Nichols and A Scheer. 2006. Cellular imaging in drug discovery. Nat Rev Drug Discovery 7: 591–607.

Lavis LD and RT Raines. 2008. Bright ideas for chemical biology. ACS Chem Biol 3: 142–55.

Law B and CH Tung. 2009. Proteolysis: a biological process adapted in drug delivery, therapy, and imaging. Bioconjug Chem 20(9): 1683–95.

Loving GS, M Sainlos and B Imperiali. 2010. Monitoring protein interactions and dynamics with solvatochromic fluorophores. Trends Biotechnol 28: 73–83.

Ludwig JA and J N Weinstein. 2005. Biomarkers in cancer staging, prognosis and treatment selection. Nat Rev Cancer 5: 845–56.

Malumbres M and M Barbacid. 2001. To Cycle or not to cycle: a critical decision in cancer. Nat Rev Cancer 1, 222.

Malumbres M and M Barbacid. 2009. Cell cycle, CDKs and cancer: a changing paradigm. Nat Rev Cancer 9(3): 153–66.

Massoud TF and SS Gambhir. 2003. Molecular imaging in living subjects: seeing fundamental biological processes in a new light. Genes Dev 17(5): 545–80.

Miyawaki A, J Llopis, R Heim, JM McCaffery, JA Adams, M Ikura and RY Tsien. 1997. Fluorescent indicators for Ca2+ based on green fluorescent proteins and calmodulin. Nature 388: 882–7.

Moore A, WZ Medarova, A Potthast and G Dai. 2004. *In vivo* targeting of underglycosylated MUC-1 tumor antigen using a multimodal imaging probe. Cancer Res 64: 1821–1827.

Morris MC. 2010. Fluorescent Biosensors of Intracellular Targets: from Genetically-encoded Reporters to Modular Polypeptide Probes. Cell Biochem Biophys 56: 19–37.

Ohnishi S, SJ Lomnes, RG Laurence, A Gogbashian, G Mariani and JV Frangioni. 2005. Organic alternatives to quantum dots for intraoperative near-infrared fluorescent sentinel lymph node mapping. Molecular Imaging 4: 172–181.

Pierce MC, DJ Javier and R Richards-Kortum. 2008. Optical contrast agents and imaging systems for detection and diagnosis of cancer. Int J Cancer 123: 1979–1990.

Reshetnyak YK, L Yao, S Zheng, S Kuznetsov, DM Engelman and OA Andreev. 2010. Measuring Tumor Aggressiveness and Targeting Metastatic Lesions with Fluorescent pHLIP. Mol Imaging Biol.

Sahai E. 2007. Illuminating the metastatic process. Nature Rev Cancer 7: 737–749.

Schrama D, R Reisfeld and J Becker. 2006. Antibody targeted drugs as cancer therapeutics. Nat Rev Drug Discovery 5: 147–159.

Slakter JS, LA Yannuzzi, DR Guyer, JA Sorenson and DA Orlock. 1995. Indocyanine-green angiography. Curr Opin Ophthalmol 6(3): 25–32.

Tsien RY. 2005. Building and breeding molecules to spy on cells and tumors. FEBS Lett 579(4): 927–32.

Tung CH. 2004. Fluorescent peptide probes for *in vivo* diagnostic imaging. Biopolymers. 76(5): 391–403.

Urano Y, D Asanuma, Y Hama, Y Koyama, T Barrett, M Kamiya, T Nagano, T Watanabe, A Hasegawa, PL Choyke and H Kobayashi. 2009. Selective molecular imaging of viable cancer cells with pH-activatable fluorescence probes. Nat Med 15: 104–109.

Wang H, E Nakata and I Hamachi. 2009. Recent progress in strategies for the creation of protein-based fluorescent biosensors. Chem biochem 10: 2560–2577.

Weissleder R and M Pittet M. 2008. Imaging in the era of molecular oncology. Nature 452: 580–589.

Weissleder R, CH Tung, U Mahmood and A Bogdanov Jr. 1999. *In vivo* imaging of tumors with protease-activated near-infrared fluorescent probes. Nat Biotechnol 17: 375–378.

Whitfield M, LK George, GD Grant and CM Perou. 2006. Common markers of proliferation. Nat Rev Cancer 6: 99–106.

Willmann JK, N van Bruggen, LM Dinkelborg and SS Gambhir. 2008. Molecular imaging in drug development. Nature Reviews Drug Discovery 7: 591–607.

Zhang J, RE Campbell, AY Ting and RY Tsien RY. 2002. Creating new fluorescent probes for cell biology. Nat Rev Mol Cell Biol 3(12): 906–18.

7

Electrical and Electrochemical Immunosensor for Cancer Study

Seung Yong Lee[1] and Seung Yong Hwang[2,*]

ABSTRACT

In recent decades, interest in health has shown a dramatic increase due to remarkable advances in development of biomedical and clinical applications. Cancer continues to be one of the leading causes of mortality each year; hence, research for development of various medical technologies for use in cancer diagnosis and treatment is ongoing. High throughput screening for use in production and analysis of various types of information in the biosensor field is currently under rapid development. The main technology of cancer sensor systems is the sensing biochip. Development of point-of-care testing (POCT) leads to development of small detection devices, which offer the advantages of rapidity, ease of handling, small volume of samples, and high sensitivity and specificity. Despite these advances, the expense incurred on cancer patients is considerably high and a cure has yet to be found. Use of a small microbiochip in an electrical detection system may make diagnostics more readily accessible to point-of-care testing facilities. Use of the biosensor has

[1]Department of Bio-Nano Technology, Hanyang University, Ansan, Gyeonggi-do, Korea;
E-mail: three2k@hanmail.net
[2]Division of Molecular and Life Science, College of Science & Technology, Hanyang University
& GenoCheck Co. Ltd., Ansan, Gyeonggi-do, Korea; E-mail: syhwang@hanyang.ac.kr
*Corresponding author

List of abbreviations after the text.

allowed for safe, effective, and easy detection of samples. Systems for measurement of electrical signals utilize chemical/biological reactions, pH, temperature, and detection in mass by measurement of changes in electrical signals. The electrochemical reaction is directly related to electrical and electrochemical signals and analog signals, such as light and mass. Therefore, electrical and electrochemical detection methods are applied in development of biosensors, because the signal change step is very simple, with high sensitivity, and can be used with a small detection device. Electrochemical measurements can involve use of analytical methods, as well as development of new sensors, membrane production capabilities, and development of new battery and capacitor materials; molecular electronic device development, also in the field of electrochemistry, can include use of polymers, biotechnology, inorganic chemistry, materials chemistry, medicine, pharmacy, and electronics, and plays a pivotal role in many areas.

As a result, high throughput methods using electrical and electrochemical detection methods have been developed for use in cancer study, and the information provided here can be expected to serve as a useful guide for researchers designing similar experiments. This experiment can be used as an alternative to currently-used methods. Compared with the current cutting edge system, integrated lab-on-a-chip tumor sensing systems will lead to innovation in cancer diagnosis.

CANCER STUDY

General Study of Cancer

Cancer (medical term: malignant neoplasm) is a type of tumor. Tumors can be malignant or benign. Malignant tumors have three main characteristics. The first characteristic is uncontrolled growth through proliferation beyond growth of normal cells. Another characteristic is invasion, which involves intrusion upon, and then destruction of adjacent tissues. The third feature is metastasis; for instance, spread of cancer cells to other locations in the body via the lymph or blood. These three malignant properties of cancerous tumors differentiate them from benign tumors, which are self-limited, and do not invade or metastasize.

Cancer is primarily an environmental disease, with 90–95% of cases due to environmental factors, including lifestyle; 5–10% is the direct result of heredity. Common environmental factors leading to cancer include the following: tobacco (25–30%), diet and obesity (30–35%), infections (15–20%), radiation, stress, lack of physical activity, and environmental pollutants. These environmental factors cause or enhance abnormalities in the genetic material of cells. Hereditary or acquired abnormalities in these regulatory genes can lead to uncontrolled cell growth, and development of cancer.

The presence of cancer can be suspected on the basis of symptoms, or findings on radiology. However, definitive diagnosis of cancer requires microscopic examination of a biopsy specimen. Most cancers can be treated by chemotherapy, radiotherapy, and surgery (Anand et al. 2008).

According to data for some developed countries, including the United States, Great Britain, Japan, and Korea, various types of cancer have been observed according to cultural differences and dietary habits (Fig. 7.1). The aim of this chapter is to conduct a comparative study of cancer incidence

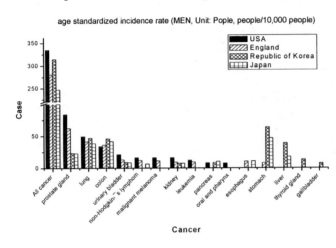

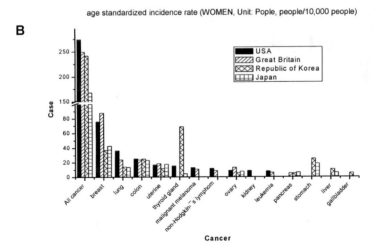

Figure 7.1. International comparison of cancer in 2008. Data for some developed countries, including the United States, Great Britain, Korea, and Japan; various types of cancer have been observed according to cultural differences and dietary habits. **(A)** men, **(B)** women.

based on international statistics, excluding some types of cancer, such as skin and orphan cancer.

According to the International Agency for Research on Cancer (IARC)—the affiliated organization of the World Health Organization (WHO)—and the *Journal of the National Cancer Institute* (JNCI), the causes of cancer are largely associated with environmental elements, as shown below (Fig. 7.2).

A   **International Agency for Research on Cancer (IARC)**

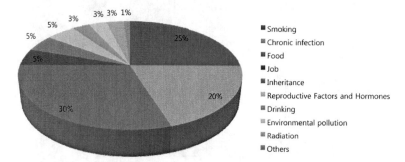

B   **The Journal of the National Cancer Institute (JNCI)**

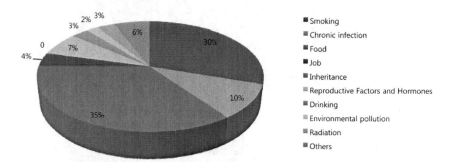

Figure 7.2. Factors contributing to cancer. (A) Cancer is largely associated with environmental elements, including food (30%), smoking (25%), and acute hepatitis (20%)—IARC, (B) Cancer is mainly associated with environmental elements, including food (35%), smoking (30%), and acute hepatitis (10%)—JNCI.

General Study of Cancer Diagnosis

Current diagnostic methods are based on patient history and physical examination. X-ray diagnosis of lung cancer or myeloma uses radiograph or CT for black and white images; methods for diagnosis of intestinal cancer include detection by observation of contrast medium using different shades for diagnosis. In particular, observation of gastric and colorectal cancer utilizes double contrast methods, such as evaluation of the status of the mucosa in early gastric cancer or colorectal cancer.

Regarding cellular diagnosis, since detection of cellular properties of malignancy in smears of uterine secretions was first introduced, methods for diagnosis and early diagnosis of cervical cancer have shown dramatic improvement. The current method for cellular diagnosis of cervical cancer has used several types of organ secretions, including prostate, urinary tract, lung, pancreas, thyroid, and breast. Pathologic microscopic examination of phyton by biopsy is used for confirmation of the diagnosis of cancer. X-ray methods, endoscopy, cellular diagnosis, and biopsy, are the main diagnostic methods used in diagnosis of cancer; other methods, including ultrasonic wave and isotope scanning CT, are used for early clinical diagnosis of pancreatic, liver, and thyroid cancer.

Recent research by Seetharaman Balasenthil et al. showed that plasma biomarkers related to cellular movement, morphology, and development can be used in a microarray system for diagnosis of pancreatic cancer. (Balasenthil et al. 2011). Abba et al. 2010 also reported on 42 genes related to breast cancer diagnosis. And, using 5760 human genes for exploration of aneuploidy, Rantala et al. exploited a 177 specific gene sorting cell spot microarray method, which can be controlled by several mechanisms, and provided evidence for division of cells into normal cells and breast cancer cells. (Rantala et al. 2010). Madu emphasized the importance of development of highly sensitive and specific biomarkers for prostate cancer (Madu and Lu 2010). These studies provide strong support for use of microarray experiments for determining new biomarkers in cancer studies.

Cancer Study Using Proteomic Techniques

Proteomic techniques are important in cancer diagnosis. According to reports from the U.S. Food and Drug Administration (FDA), over 95% of currently licensed drugs target proteins, such as interferon-alpha, which is used in therapeutics of hepatitis. Proteomic methods provide advanced determination of factors for cancer prevention, and those prepared according to the characteristics of each cell unit can be regarded as personalized treatment.

The first decades of diagnosis derived high cure rates and complete recovery in ovarian cancer; however, 80% of patients were already in advanced stages of cancer. Therefore, patients in the terminal stage underwent surgical or pharmacologic therapy, despite the fact that the 5-yr survival rate was 35% or less. In other words, early diagnosis has an impact on patient survival; there is no further need to emphasize this fact. In addition, presence of cancerous tissue often leads to other diseases.

In general, proteomics research techniques use electrospray ionization (ESI), matrix-assisted laser desorption/ionization (MALDI), and surface-enhanced laser desorption/ionization (SELDI). Matrix-assisted laser desorption/ionization (MALDI) is a soft ionization technique used in mass spectrometry, allowing for analysis of biomolecules (biopolymers, such as proteins, peptides, and sugars) and large organic molecules (such as polymers, dendrimers, and other macromolecules), which tend to be fragile and fragment when ionized by more conventional ionization methods. SELDI is typically used with time-of-flight mass spectrometers and is used in detection of proteins in tissue samples, blood, urine, or other clinical samples. Comparison of protein levels between patients with and without a disease can be used for biomarker discovery (Li et al. 2002). Electrospray ionization (ESI) is a technique used in mass spectrometry for production of ions. Use of this technique can overcome the propensity of these molecules to fragment when ionized; therefore, it is particularly useful in production of ions from macromolecules (Fenn et al. 1989) (Table 7.1).

Table 7.1. Cancer Biomarker. Table 7.1 shows the basic types of cancer biomarkers. Under the formation of a small cancer, the levels of some biomarkers increase; therefore, limits of detection (LOD) of the detection methods are important for early screening of a small cancer. It shows the thresholds of basic cancer biomarkers in human serum.

Cancer	Biomarker	Normal value
Liver cancer	AFP	<5.4 ng/ml
Colorectal and pancreatic cancer	CEA	< 2.5 ng/ml (nonsmokers)
		< 5 ng/ml (smokers)
Ovarian cancer	CA 125	< 35 units/ml
Nonseminomatous germcell tumors	β-hCG	< 5 mIU/ml
Pancreatic cancer	CA 19-9	< 37 units/ml
Breast cancer	CA 27.29	< 38 units/ml
Prostate cancer	PSA	< 4 ng/ml

Masilamani et al. contributed to the development of methods for early diagnosis of cancer using various biochemical methods, including fluorescence emission spectra Group (FES) and stroke shift spectra (SSS). Based on these methods, they conducted research on feasibility of simple, non-invasive, and inexpensive protocol methods through spectral analysis of urine (Masilamani et al. 2010). Liu et al. studied measurement of cancer diagnosis through serum samples for comparison of data from 80 cervical cancer patients and 80 healthy volunteers. Use of these methods demonstrated problems associated with established biomarkers and the necessity for new biomarkers and development of proteomics techniques for detection (Liu et al. 2010). Through comparative analysis of clinical blood samples by ELISA (Enzyme-linked immunosorbent assay), He et al. demonstrated cancer diagnosis from serum protein using a liquid chromatography-coupled electrospray ionization tandem mass spectrometry (MS/LC-MS) technique. The group also performed *in vitro* and *in vivo* experiments for analysis of three identified proteins from 97 samples in a cell line model experiment comparing data from a nude mouse model experiment (He et al. 2010). These results support the need for conduct of a multifaceted analysis for development of biomarker applications.

High throughput screening for production and analysis of various types of information in the biosensor field is under rapid development. Detection of target proteins using antigen-antibody reactions is the main technology used in cancer sensor systems. In addition, study or selection of various biomarkers as a new access method of proteomics, which is limited by protein amount, hydrophobicity, and molecular weight. Currently, development of portable protein biochip systems for multiple cancer diagnosis is one of the hot topics in this field.

Table 7.2. Key features of Cancer Diagnosis.

1. There are various types of cancer; however, many types of cancers are easier to treat and cure if they are found early.
2. Traditional cancer diagnosis has been dependent on symptoms revealed by physical examination, radiology, and patient history.
3. Genetic-based cancer diagnosis utilizes various specific biomarkers.
4. Genomics technologies, including microarray, provide strong support for determination of new biomarkers in cancer studies.
5. Proteomic methods for cancer diagnosis utilize mass spectroscopy for advanced identification of factors for cancer prevention.

ELECTRICAL AND ELECTROCHEMICAL IMMUNOSENSORS

General Study of Biosensors

Biosensors, through an electrical detection system, detect a specific electrical change of the target biomaterials (e.g. DNA, Protein, etc.) when there is cohesion between probe materials of detection parts. A DNA microarray is a multiplex technology used in molecular biology. It consists of an arrayed series of thousands of microscopic spots of DNA oligonucleotides, called features, each containing picomoles (10^{-12} moles) of a specific DNA sequence, known as probes (or reporters). These can be a short section of a gene or other DNA element that is used in hybridization of a cDNA or cRNA sample (called a target) under high-stringency conditions. Probe-target hybridization is usually detected and quantified by detection of fluorophore-, silver-, or chemiluminescence-labeled targets for determination of relative abundance of nucleic acid sequences in the target. As a result, use of arrays has resulted in a dramatic acceleration of many types of investigation (Lee et al. 2010) (Fig. 7.3).

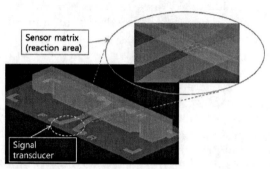

Figure 7.3. Schematic model of a general biochip sensor. The three main components of the biochip are the biosensor, sensor matrix, and signal transduction part. Modified from Ko et al. 2008.

Microbiochips can be applied in many ways, including drug screening, disease diagnosis, and analysis of environmental pollution. Currently, active areas of research include nanotechnology, including bio-MEMS (Micro electric mechanical system), μ-TAS (Total analysis system), microfluidics, and biotechnology, including treatment of integrated nanobiomaterials and study of microbiochips. In particular, the biosensor has been in the spotlight as a real time and simple detection method for use in diagnosis of disease in the field.

A biosensor is an analytical device used for detection of an analyte, which combines a biological component with a physicochemical detector component. A biosensor is a simple diagnostic device for use in detection and analysis of various physiologically active substances and chemical materials in real time, and can be subdivided into target materials, such as DNA, enzymes, antibodies, toxicants, and cells. Immunosensors using specific binding between antigen and antibody have demonstrated better specificity and sensitivity than other analytical methods. New technology for use in performance of immunoassays has been developed. Electrical and electrochemical detection between antigen and antibody reactions is one of the new technologies. Detection of electrical and electrochemical signals is relatively simple and easy to manage, and requires a minimal amount of detection equipment, so that electrical and electrochemical detection devices could be used at once in sample preparation, reaction, and detection. Based on these results, potential implementation of point-of-care testing (POCT) has been demonstrated in recent research.

A Lab-On-a-Chip (LOC) is a device that integrates one or several laboratory functions on a single chip of only millimeters to a few square centimeters in size. LOCs deal with the handling of extremely small fluid volumes, down to less than picoliters. Microfluidics is a broader term that also describes mechanical flow control devices, like pumps and valves, or sensors, like flow meters and viscometers. However, strictly considered, "Lab-on-a-Chip" generally indicates the scaling of single or multiple lab processes down to chip-format. The term "Lab-on-a-Chip" was introduced later, when it turned out that µTAS technologies were more widely applicable than only for analytical purposes.

General Study of Electrical and Elcetrochemical Immunosensors

Electrical signals detect voice (frequency, intensity, and language), image (color, light and shade, and movement), or differences of physical, chemical, and biological reactions using electrical properties. These signals are based on membrane potential, which is stimulated by an action potential under special conditions. In biological systems, application of excitable cells can be used in study and detection of functions in the human body. The biosensor requires simple electrodes for acquisition of biosignals. Electrodes are necessary, because electrical conduction is detected by ions in the detection system. Electrochemistry is a branch of chemistry involving the study of chemical reactions that take place in a solution at the interface of an electron conductor (a metal or a semiconductor) and an ionic conductor (the electrolyte), and which involves electron transfer between the electrode and the electrolyte or species in solution. Chemical reactions involving transfer of electrons between molecules are called oxidation/reduction (redox) reactions. In general, for an understanding of each process, electrochemistry deals with situations where oxidation and reduction reactions are separated in space or time, connected by an external electric circuit.

Electrochemical measurements have recently been used in both analytical methods and in development of new sensors, membrane production capabilities, and in development of new battery and capacitor materials; molecular electronic device development, also in the field of electrochemistry, can be used in polymers, biotechnology, inorganic chemistry, materials chemistry, medicine, pharmacy, and electronics, and plays a pivotal role in many areas. Electrochemical measurement has been used increasingly in cycle voltammetry, polarography, impedance spectroscopy, and oxidation of various electronic states and systematic analysis of electrochemical reaction mechanisms.

The system for measurement of electrical signals includes chemical/ biological reaction pH, temperature, and detection in mass by measurement of electrical signal change. Electrochemical reaction is directly related to electrical and electrochemical signals and analog signals, such as light and mass. Therefore, electrical and electrochemical detection methods are applied for biosensors, because the signal change step is very simple, with high sensitivity, and can be used with a small detection device.

Electroanalytical methods are used for measurement of the potential (volts) and/or current (amps) in an electrochemical cell containing an analyte. Concentration of active species, equilibrium constants, reaction mechanisms, as well as electron transfer reactions occurring on the electrode surface, and adsorption of a series will bring forth a significant amount of information on this phenomenon.

Electrical and Electrochemical Immunosensors for Diagnosis

Typically, electrical and electrochemical experiments have detected one or more, such as a difference of potential, charge, current or time. Each experimental response is dependent on excitation signals for stimulation. Results obtained can provide significant information for use in description of various forms using variables. Electrochemical detection methods include the following: linear sweep voltammetry, cyclic voltammetry, chronoamperometry, chronocoulometry, chronopotentiometry, polarography, and electrochemical impedance. Regarding these methods, Dtantiev et al. developed methods for measurement of two immunochemical sensors (Immunoenzyme electrodes) for comparison of 4-dichlorophenoxyacetic acid (2,4-D) and 2,4,5-trichlorophenoxyacetic acid (2,4,5-T). They utilized an assay for monitoring of free pesticide and pesticide-peroxidase for recording of peroxidase activity of immune complexes on a fixed graphite electrode (Dzantiev et al. 1996).

Sadik and Van Emon described the basic electrochemical immunoassay technology, including information on electrochemical detection based immunoassay methods for analysis of environmental samples. Immunosensing systems based on conducting electroactive polymers (CEPs) are more rapid, sensitive, and inexpensive than traditional environmental immunoassays. (Sadik and Van Emon 1996). Wang et al. manufactured disposable electrochemical immunosensors based on potentiometric stripping analysis of metal tracers using a verified assay format of entire on-chip. In planning their experiments, they decided on adoption of easy stripping voltammetric immunoassays and evaluation of decentralized testing on-chips. Results provided affirmation for use of this on-chip operation in decentralized (clinical and environmental) applications (Wang et al. 1998). Dijksma et al. read a paper on continuous development of electrochemical immunosensors for use in detection of interferon-γ (IFN-γ). According to their paper, cysteine or self-assembled monolayers (SAMs) of acetylcysteine have electropolished polycrystalline Au electrodes.

Based on this information, they maintained that a plot of the real (Z') and an imaginary (Z") component of impedance provide adjusted information on the process (Dijksma et al. 2001). Authier et al. reported on their study of electrochemical DNA detection methods, which identified sensitive quantification of amplified 406-base pair human cytomegalovirus DNA sequences (HCMV DNA) (Authier et al. 2001). Wang et al. performed amplification of enzyme-based bioaffinity electrical sensing of DNA and proteins using carbon nanotubes (CNTs). These experiments led to improved sensitivity by combination of CNTs amplifiers and transducers in detection of proteins and DNA for polymerase chain reaction (PCR)-free DNA assay. (Wang et al. 2004). Yang et al. developed label-free electrochemical impedance immunosensors for Escherichia coli (E. coli) O157:H7 using anti-E. coli antibodies on indium-tin oxide interdigitated array (IDA) microelectrodes. In particular, binding of E. coli cells was monitored using two-electrode electrochemical impedance spectroscopy in the presence of $[Fe(CN)6]^{3-/4-}$ without enzymatic amplification (Yang et al. 2004). Chen et al. have developed a new immunosensor, which allows for direct attachment of receptor proteins on permeable gold film. According to the results, this experiment proved that porous nanostructure gold film has the capability of adsorption of protein on the surface through an increase in the electronics potential resistance response over time (Chen et al. 2005).

Development of an electrochemistry system is in progress in various fields of science and technology. Performance and application of basic science applications has narrowed the gap between modern research, and developmental trends in areas of electrochemical systems application have been increasingly extended. In particular, the recent nanotechnology, where new materials are being developed for ultra-fine electrode electric chemistry, is a reminder of that potential (Fig. 7.4).

ELECTRICAL AND ELECTROCHEMICAL IMMUNOSENSORS FOR CANCER STUDY

Immunosensors for Diagnosis

An immunoassay is a biochemical test that measures the presence or concentration of a substance in solutions that frequently contain a complex mixture of substances. Immunoassay methods are frequently employed for assay of analytes in biological liquids, such as serum or urine. Such assays

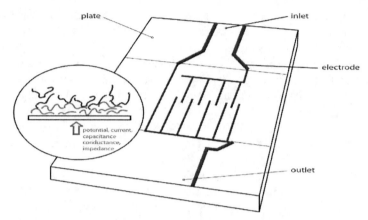

Figure 7.4. The model of general electric and electrochemical biochips. Biochips, which consist of an electrochemical system, use potential, current capacitance, conductance, and impedance for induction of electron-transfer resistance.

Table 7.3. Key features of Biosensors.

1. A biosensor is a simple diagnostic device used for detection and analysis of various physiologically active substances and chemical materials in real time, and can be targeted toward specific molecules and materials.
2. Advantages of biosensors include reduction of sample and reagent, rapid reaction and detection, automation and portability, ease of use, high throughput, improved analysis accuracy and sensitivity, etc.
3. Disadvantages of biosensors include increase of machine size, limit of microfluidics, solubility, and flexibility.
4. Biosensors can be applied in many ways, including drug screening, disease diagnosis, and analysis of environmental pollution.
5. Biosensors can detect targets according to specific molecular sequences or structural features and provide the advantages of miniaturization, screening, and low cost.

are based on the unique ability of an antibody to bind with high specificity to one or a very limited group of molecules. In the early days, researchers used this method for protein detection and quantitation; however, in recent years, it has been used for development of antibody molecules, analysis of carbohydrates, lipids, and various microorganisms. In addition to binding specificity, the other key feature of all immunoassays is a means for production of a measurable signal in response to specific binding. Historically, this was accomplished by measurement of a change in certain physical characteristics, such as light scattering or changes in refractive index. Nevertheless, most immunoassays today are dependent on the use of an analytical reagent that is associated with a detectable label. A large variety of labels have been demonstrated, including radioactive elements used in radioimmunoassays; enzymes; fluorescent, phosphorescent, and chemiluminescent dyes; latex and magnetic particles; dye crystalites, gold, silver, and selenium colloidal particles; metal chelates; coenzymes; electroactive groups; oligonucleotides, stable radicals, and others. Such labels serve in detection and quantitation of binding events, either after separation of free and bound labeled reagents or by designing the system in such a way that a binding event affects a change in the signal produced by the label. Immunoassays in which the signal is affected by binding can often be run without a separation step. (Fig. 7.5).

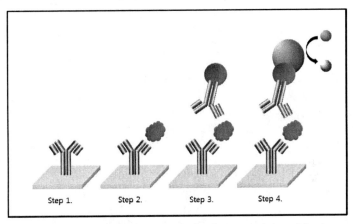

Step 1.   Step 2.   Step 3.   Step 4.

Figure 7.5. Model of general immunoassay. Analytes are detected by immunoassay. Immunoassays are chemical tests used for detection or quantification of a specific substance, the analyte, in a blood or body fluid sample, using an immunological reaction.

Recently, protein detection technology has been developed by introduction of immunoanalysis, fusion with nanotechnology, and bio-barcode systems at femtogram (fg) per milliliter concentration. This new technology allows for maximum sensitivity and ability of multiplex analysis with protein arrays for high-throughput protein analysis. Attributes of immune reaction include build up of special complexes between antigens and antibodies. This phenomenon can make possible the use of markers, such as isotopes, fluorescence, and enzymes in immunoanalysis. In particular, because radioimmunoassay analysis can detect ultra trace amounts, such as picogram (10^{-12}g), the assay should be performed carefully in order to avoid contamination from radio-isotopes or radioactivity. As a result of their simple and fast methodologies, immunosensors are quite popular in the biosensing arena.

The foundation of immunosensors is not only antibody-antigen reactions, but also detection of membrane potentials and electrodes directly or by use of chemically amplified markers on the antibody membrane. In immunosensors, electric or optic signals are adopted for occurrence of electrical signals, such as electrodes or semiconductors. These analytical systems have the advantage of changing electrical signals to antigen-antibody reactions. Two materials will be used in future transducers; an electrode is a popular transducer, and a semiconductor has the advantages of economical mass production and miniaturization.

Point-of-Care Testing (POCT)

Point-of-care testing (POCT) involves clinical examination near the patient. POCT is an all clinical testing technique that is used outside the central clinical system. Development of POCT leads to development of small detection devices that offer the advantages of rapidity, ease of handling, small volume of samples, and high sensitivity and specificity. These developments could result in derivation of many types of advantages, such as inexpensive diagnosis, increased patient satisfaction, and reduced test time, error rate, and hospitalization. POCT devices are used widely with electrical and electrochemical detection methods. Preventive health care in consumer self-testing is an important argument, and health care and promotion have resulted in commercialization of a variety of self-help devices for detection of blood sugar, pregnancy, blood, urine, stool, and ingredients. These innovative devices are non-invasive, compact, and portable, and the home care service is available by approval and its use is expected to increase due to ageing of the population (Kost 2002).

Electrical and Electrochemical Biosensors for Cancer Study

Recently, electrical and electrochemical biosensors have been studied in many fields of application. Michael Wilson has developed electrochemical immunosensors that are capable of detection of two different analytes. The ELISA method was used in this study. Capture antibodies were immobilized on a three dimensional porous IrOx matrix by covalent attachment using silane coupling chemistry; analytes were then introduced in the sensor. AP (alkaline phosphatase)-labeled antibodies were then bound to the electrode-bound analytes. Finally, analytes were detected by electrochemical oxidation of alkaline phosphatase-generated hydroquinone using Hydroquinone diphosphate (HQDP), a novel AP substrate. (Wilson 2005). Zheng's group has developed a nanowire sensor device for use in detection of various cancer markers by a highly sensitive, label-free, multiplexed electrical detection method. As they also measured targets using atomic force microscopy (AFM), results from the nanowire sensor device were validated (Zheng et al. 2005). Ibtisam Tothill emphasized the importance of point-of-care diagnostic devices for rapid detection and analysis of cancer markers with high sensitivity and selectivity. Molecular profiles of patients have been studied using molecular tools (e.g. genomic and proteomic techniques), and these methods, united with bioinformatics tools, are used to find and elucidate biomarkers of the new disease. However, the task of finding only one ultra-specific and sensitive marker for a disease is very difficult. Because the level of biomarkers in human biological fluids can vary under different disease conditions and stages, a number of molecular markers are usually measured for cancer diagnosis. (Tothill 2009). Mani et al. have increased the sensitivity and signal amplification for the target using nanoparticles coated with HRP-labeled secondary antibodies (Mani et al. 2009). Bangar et al. have performed studies in the field of conduction of polymer nanowire based immunosensors. The aluminal template was used in fabrication of Polypyrrole (Ppy) nanowires. The CA 125 biomarker, which was used in this study, is clinically approved for monitoring of the response to treatment and prediction of prognosis after treatment. It is especially useful for detection of recurrence of ovarian cancer (Bangar et al. 2009). Rusling et al. have also achieved signal amplification and an increase in sensitivity for the target using the single-wall carbon nanotube (SWNT), which is coated with HRP-labeled secondary antibodies. In order to extend an application of this platform, they recently studied another platform using multi-labeled secondary antibody labeled particles instead of single-wall carbon nanotubes (SWNT) to obtain an improved sensitivity and signal (Rusling et al. 2009). Yun et al. developed highly aligned multi-wall carbon nanotube electrodes for electrochemical impedance measurement of prostate cancer cells in the fluidic channel. Based on the impedance results, this device can distinguish different kinds of solution. They also suggested that modification of the gold functionalized carbon nanotube electrode with biomaterials that can recognize the target, such as antibodies and aptamers, could be very useful for cancer diagnosis (Yun et al. 2007). Ho et al. have developed an electrochemical immunoassay system for detection of carcinoembryonic antigen (CEA). Carbon nanoparticles (CNP)/poly(ethylene imine) (PEI) coated with anti-CEA antibodies were immobilized onto the electrode. (Ho et al. 2009). Maeng et al. developed a microbiochip that is based on an electrical detection system that can be used for detection of AFP antigen. Using this system, with the simple structure of the microfilter, microbeads were efficiently fixed, and AFP could be detected at concentrations as low as 1 ng/mL. These results indicate that this system would be adequate for use in clinical diagnosis (Maeng et al. 2008). Ko et al. reported on successful development and operation of the integrated multiplex electro-immunosensing system. In addition, the electrical signal that corresponds to the immunocomplex was amplified by use of a silver enhancer and the electrical signal was successfully measured using a PC-based system. This multiplex electro-immunosensing system can be applied widely to various cancer biomarkers by use of the appropriate antibodies or bioreceptors (Ko et al. 2008) (Fig. 7.6).

Study of early diagnosis of cancer using electrochemical biosensors has increased as part of an effort to develop a rapid and easy kit product for use with a portable diagnostic device, which is not yet practically available. This study is amplified based on multiplex ligation dependent probe amplification (MLPA). In order to integrate all processes, a combination of innovative research and process steps using special techniques from different project partners (ranging from microfluidics to interfacing, miniaturization, and integration techniques) will be required. Compared with the current cutting edge system, an integrated portable lab-on-a-chip tumor sensing system will open the door to a new era in cancer diagnosis (Fig. 7.7).

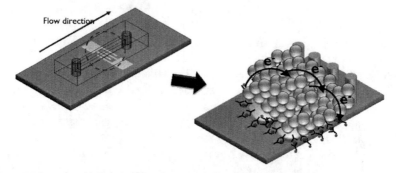

Figure 7.6. Integrated lab-on-a-chip tumor sensing system. Integrated biosensor for complex detection, such as potential, current, capacitance, conductance, and impedance from existing single detection methods, which is only possible for use in single detection. Modified from Maeng et al. 2008.

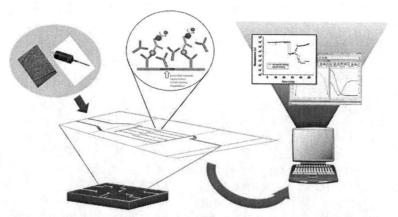

Figure 7.7. Multiplex electro-immunosensing system. Integrated multiplex electro-immunosensing system uses immunocomplexes, such as appropriate antibodies or bioreceptors.

Table 7.4. Key features of Electrical and Electrochemical Immunosensors.

1. Electrical and electrochemical immunoassay is a type of technique using electron transfer or redox reactions in the sensor.
2. Electrical and electrochemical measurements have recently been used in analytical methods for biological reactions, and in development of new sensors, membrane production capabilities, and new battery and capacitor materials.
3. Biosensor systems with electrical and electrochemical techniques are more rapid, sensitive, and inexpensive than traditional assays.
4. These sensors have various applications, such as in integrated tumor sensing systems or multiplex electron sensing systems.
5. Special techniques from different project partners (miniaturization, and integration techniques) are required for post-technology of biosensors.

APPLICATIONS TO OTHER AREAS OF HEALTH AND DISEASE

Biosensors comprise one of the most interesting technologies for use in rapid sensing of small quantities of materials in the clinic and in food. Electrochemical sensors detect bio-specific recognition elements and convert them into intelligible electrical impulses. These sensors are actively used because the required equipment is small in scale. Recently, use of biosensor principles in conjunction with semiconductor technology has led to miniaturization and mass production. As the population ages, biosensors are needed for use in rapid detection and diagnosis of disease. In addition, portable miniature biochips, based on microfluidic control techniques are also being studied. Electrochemical sensors can be used anywhere in the modern world and have applications in industry, the environment, and the clinic. Electrochemical sensors must be able to deliver real-time information and detect targets without sampling the target material. In addition, sensors can operate in extreme environments, depending on the electrolytes used in the device. The two types of electrical sensors can conduct electrochemical measurements of electric current, voltage, or impedance. Sensitivity, selectivity, and stability of a sensor are affected by temperature, pressure, and the chemical environment.

Table 7.5. Summary points.

• Cancer is a type of tumor. Characteristics of cancer include uncontrolled growth, invasion, and metastasis. Currently, genetic and proteomic methods are being actively studied for use in cancer diagnosis. Genetically based cancer diagnosis utilizes a variety of specific biomarkers and microassay methodologies. Proteomic methods for cancer diagnosis provide advanced identification of factors for cancer prevention by mass spectrometry.
• A biosensor is a simple diagnostic device for use in detection and analysis of various physiologically active substances and chemical materials in real time, and can be targeted toward specific materials. It can detect a target by specific molecular sequences or structural features and provides the advantages of miniaturization, screening, and low cost.

Table 7.5. Contd....

Table 7.5. Contd....

- Electrical and electrochemical measurements have recently been used in analytical methods for biological reactions. Typically, electrical and electrochemical experiments have detected one or more changes, such as a difference in potential charge, current, or time.
- Biosensor systems based on electrical and electrochemical techniques are more rapid, sensitive, and inexpensive than traditional assays.
- Biosensors could provide a useful tool for point-of-care testing (POCT) in the field, in association with different research topics.

Table 7.6. Key terms.

- Biomarker: A biomarker, or biological marker, a biochemical feature or fact that can be an indicator of a biological state and used to measure the progress of disease or the effects of treatment.
- Genomics: Genomics is a discipline in genetics concerning the study of the genomes of organisms. The aim of this genetic pathway, and functional information analysis is to elucidate its effect on, place in, and response to the entire genome's networks.
- Proteomics: The proteome is the entire complement of proteins, including the modifications made to a particular set of proteins, produced by an organism or system. Proteomics is the large-scale study of proteins, particularly their structures and functions.
- Cancer diagnosis: Cancer is a class of diseases in which a group of cells display uncontrolled growth, invasion that intrudes upon and destroys adjacent tissues, and sometimes metastasis, or spreading to other locations in the body via the lymph or blood. Most cancers are initially recognized either because signs or symptoms appear or through diagnostic screening.
- Electrochemistry: Electrochemistry is a branch of chemistry that studies chemical reactions which take place in a solution at the interface of an electron conductor (a metal or a semiconductor) and an ionic conductor (the electrolyte), and which involve electron transfer between the electrode and the electrolyte or species in solution
- Biosensor: A biosensor is an analytical device that converts a biological response and combines a biological component with a physicochemical component.
- Immunoassay: An immunoassay is a biochemical test using an immune reaction for measurement or quantification of a substance, an analyte, in a body fluid sample.
- Immunosensor: An immunosensor is a type of biosensor for use in detection of response by a specific immunological reaction.
- Lab-on-a-chip (LOC): A lab-on-a-chip is a miniaturized device that has the ability to execute laboratory operations.
- Point-of-care testing (POCT): Point-of-care testing (POCT) is a type of medical testing at the bedside, near patients, and for decentralized testing provided by clinical operators immediately to the patient. This increases the likelihood that the patient, physician, and care team will receive the results on a timely basis.

ABBREVIATIONS

AFM	:	atomic force microscopy
AP	:	alkaline phosphatase
CEA	:	carcinoembryonic antigen
CEP	:	conducting electroactive polymers

CNP	:	carbon nanoparticle
CNT	:	carbon nanotubes
E. coli	:	Escherichia coli
EDC	:	N-(3-dimethylaminopropyl)-N'-ethylcarbodiimide hydrochloride
ELISA	:	enzyme-linked immunosorbent assay
ER	:	emergency room
ESI	:	electrospray ionization
FDA	:	Food and Drug Administration
FES	:	fluorescence emission spectra
fg	:	femtogram
HCMV	:	human cytomegalovirus
HQDP	:	hydroquinone diphosphate
IARC	:	International Agency for Research on Cancer
ICU	:	Intensive care unit
IDA	:	interdigitated array
IFN-γ	:	interferon-γ
JNCI	:	The Journal of the National Cancer Institute
LOC	:	lab-on-a-chip
MALDI	:	matrix-assisted laser desorption/ionization
MALPA	:	multiplex ligation dependent probe amplification
MEMS	:	micro-electro-mechanical system
MS/LC-MS	:	liquid chromatography-coupled electrospray ionization tandem mass spectrometry
OR	:	operating room
PCR	:	polymerase chain reaction
PDMS	:	polydimethylsioxane
PEI	:	poly(ethylene imine)
POCT	:	point-of-care testing
Ppy	:	polypyrrole
Redox	:	oxidation/reduction
SAM	:	self-assembled monolayers
SSS	:	stroke shift spectra
SWNT	:	single-wall carbon nanotube
μ-TAS	:	micro-total analysis systems
WHO	:	World Health Organization

REFERENCES

Abba MC, E Lacunza, M Butti and CM Aldaz. 2010. Breast cancer biomarker discovery in the functional genomic age: a systematic review of 42 gene expression signatures. Biomark Insights 5: 103–118.

Anand P, AB Kunnumakkara, C Sundaram, KB Harikumar, ST Tharakan, OS Lai, B Sung and BB Aggarwal. 2008. Cancer is a Preventable Disease that Requires Major Lifestyle Changes. Pharm Res. 25: 2097–2116.

Authier L, C Grossiord and P Brossier. 2001. Gold nanoparticle-based quantitative electrochemical detection of amplified human cytomegalovirus DNA using disposable microband electrodes. Anal Chem 73: 4450–4456.

Balasenthil S, N Chen, ST Lott, J Chen, J Carter, WE Grizzle, ML Frazier, S Sen and AM Killary . 2011. A migration signature and plasma biomarker panel for pancreatic adenocarcinoma. Cancer Prev Res (Phila) 4: 137–49.

Bangar MA, DJ Shirale, W Chen, NV Myung and A Mulchandani. 2009. Single conducting polymer nanowire chemiresistive label-free immunosensor for cancer biomarker. Anal Chem 81: 2168–2175.

Chen Z, J Jiang, G Shen and R Yu. 2005. Impedance immunosensor based on receptor protein adsorbed directly on porous gold film. Analytica Chimica Acta 553: 190–195.

Dijksma M, B Kamp, JC Hoogvliet and WP van Bennekom. 2001. Development of an electrochemical immunosensor for direct detection of interferon-gamma at the attomolar level. Anal Chem 73: 901–907.

Dzantiev BB, AV Zherdev, MF Yulaev, RA Sitdikov, NM Dmitrieva and I Yu Moreva. 1996. Electrochemical immunosensors for determination of the pesticides 2,4-dichlorophenoxyacetic and 2,4,5-tricholorophenoxyacetic acids. Biosensors and Bioelectronics 11: 179–185.

Fenn JB, M Mann, CK Meng, SF Wong and CM Whitehouse. 1989. Electrospray ionization for mass spectrometry of large biomolecules. Science 246: 64–71.

He Y, X Wu, X Liu, G Yan and C Xu. 2010. LC-MS/MS analysis of ovarian cancer metastasis-related proteins using a nude mouse model: 14-3-3 zeta as a candidate biomarker. J Proteome Res 9: 6180–90.

Ho JA, YC Lin, LS Wang, KC Hwang and PT Chou. 2009. Carbon nanoparticle-enhanced immunoelectrochemical detection for protein tumor marker with cadmium sulfide biotracers. Anal Chem 81: 1340–1346.

Ko YJ, JH Maeng, Y Ahn, SY Hwang, NG Cho and SH Lee. 2008. Microchip-based multiplex electro-immunosensing system for the detection of cancer biomarkers. Electrophoresis. 29: 3466–3476.

Kost GJ. 2002. Guidelines and principles for point-of-care testing. pp. 3–12. *In:* Principles & practice of point-of-care testing. Lippincott Williams & Wilkins. Hagerstwon, MD.

Lee JH, YD Han, SY Song, D Kim and HC Yoon. 2010 Biosensor for organophosphorus pesticides based on the acetylcholine esterase inhibition mediated by choline oxidase bioelectrocatalysis. BioChip J 4: 223–229.

Li J, Z Zhang, J Rosenzweig, YY Wang and DW Chan. 2002. Proteomics and bioinformatics approaches for identification of serum biomarkers to detect breast cancer. Clin Chem 48: 1296–1304.

Liu C, C Pan, J Shen, H Wang, L Yong and R Zhang. 2010. Discrimination analysis of mass spectrometry proteomics for cervical cancer detection. Med Oncol. 28: 556–559.

Madu CO and Y Lu. 2010 Novel diagnostic biomarkers for prostate cancer. J Cancer 1: 150–177.

Maeng JH, BC Lee, YJ Ko, W Cho, Y Ahn, NG Cho, SH Lee and SY Hwang. 2008. A novel microfluidic biosensor based on an electrical detection system for alpha-fetoprotein. Biosens Bioelectron 23: 1319–1325.

Mani V, BV Chikkaveeraiah, V Patel, JS Gutkind and JF Rusling. 2009. Ultrasensitive immunosensor for cancer biomarker proteins using gold nanoparticle film electrodes and multienzyme-particle amplification. ACS Nano 3: 585–594.

Masilamani V, T Vijmasi, M Al Salhi, K Govindaraj, AP Vijaya-Raghavan and B Antonisamy. 2010. Cancer detection by native fluorescence of urine. J Biomed Opt 15: 057003

Rantala JK, H Edgren, L Lehtinen, M Wolf, K Kleivi, HK Vollan, AR Aaltola, P Laasola, S Kilpinen, P Saviranta, K Iljin and O Kallioniemi. 2010. Integrative functional genomics analysis of sustained polyploidy phenotypes in breast cancer cells identifies an oncogenic profile for GINS2. Neoplasia 12: 877–888.

Rusling JF, G Sotzing and F Papadimitrakopoulosa. 2009. Designing nanomaterial-enhanced electrochemical immunosensors for cancer biomarker proteins. Bioelectrochemistry 76: 189–194.

Sadik OA and JM Van Emon. 1996. Applications of electrochemical immunosensors to environmental monitoring. Biosens Bioelectron 11: i–xi.

Tothill IE. 2009 Biosensors for cancer markers diagnosis. Semin Cell Dev Biol 20: 55–62.

Wang J, B Tian and KR Rogers. 1998. Thick-film electrochemical immunosensor based on stripping potentiometric detection of a metal ion label. Anal Chem 70: 1682–1685

Wang J, G Liu and MR Jan. 2004. Ultrasensitive electrical biosensing of proteins and DNA: carbon-nanotube derived amplification of the recognition and transduction events. J Am Chem Soc 126: 3010–3011.

Wilson MS. 2005. Electrochemical immunosensors for the simultaneous detection of two tumor markers. Anal Chem 77: 1496–1502.

Yang L, Y Li and GF Erf. 2004. Interdigitated Array Microelectrode-based Electrochemical Impedance Immunosensor for Detection of Escherichia coli O157:H7. Anal Chem 76: 1107–1113.

Yun YH, Z Dong, VN Shanov and MJ Schulz1. 2007. Electrochemical impedance measurement of prostate cancer cells using carbon nanotube array electrodes in a microfluidic channel. Nanotechnology 18: 465505

Zheng G, F Patolsky, Y Cui, WU Wang and CM Lieber. 2005. Multiplexed electrical detection of cancer markers with nanowire sensor arrays. Nat Biotechnol 23: 1294–1301.

Multifunctional Nanobiosensors for Cancer

Dai-Wen Pang[1,*] and Er-Qun Song[2]

ABSTRACT

Nanoscience and nanotechnology are becoming more and more applicable in biomedical research, especially in human disease diagnosis and therapy. Of the diseases, cancer has become the second one resulting in death, surpassing cerebrovascular diseases due to lack of early disease detection methods, poor drug bioavailability and non-specificity, and inability to monitor therapeutic responses. Nanobiotechnology combining nanotechnology with biotechnology has led to a new strategy for cancer imaging and therapy. In this way, promising approaches of earlier detection and therapy of cancer using nanobiosensors have emerged in the recent years. Recently, multifunctional nanobiosensors (MFNBs) constructed by using a wide range of materials, such as polymers, metals, semiconductors, etc., which integrate imaging, diagnostic, therapeutic or monitoring components into a single system, have gained the most attention. This chapter highlights recent progress in the design and engineering of MFNBs with unique optical, magnetic

[1]Key Laboratory of Analytical Chemistry for Biology and Medicine (Ministry of Education), College of Chemistry and Molecular Sciences, Research Center for Nanobiology and Nanomedicine (MOE 985 Innovative Platform), State Key Laboratory of Virology, Wuhan University, Wuhan, 430072, People's Republic of China; E-mail: dwpang@whu.edu.cn
[2]Key Laboratory of Luminescence and Real-Time Analysis of the Ministry of Education, College of Pharmaceutical Sciences, Southwest University, Chongqing, 400715, People's Republic of China; E-mail: eqsong@swu.edu.cn
*Corresponding author

List of abbreviations after the text.

and electrical properties for multi-modal imaging, indentifying and locating the cancer cells, and carrying imaging and therapeutic agents for diagnosis and drug delivery to tumor *in vitro* and *in vivo*. Not limited to cancer, these MFNBs also have broad applications in many other areas of health and disease, such as atherosclerosis, which may ultimately facilitate the realization of personalized medicine in the near future.

INTRODUCTION

Cancer is a disease with widespread occurrence, high death rate and recurrence. According to the data from the agencies of United States Centers for Disease Control and American Cancer Society, cancer is becoming the second leading cause of death, surpassing the cerebrovascular diseases due to the above-mentioned traits of cancer. It is estimated that one out of four deaths is attributed to cancer in the United States. Survival of a cancer patient depends largely on early detection, drugs and surgery. However, the yearly cancer death rate has not significantly decreased despite the use of more powerful diagnostic tools, more effective drugs and more consummate surgical techniques for recent several decades. This phenomenon could be explained by the following reasons: one is that the diagnosis for cancer is usually not early enough when the primary tumor has metastasized and invaded other organs, which is beyond surgical intervention; another is that the current used therapy methods for cancer lack specificity toward cancer tissue; the last one is due to the easy recurrence of cancer. Therefore, the development of technology that is specific, reliable and handy for detecting cancers at early stages functioning as the first-line guidance is of utmost importance, the development of new drugs targeting cancer tissue with minimal side effect, surgical techniques that only selectively removes diseased tissues without causing collateral damage, and techniques for monitoring therapeutic responses in real-time is an inevitable task for cancer researchers.

Recently the development of nanotechnology and biotechnology, and the cross-disciplinary integration of nanotechnology, biology, chemistry, medicine, engineering, and photonics provide the potential to offer solutions to many of the current challenges in cancer diagnosis and therapy. Figure 8.1 shows the application of nanobiomedical technology in cancer research. In particular, the development of multifunctional nanobiosensors (MFNBs) which integrate several properties into a single nanoscale system can provide both structural and metabolic information specifically from diseased sites, thus leading to significantly improved imaging techniques for the detection of a variety of human cancers and monitoring of the hidden metastasis (Gindy and Prud'homme 2009). The basic rationale is that MFNBs are fabricated by using nanometer-sized materials (such as polymers,

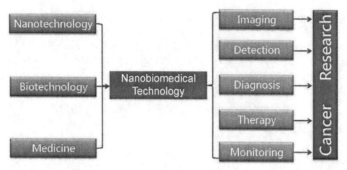

Figure 8.1. The application of nanobiomedical technology in cancer research. Schematic diagram for the combination of nanotechnology with biotechnology and medicine and its application in cancer research through imaging, detection, diagnosis, therapy, and monitoring.

metals, semiconductors, etc. as shown in Fig. 8.2) which have novel optical, electronic, magnetic, and structural properties that are often not shown at an individual molecule or bulk scale due to the surface area and quantum effects of nanomaterials, and nanoparticles offer a wide range of surface functional groups allowing chemical conjugation to multiple diagnostic and therapeutic agents. These engineered multifunctional systems are intended to integrate therapeutic and diagnostic or monitoring components to meet the needs of cancer treatment, such as early disease diagnosis, better drug bioavailability and specificity, better ability to monitor therapeutic responses in real-time, and localized therapeutic approaches such as photothermal and magnetic hyperthermia therapies which have already shown promising anticancer efficacy.

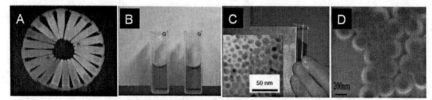

Figure 8.2. Commonly used nanomaterials. Pictures of typical nanomaterials: **(A)**, quantum dots; **(B)**, gold nanoparticles; **(C)**, nano-γ-Fe$_2$O$_3$; **(D)**, polymer.

Color image of this figure appears in the color plate section at the end of the book.

Recent research has developed biofunctionalized nanoparticles that are covalently linked to biological molecules such as peptides, proteins, nucleic acids, or small-molecule ligands. Medical applications have also appeared, e.g. the use of superparamagnetic iron oxide nanoparticles (IONs) as a contrast agent for lymph node prostate cancer detection and the use of polymeric nanoparticles for targeted gene delivery to tumor vasculatures.

New technologies by using semiconductor nanoparticles are also under intense development for the research of cancer diagnosis and metastasis. In this chapter, current examples of multifunctional systems (referring to MFNBs here), where two or more components are cooperatively integrated to improve the application potential in cancer research are discussed.

WHAT IS MFNB?

Conceptually, a biosensor is an analytical device that uses specific biochemical reactions to detect bio/chemical compounds usually by electrical, thermal or optical signals according to the recommendations of IUPAC in 1992. A biosensor consists of three parts: the sensitive biological element, the transducer and the detector element. Biosensors have been under development for decades and research in this field has become very popular in recent years. Although biosensors are used for several clinical applications, few biosensors have been developed for cancer-related clinical testing. The emergence of nanotechnology is opening a new field for the development of nanobiosensors with submicron-sized dimensions that are suitable for intracellular measurements. So what is a nanobiosensor? Uptodate, there is no unified definition for a nanobiosensor. Literally, nanobiosensor could be explained as a biosensor with dimensions on the nanometer scale or a biosensor fabricated with nanoscale materials, the similar sizes as the biological vesicles or molecules in human body. Nanobiosensors are a relatively new class of biosensing and imaging devices that serve for early cancer detection in body fluids such as the blood and serum, for analytical measurements in individual living cells such as the cell reaction when they are treated with a drug or invaded by a biological pathogen, which have the ability to sense individual chemical species in a specific location within a cell. Nanobiosensors of various types have been reported in the literature over the past decades. Some of the nanobiosensors have been used for cancer research. For examples, Chiu and Huang summarized the recent researches of aptamer-functionalized nanobiosensors for cancer imaging and detection (Chiu and Huang 2009). Quantum dots (QDs)-based optical nanobiosensors have been used for immunofluorescent labeling of breast cancer marker Her2 and tracking metastatic tumor cell extravasation (Chen et al. 2009; Chen et al. 2008). However, the developed mono-functional nanobiosensors cannot satisfy requirement of early cancer diagnosis, targeting therapy and monitor the therapeutic response in real- time in cancer research and development. Thanks to the availability of nanoparticles, several different detection signals can be obtained within a single nanoparticle and multiple diagnostic and therapeutic agents can be encapsulated, covalently attached, or adsorbed onto nanoparticles, which affords a good platform for developing MFNBs that could be used for multi-modal imaging of cancer, detection and manipulation of cancer cells, and simultaneous targeting, imaging and treatment of cancer, a major goal in cancer research and development.

MFNB FOR CANCER RESEARCH APPLICATION

The continuous progression of death rate associated with cancer disease necessitates the development of multifunctional intelligent nanodevice that combines several properties into a single system with the capability of diagnosis (detecting and visualizing cancer cells), therapy (targeted drug delivery to killing cancer cells with minimal side effects) and monitoring of treatment effects (multimodal imaging for occult metastases), ultimately facilitating in the prevailing battle against cancer. Thus, the development of MFNBs which incorporate diagnostic and therapeutic properties, as well as specific targeting capability, is a continuous topic of research (as shown in Fig. 8.3). Currently, these kinds of MFNBs are usually fabricated based on polymeric nanoparticles, magnetic nanoparticles (MNPs), QDs, gold nanoparticles and so on by carrying therapy drugs (chemotherapy and radiation drugs), specific targeting agents (antibody, peptide, aptamer) and sometimes cell-penetrating agents (usually peptide). In this section, the recent ideas and applications of these MFNBs for cancer research will be discussed.

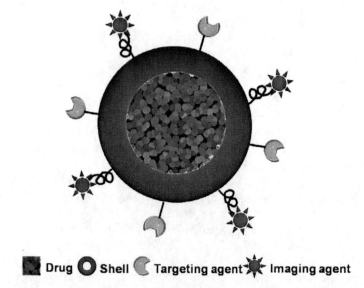

■ Drug ● Shell ◖ Targeting agent ✳ Imaging agent

Figure 8.3. The schematic diagram of a multifunctional nanobiosensor. Schematic diagram of a typical multifunctional nanobiosensor with the functions of targeting, imaging, and therapy.

Imaging and Chemotherapy Drug Delivery

By now, many new chemotherapy drugs have been produced and marketed, such as doxorubicin (Dox), cisplatin, camptothecin and so on. However, most of the anticancer drugs have low therapeutic efficacies for cancers and many side effects due to the fact that they are small molecules and have no targeting properties. Polymeric nanoparticles have been applied as effective drug delivery systems to enhance the therapeutic efficacy and reduce the side effects of drugs by improving the solubility of poorly soluble drugs and increase drug half-life and specificity to the target site due to the enhanced permeability and retention effect. Early efforts toward MFNBs for integrated drug delivery and imaging focused on combining polymeric drug carriers with organic fluorescent dyes for visualization, which are generally applied in vitro. For an example, Huang et al. designed organic dye fluorescein isothiocyanate (FITC) modified polymer micelles loading with Dox for imaging and killing the liver cancer HepG2 cells (Huang et al. 2007). QDs and MNPs have the natural advantages of serving both as an imaging agent and as a drug carrier *in vitro* and *vivo* due to their fluorescence/ magnetism properties and large surface-to-volume ratio. Bagalkot et al. designed quantum dot-aptamer (Apt)-doxorubicin (QD-Apt-Dox) MFNBs by functionalizing the surface of QDs (donor) with an aptamer into which the Dox (acceptor) intercalated to simultaneously image and deliver anticancer drugs to prostate cancer cells, and sense drug delivery based on a fluorescence resonance energy transfer (FRET) mechanism (Bagalkot et al. 2007). Piao et al. used Dox-loaded hollow magnetic nanocapsules to incubate with SKBR3 breast cancer cells for magnetic resonance imaging (MRI) and growth inhibition of the cancer cel (Piao et al. 2008). For better stability and biocompatibility, γ-Fe$_2$O$_3$ nanoparticles and Dox were encapsulated into biodegradable and biocompatible membrane made of poly(trimethylene carbonate)-b-poly(L-glutamic acid) by one-step nanoprecipitation to produce MFNBs with functions of simultaneous cancer MRI and treatment. Moreover, the feasibility of controlled drug release by radio frequency magnetic hyperthermia was demonstrated, showing the viability of the concept of magneto-chemotherapy (Sanson et al. 2011).

Besides the single-modal nanoparticles based MFNBs for imaging and drug delivery, the hybrid nanostructures also hold these functions. The multifunctional chitosan-gold nanorod hybrid nanobiosensors with encapsulated anticancer drug cisplatinand and fluorescent tag attached to the surface have been successfully developed based on a simple nonsolvent-aided counterion complexation method by Guo and co-workers (Guo et al. 2010). Their results demonstrated that the hybrid MFNBs were very promising biocompatible carriers for loading and delivery of anticancer drugs to human colorectal cancer cells and could be utilized as contrast agents for real-time dark-field and fluorescence imaging (FI) for cancer cells. The combo of QDs and MNPs is another type of nano-hybrid, commonly serving as MFNBs for drug delivery and imaging agent more recently. For an example, Cho et al. developed the MFNBs by embedding superparamagnetic nano-Fe_3O_4 nanoparticles inside a spherical polystyrene matrix, loading with chemotherapeutic agent paclitaxel for simultaneous prostate cancer cells diagnosis and treatment. The results of *in vitro* and *in vivo* experiments show the potential for preclinical applications (Cho et al. 2010).

Imaging and Photoactivated Therapy Drug Delivery

For cancer treatment, photoactivated therapy has emerged as an important area in preclinical research and clinical practice. Photodynamic therapy (PDT) involving a combination of photosensitizers and light to treat cancers is the commonly used photoactivated therapy, with the advantages that the treatment can be localized as destruction takes place only under the irradiation of light and is less invasive than surgery. Upon irradiation, the photosensitizers (such as porphyrinic origin) transfer energy to molecular oxygen, producing singlet oxygen or other reactive oxygen species, which leads to the irreversible destruction of adjacent diseased cells and tissues. However, PDT has disadvantage: limited tumor selectivity of PDT agents. Recently, the development of MFNBs comprising of PDT, targeting and imaging agents to achieve the diagnosis and treatment of tumor cells simultaneously may overcome the various disadvantages of small molecule photosensitizers similar to the chemotherapy drugs. IONs were usually used as nanoplatform for simultaneous imaging and PDT. For example, a light-activated theragnostic MFNB has been developed by Reddy and co-workers (Reddy et al. 2006). These MFNBs have a polyacrylamide core and contained Photofrin (commercial PDT agent), ION (MRI agent), Alexa Fluor 594 (fluorophore), F3-peptide (tumor vascular targeting peptide), and poly(ethylene glycol) (for increase of circulation time). FI shows that these MFNBs were specifically internalized and concentrated within the breast cancer MDA-MB435 cells nuclei, while the MRI revealed the tumors clearly when tested with a mouse bearing glioma brain tumors. Moreover, the photoactivation of the MFNBs brought high cytotoxicity to cancer cells and a significantly increased survival time of the nanbiosensors resulted in significant therapeutic benefit when guiding the laser light through a fiber optic applicator into the brain tumor site. It was considered that the ability to induce cancer cell death of MNPs conjugated photosensitizer nanocomposites would be weakened due to the fluorescence quenching by MNPs. To solve this problem, the synthesis of MNPs/polymer core/shell nanocomposites with attached fluorophore and anticancer drugs would be a choice. Lai et al. synthesized a MFNBs comprising of Fe_3O_4/SiO_2 core/ shell nanocomposite and a functionalized iridium complex via a reverse-microemulsion system for simultaneous MRI, phosphorescence imaging and PDT to human cervical cancer Hela cells (Lai et al. 2008).

Recently, QDs serving as either photosensitizers themselves or as the energy donor for activation of another photosensitizer have been employed in PDT. The energy transfer between QDs and cell molecules potentially could generate reactive oxygen species to induce apoptosis in cells. Compared to conventional photosensitizers, QDs can be tuned to emit in the NIR regions, which can be useful in PDT for deep-seated tumors since NIR is not scattered and absorbed by tissue. Even though QDs can generate singlet oxygen, however, the quantum yield of QD-generated singlet oxygen is very low compared to classic photosensitizer. Tsay et al. synthesized QD-photosensitizer MFNBs to increase the high steady-state level of singlet oxygen by the indirect activation of photosensitizers through the FRET from the QDs to photosensitizers, which overcome the trouble to a large extent. In addition, these QDs based multifunctional nanoconjugates have the ability for optical imaging cancer cell due to their fluorescence property (Tsay et al. 2007).

Photothermal therapy (PTT) is another kind of photoactivated therapy, which has gained a great deal of attention in recent years. PTT utilizes the large absorption cross section of materials in the NIR region to absorb radiation that is converted efficiently into heat to induce cell death. Nanomaterials, such as gold nanoparticles, MNPs, etc., can act as intrinsic therapeutic and imaging agents. Plasmon-resonant gold nanoshells exhibiting both absorption and scattering in the NIR have served as MFNBs for molecular imaging and photoactivated therapy. Gobin et al. successfully demonstrated the multifunctional abilities of gold nanoshells for increased optical coherence tomography imaging of tumors *in vivo* and for treating the tumors based on photothermal ablation in a mouse model (Gobin et al. 2007). Gold nanorods absorb NIR light owing to their longitudinal resonance ascribed to their aspect ratio. Huang et al. reported *in vitro* oral epithelial cancer cell imaging and photothermal therapy using gold nanorods, which were synthesized via seed-mediated growth and conjugated to anti-epidermal growth factor receptor monoclonal antibodies (Huang et al. 2006). Their results show the strongly scattered red light from gold nanorods in the dark field from the malignant cells, and the photothermal destruction of the cancer cell. Gold nanocubes, a new kind of gold nanomaterial with unique optical properties of the high photoluminescence quantum yield and a remarkably enhanced extinction band were synthesized and these MFNBs gained successfully application for human liver cancer cells optical imaging and PTT (Wu et al. 2010). Besides the functions of imaging, and carrying drugs as mentioned above, the MNPs can be used for cancer treatment by hyperthermia due to their sensitivity to radio frequency radiation. Xu et al. used CdSe/ZnS QDs and Fe_3O_4 MNPs to construct highly biocompatible MFNBs which were successfully demonstrated for both treatment of human pancreatic cancer due to the high-efficiency radio radiation absorption by MNPs and the monitoring of apoptotic process of cancer cells based on fluorescence optical property of QDs (Xu et al. 2010)

Multimodal Imaging of Cancer

The early diagnosis and accurate surgery could increase the survival rate of patients with cancer disease, which depends on the development of imaging techniques to a great extent. Current imaging techniques such as MRI, positron emission tomography (PET), and computed tomography (CT) are very important in the diagnosis of various diseases. Each imaging modality has its own merits and deficiencies, that is modalities with high sensitivity have relatively poor resolution while those with high resolution have relatively poor sensitivity, and none of them can possess all the required capabilities for perfect imaging. For example, MRI and CT have the merits of being noninvasive techniques for *in vivo* imaging and three-dimensional tomography, but they are limited by low target sensitivity. On the other hand, radioactive imaging techniques such as PET have very high target sensitivity but poor spatial resolution. Other optical imaging methods such as FI have relatively good sensitivity but suffer from low tissue penetration depths. Recently, the combination of different modalities into a single system for multi-modal imaging, has been developing, which seems to compensate for the deficiencies of single imaging modalities to improve the diagnosis and treatment of diseases in their earliest stages by providing far more comprehensive data to clinicians. For example, the simultaneous use of PET, for its highly sensitive functional imaging, and CT, for its ability to provide clear anatomical information, has been demonstrated for the early detection of cancer. Nanoparticles with extremely small size and their exceptional physical and chemical properties can afford imaging techniques with enhanced signal sensitivity, better spatial resolution, and the ability to transfer information about biological systems at the molecular and cellular levels. However, despite such remarkable progresses in the utilization of nanoparticles for applications in the biomedical science, most of the currently developed nanoparticle probes are limited to a single imaging modality. Therefore, if nanoparticles with different imaging modalities could be combined into a single system, then multi-modal imaging can be achieved (shown in Fig. 8.4). According to current research, there are several kinds of commonly used methods for fabricating multimodal-imaging nanobiosensors (Fig. 8.5). One is via the covalent bond conjugation by using a variety of cross-linker molecules, another is based on the epitaxial

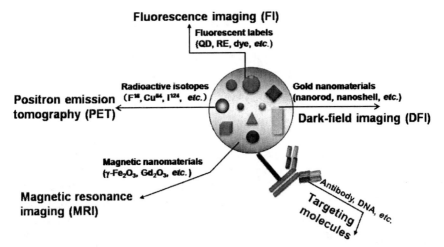

Figure 8.4. The schematic diagram of a multimodal imaging nanobiosensor. Schematic diagram of a multimodal imaging nanobiosensor fabricated by integrating optical tags, radioactive isotopes, magnetic nanoparticles, and targeting molecules. Here, QD refers to quantum dot and RE refers to rare earth.

Color image of this figure appears in the color plate section at the end of the book.

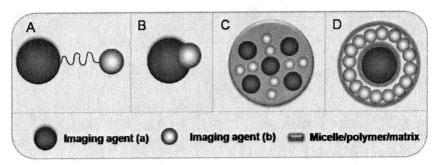

Figure 8.5. The schematic diagram of the fabrication strategy of multimodal imaging nanbiosensor. Schematic diagram for the fabrication of multimodal imaging nanbiosensor by different methods: **(A)**, covalent bonding; **(B)**, epitaxial growth; **(C)**, encapsulation/embedding; **(D)**, self-assembly.

Color image of this figure appears in the color plate section at the end of the book.

growth strategy by which a secondary component is epitaxially grown on the primary nanoparticle, the third is encapsulation or embedding different contrast agents into silica or polymer nanosphere or matrix, and the last is based on the self-assembly method.

The current contrast agents for MRI perform negative contrast, or positive contrast depending on the agent used. IONs prevailed among negative contrast agents. Therefore, the IONs serve as a core platform for the addition of other functional imaging moieties. Combining the excellent three dimension spatial resolution of MRI with the high sensitivity of FI should serve to overcome the shortcomings of each technology, which is the commonly employed strategy in surgery. One of the well-studied examples is the nanobiosensors consisting of an optically detectable NIR dye (Cy5.5) conjugated to a MRI-detectable ION offer MRI-optical dual-modal imaging for the preoperative MRI and intraoperative optical delineation of brain tumors (Kircher et al. 2003). Although this type of nanobiosensor works well, there are potential disadvantages such as photobleaching due to the usage of organic dye and rapid fluorescence quenching by MNPs. Then, a new more robust and advanced nanobiosensor with the merit of anti-photobleaching by the encapsulation of fluorophore conjugated polymers and IONs in phospholipid micelles are proposed for more stable optical signal and enhanced MR signal (Howes et al. 2010). In addition, the combination of MNPs with QDs to obtain MR and fluorescence multimodal-imaging nanobiosensors is another effective approach to avoid the photobleaching, which has been achieved for imaging the cancer cells and tumor bearing in a animal based on MR-NIRF dual-modal imaging (Kim et al. 2008). Positive contrast agents are mainly metal ions chelates, such as Gd^{3+} and Mn^{2+} chelates. Examples of Gd based multi-modal positive contrast agents have been reported. For an example, a dendrimer based G6-Cy5.5-Gd dual-modal imaging MFNB was constructed through chemistry conjugating for the efficient visualization of sentinel lymph nodes in mice by both MRI and FI modalities *in vivo* by Talanov et al. (Talanov et al. 2006). However, due to the drawbacks of being nonspecific to target, quick removal by renal excretion, and short accumulation, the metal ion chelates have limitations. Gd-based nanoparticles such as gadolinium oxide, gadolinium fluorides have been employed for fabricating MR-opical dual-modal imaging nanobiosensors. The hybrid MFNB synthesized by encapsulating Gd_2O_3 cores within a polysiloxane shell which carries organic dye were applied as contrast agents for both *in vivo* FI and MRI (Bridot et al. 2007).

MRI-PET dual-modal imaging has the potential for providing better spatial resolution with anatomical information and also improved signal sensitivity. Mn-doped IONs were integrated with radioactive iodide ions (^{124}I) to fabricate MRI-PET dual-mode nanobiosensors for imaging sentinel lymph node which is used as a route for the metastasis of malignant cancer cells (Choi et al. 2008). In addition to the IONs and metal ions based MRI-FI and MRI-PET dual-imaging modalities, the newly developed superparamagnetic FePt nanoparticles combined with other materials forming hetero-structured MFNBs can also afford multi-modal imaging. Both MRI and CT signals were found in tumor bearing animal after tail vein injection of the anti-HER2 antibody conjugated FePt nanobiosensors (Chou et al. 2010). The development of dual-modal PET-NIRF imaging extended the range of multi-modal imaging. Lin et al. load Arg-Gly-Asp peptide,

Cy5.5 dye and ^{64}Cu agent simultaneously onto heavy chain ferritins to produce MFNBs with both PET and NIRF functionalities for tumor imaging *in vivo* (Lin et al. 2011).

Magnetic Manipulation Plus Optical Imaging for Cancer Cells

As mentioned above, the fluorescent-magnetic MFNBs could be served as multi-modal MR-optical imaging agents for cancer *in vitro* or *in vivo* and simultaneous imaging and therapy, which is showing promising potential for early diagnosis of cancer or as a useful tool for an intraoperative guide to provide accurate delineation between the targeted and surrounding tissues. Moreover, besides their function as contrast agents, drug carrier, the fluorescent-magnetic MFNBs can also be used as tools for separation, manipulation and imaging simultaneous of target subjects, which makes them very promising in fields concerning the early diagnosis, selective eliminating of targeted carcinoma cells and targeting therapy since they could be controlled by an external magnetic field. For fabrication of fluorescent-magnetic MFNBs, QDs and MNPs are the common used materials. Wang et al. employed thiol and carboxy contained nano-γ-Fe$_2$O$_3$ nanoparticles reacting with CdSe/ZnS QDs based on the thiol-metal bonds to form the fluorescent-magnetic nanocomposites. After anti-cycline E antibodies coupled on their surface, the formed fluorescent-magnetic MFNBs were used to separate and image MCF-7 breast cancer cells from serum solutions (Wang et al. 2004). In the last several years, Pang's group have been synthesizing a series of different ligand molecules (such as folate, avidin, lectin, antibody, etc.) modified MFNBs by embedding CdSe/ZnS QDs and nano-γ-Fe$_2$O$_3$ into styrene/acrylamide copolymer nanospheres simultaneously to capture, separate, detect, and image several different types of cancer cells (as shown in Fig. 8.6) (Xie et al. 2005, 2007; Song et al. 2011). More recently, they used monoclonal antibody-coupled MFNBs, with the help of a magnet and a fluorescence microscope, to sensitively detect and isolate multiple types of target tumor cells (human leukaemia and prostate carcinoma cells) at concentrations as low as 0.01% in mixed cell samples, which is very promising for early detection of cancers (Song et al. 2011).

APPLICATIONS TO OTHER AREAS OF HEALTH AND DISEASE

Besides application in cancer research, MFNBs are also important tools for other areas of health and disease. Good examples are their usage in detection

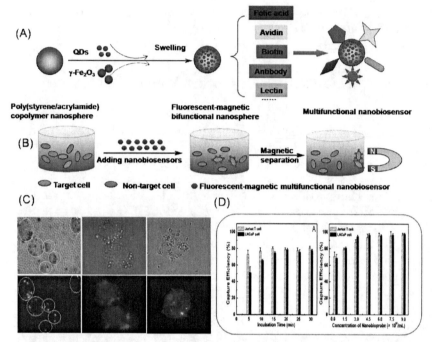

Figure 8.6. The fabrication and application of fluorescent-magnetic multifunctional nanobiosensor. Schematic diagrams for **(A)** fabrication of a fluorescent-magnetic multifunctional nanobiosensor and; **(B)** separation of cells with fluorescent-magnetic multifunctional nanobiosensors; **(C)** Capture and imaging of human breast cancer cells (left panel), human leukaemia cells (middle panel), and human prostate carcinoma cells (right panel). The top row for bright field images; the bottom row for fluorescent images. **(D)** The efficiency of fluorescent-magnetic multifunctional nanobiosensors to capture target cells. QDs: quantum dots. Reproduced with permission from References (Xie et al. 2005; 2007; Song et al. 2011). Copyright 2005 Wiley-VCH Verlag GmbH & Co. KGaA and copyright 2011 American Chemical Society.

Color image of this figure appears in the color plate section at the end of the book.

and imaging of atherosclerosis. Atherosclerosis is a disease in which plaque builds up inside the arteries, whose occurrence rate is increasing in recent years due to people's bad habits. Atherosclerosis can affect any artery in the body, including arteries in the heart, brain, arms, legs, and pelvis, and as a result, different diseases may develop based on which arteries are affected. The early diagnosis and clearly imaging of atherosclerosis is very vital for prevention and therapy of diseases caused by atherosclerosis. Nonetheless, the developed nanobiotechnology may have the potential to solve the problems. One of the approaches to identify suspect lesions is using MNPs to image macrophages. Recently, the emergence multi-modal imaging techniques can enable comprehensive information for diagnosis of atherosclerosis. People have utilized MFNBs (fluorophore derived

Table 8.1. Key Features of cancer. This table lists the key facts of cancer diseases including the definition, effect factor, people related, clinical treatment, and the relationship between cancer and nanotechnology.

1. Cancer is a kind of disease, with the feature of uncontrolled growth and spread of abnormal cells, which is caused by both external factors (tobacco, chemicals, radiation, etc.) and internal factors (inherited mutations, hormones, etc.).

2. The reports from National Vital Statistics shows that from 2002 to 2006 the occurrence of cancer in white people was 470.6, in black people 493.6, in Asians 311.1, and Hispanics 350.6 (per 100,000 persons), indicating that cancer is widespread among all races.

3. Worldwide 1,301,867 new cases of breast cancer were diagnosed, 464,854 deaths were caused by breast cancer, and more than 4.4 million women were diagnosed with breast cancer in 2007.

4. The risk of developing cancer increases with the age; more than 70% cancer patients are 55 years old or older.

5. Cancer may be cured by the technologies of surgery, radiation, chemotherapy, photodynamic therapy, photothermal therapy, and etc.

6. Nanotechnology, an interdisciplinary field concerning chemistry, physics, materials, engineering, biology, and medicine, which makes use of the unique chemical and physical properties of nanoscale (1–100 nm) materials, is demonstrating a promising potential for cancer diagnosis and treatment.

IONs) to investigate atherosclerotic lesions and to detect the intravascular thrombi by MR/optical dual-modal imaging approach (McCarthy et al. 2009). Cormode et al. created multimodality imaging nanobiosensors by combining gold nanoparticles, IONs, QDs, and fluorescence tag with high density lipoprotein mimicking. Then, based on the CT, MRI, and FI techniques, the *in vivo* imaging of atherosclerosis was successfully achieved by employing the multimodality nanobiosensors (Cormode et al. 2008).

CONCLUSION

As discussed in this chapter, nanobiomedical technology combining nanotechnology, biotechnology, and medicine has shown a tremendous potential in cancer and other human disease research. Especially, MFNBs constructed by integrating different types of nanomaterials (MNPs, QDs, nanogold, nanopolymers, and so on) with different functions (imaging, diagnosis, therapy, and monitoring) based on different fabrications are playing an increasing role in the research of early diagnosis, targeted therapy, and treatment monitoring of cancers. It can be envisioned that the development of nanotechnology, biotechnology, and cancer research will facilitate the prevention, diagnosis, and treatment of human cancers in the future in the clinic. However, we still have a long way to go before it can be used in the clinic, for example, the biosafety of nanotechnology to human beings should be intensively and systematically investigated, which will be highly focused on over the next few decades.

DEFINITIONS

- *Magnetic resonance imaging (MRI)*: is a non-invasive medical imaging technique by measuring proton spin relaxations to visualize the pathological or other physiological alterations of soft tissues inside the body.
- *Computed tomography (CT)*: a medical imaging technique that uses X-ray scanning, and computes to generate a three-dimensional image of the relatively dense or opaque structures inside a body, such as bone, vessels, bowel, and etc.
- *Positron emission tomography (PET)*: is a nuclear medicine imaging technique by measuring the gamma rays signals from positron-emitting radioactive isotopes (such as ^{64}Cu, ^{144}I) to produce a low spatial resolution but high-sensitivity image of functional processes in the body.
- *Superparamagnetism*: is a property of nanoparticles, with which nanoparticles become ferromagnetic in the presence of an external magnetic field but lose magnetization when the magnetic field is removed.
- *Nanoparticle*: refers to the particle with at least one dimension less than 100 nanometers.
- *Nanotechnology*: refers to the technology of manipulating individual atoms and molecules, creating new materials and structures from the bottom to the top with designing properties by controlling structure.
- *Quantum dots*: are often semiconductor nanocrystals with quantum-confinement properties such as size-tunable light emission and often composed of II-VI or III-V elements.
- *Biomarker*: is anything (such as bacterium, biomolecule, drug, inorganic ion, and etc.) that can be used as an indicator of a particular disease and its behavior or some other physiological state of an organism.

SUMMARY POINTS

- Nanomaterials such as MNPs, QDs and nanopolymers have novel optical, electronic, magnetic, or structural properties, and biofunctionalized nanomaterials can be usually used as biosensors, some of which are being developed for the detection of cancer, cardiovascular diseases and so on.
- MFNBs with dual/multimodal integrative properties can be fabricated by attaching moieties with targeting, imaging or therapeutic functions to nanoscale scaffolds for simultaneous imaging and therapy of cancers.

- Multi-modal imaging (MRI-FI, MRI-NIRF, MRI-CT, MRI-PET, PET-NIRF) techniques based on nanoparticles that can emit different detectable signals are being developed for molecular profiling for clinical oncology, imaging of cancer-related biomarkers, cancer diagnosis, surgical ablation, and monitoring metastasis and therapy effects.
- Fluorescent-magnetic-biotargeting MFNBs have the ability to capture, identify, isolate rare cancer cells from a mixture with a large number of coexisting cells, showing promise for early detection of cancers.
- For the application in clinics in the near future, some essential, important and troublesome issues including the biocompatibility, biosafety, *in vivo* targeting efficacy, and long term stability of MFNBs need to be made more clear.
- For MFNBs themselves, the controllable fabrication needs further exploring.

ACKNOWLEDGMENT

This work was supported by the National Basic Research Program of China (973 Program, Nos. 2011CB933600 and 2006CB933100), the Science Fund for Creative Research Groups of NSFC (20621502; 20921062), the National Natural Science Foundation of China (20833006; 21005064), and the Ministry of Public Health (2009ZX10004-107; 2008ZX10004-004).

ABBREVIATIONS

CT	:	computed tomography
Dox	:	doxorubicin
FI	:	fluorescence imaging
FITC	:	fluorescein isothiocyanate
FRET	:	fluorescence resonance energy transfer
ION	:	iron oxide nanoparticle
MNP	:	magnetic nanoparticle
MRI	:	magnetic resonance imaging
MFNB	:	multifunctional nanobiosensor
NIR	:	near-infrared
NIRF	:	near-infrared fluorescence
PDT	:	Photodynamic therapy
PET	:	positron emission tomography
PTT	:	photothermal therapy
QD	:	quantum dot

REFERENCES

Bagalkot V, L Zhang, E Levy-Nissenbaum, S Jon, PW Kantoff, R Langer and OC Farokhzad. 2007. Quantum dot-aptamer conjugates for synchronous cancer imaging, therapy, and sensing of drug delivery based on bi-fluorescence resonance energy transfer. Nano Lett 7: 3065–3070.

Bridot JL, AC Faure, S Laurent, C Riviere, C Billotey, B Hiba, M Janier, V Josserand, JL Coll, L Vander Elst, R Muller, S Roux, P Perriat and O Tillement. 2007. Hybrid gadolinium oxide nanoparticles: multimodal contrast agents for *in vivo* imaging. J Am Chem Soc 129: 5076–5084.

Chen C, J Peng, HS Xia, GF Yang, QS Wu, LD Chen, LB Zeng, ZL Zhang, DW Pang and Y Li. 2009. Quantum dots-based immunofluorescence technology for the quantitative determination of HER2 expression in breast cancer. Biomaterials 30: 2912–2918.

Chen LD, J Liu, XF Yu, M He, XF Pei, ZY Tang, QQ Wang, DW Pang and Y Li. 2008. The biocompatibility of quantum dot probes used for the targeted imaging of hepatocellular carcinoma metastasis. Biomaterials 29: 4170–4176.

Chiu TC and CC Huang. 2009. Aptamer-functionalized nano-biosensors. Sensors. 9: 10356–10388.

Cho HS, Z Dong, GM Pauletti, J Zhang, H Xu, H Gu, L Wang, RC Ewing, C Huth, F Wang and D Shi. 2010. Fluorescent, superparamagnetic nanospheres for drug storage, targeting, and imaging: a multifunctional nanocarrier system for cancer diagnosis and treatment. ACS Nano 4: 5398–5404.

Choi J, JC Park, H Nah, S Woo, J Oh, KM Kim, GJ Cheon, Y Chang, J Yoo and J Cheon. 2008. A Hybrid Nanoparticle Probe for Dual-Modality Positron Emission Tomography and Magnetic Resonance Imaging. Angew. Chem Int Ed 47: 6259–6262.

Chou SW, YH Shau, PC Wu, YS Yang, DB Shieh and CC Chen. 2010. *In vitro* and *in vivo* studies of FePt nanoparticles for dual modal CT/MRI molecular imaging. J Am Chem Soc 132: 13270–12378.

Cormode DP, T Skajaa, MM van Schooneveld, R Koole, P Jarzyna, ME Lobatto, C Calcagno, A Barazza, RE Gordon, P Zanzonico, EA Fisher, ZA Fayad and WJM Mulder. 2008. Nanocrystal core high-density lipoproteins: a multimodality contrast agent platform. Nano Lett 8: 3715–3723.

Gobin AM, MH Lee, NJ Halas, WD James, RA Drezek and JL West. 2007. Near-infrared resonant nanoshells for combined optical imaging and photothermal cancer therapy. Nano Lett 7: 1929–1934.

Guo R, L Zhang, H Qian, R Li, X Jiang and B Liu. 2010. Multifunctional nanocarriers for cell imaging, drug delivery, and near-IR photothermal therapy. Langmuir 26: 5428–5434.

Howes P, M Green, A Bowers, D Parker, G Varma, M Kallumadil, M Hughes, A Warley, A Brain and R Botnar. 2010. Magnetic conjugated polymer nanoparticles as bimodal imaging agents. J Am Chem Soc 132: 9833–9842.

Huang CK, CL Lo, HH Chen and GH Hsiue. 2007. Multifunctional micelles for cancer cell targeting, distribution imaging, and anticancer drug delivery. Adv Funct Mater 17: 2291–2297.

Huang X, IH El-Sayed, W Qian and MA El-Sayed. 2006. Cancer Cell Imaging and Photothermal Therapy in the Near-Infrared Region by Using Gold Nanorods. J Am Chem Soc 128: 2115–2120.

Kircher MF, U Mahmood, RS King, R Weissleder and LA Josephson. 2003. Multimodal nanoparticle for preoperative magnetic resonance imaging and intraoperative optical brain tumor delineation. Cancer Res 63: 8122–8125.

Lai CW, YH Wang, CH Lai, MJ Yang, CY Chen, PT Chou, CS Chan, Y Chi, YC Chen and JK Hsiao. 2008. Iridium-complex-functionalized Fe_3O_4/SiO_2 core/shell nanoparticles: a facile three-in-one system in magnetic resonance imaging, luminescence imaging, and photodynamic therapy. Small 4: 218–224.

Lin X, J Xie, G Niu, F Zhang, H Gao, M Yang, Q Quan, MA Aronova, G Zhang, S Lee, R Leapman and X Chen. 2011. Chimeric ferritin nanocages for multiple function loading and multimodal imaging. Nano Lett 2: 814–819.

Gindy ME and PK Prud'homme. 2009. Multifunctional nanoparticles for imaging, delivery and targeting in cancer therapy. Expert Opin Drug Deliv 6: 865–878.

McCarthy JR, P Patel, I Botnaru, P Haghayeghi, R Weissleder and FA Jaffer. 2009. Multimodal nanoagents for the detection of intravascular thrombi. Bioconjugate Chem 20: 1251–1255.

Piao Y, J Kim, HB Na, D Kim, JS Baek, MK Ko, JH Lee, M Shokouhimehr and T Hyeon. 2008. Wrap-bake-peel process for nanostructural transformation from β-FeOOH nanorods to biocompatible iron oxide nanocapsules. Nat Mater 7: 242–247.

Reddy GR, MS Bhojani, P McConville, J Moody, BA Moffat, DE Hall, G Kim, YEL Koo, MJ Woolloscroft, JV Sugai, TD Johnson, MA Philbert, R Kopelman, A Rehemtulla and BD Ross. 2006. Vascular targeted nanoparticles for imaging and treatment of brain tumors. Clin Cancer Res 12: 6677–6686.

Sanson C, O Diou, J Thvenot, E Ibarboure, A Soum, A Brlet, S Miraux, E Thiaudiere, S Tan, A Brisson, V Dupuis, O Sandre and S Lecommandoux. 2011. Doxorubicin loaded magnetic polymersomes: theranostic nanocarriers for mr imaging and magneto-chemotherapy. ACS nano 2: 1122–1140.

Song EQ, J Hu, CY Wen, ZQ Tian, X Yu, ZL Zhang, YB Shi and DW Pang. 2011. Fluorescent-magnetic-biotargeting multifunctional nanobioprobes for detecting and isolating multiple types of tumor cells. ACS Nano 2: 761–770.

Talanov VS, CAS Regino, H Kobayashi, M Bernardo, PL Choyke and MW Brechbiel. 2006. Dendrimer-based nanoprobe for dual modality magnetic resonance and fluorescence imaging. Nano Lett 6: 1459–1463.

Tsay JM, M Trzoss, L Shi, X Kong, M Selke, ME Jung and S Weiss. 2007. Singlet oxygen production by peptide-coated quantum dot-photosensitizer conjugates. J Am Chem Soc 129: 6865–6871.

Wang D, J He, N Rosenzweig and Z Rosenzweig. 2004. Superparamagnetic Fe_2O_3 beads–CdSe/ZnS quantum dots core–shell nanocomposite particles for cell separation. Nano Lett 4: 409–413.

Wu X, T Ming, X Wang, P Wang, J Wang and J Chen. 2010. High-photoluminescence-yield gold nanocubes for cell imaging and photothermal therapy. ACS Nano 4: 113–120.

Xie HY, C Zuo, Y Liu, ZL Zhang, DW Pang, XL Li, JP Gong, C Dickinson and WZ Zhou. 2005. Cell-targeting multifunctional nanospheres with both fluorescence and magnetism. Small 1: 506–509.

Xie HY, M Xie, ZL Zhang, YM Long, X Liu, ML Tang, DW Pang, Z Tan, C Dickinson and W Zhou. 2007. Wheat germ agglutinin-modified trifunctional nanospheres for cell recognition. Bioconjugate Chem 18: 1749–1755.

Xu Y, A Karmakar, D Wang, MW Mahmood, F Watanabe, Y Zhang, A Fejleh, P Fejleh, Z Li, G Kannarpady, S Ali, AR Biris and AS Biris. 2010. Multifunctional Fe_3O_4 cored magnetic-quantum dot fluorescent nanocomposites for RF nanohyperthermia of cancer cells. J Phys Chem C 114: 5020–5026.

9

Silicon Nanowire Biosensor for Cancer Marker

Yang-Kyu Choi[1,a,*] and Chang-Hoon Kim[1,b]

ABSTRACT

Early detection is vitally important in decreasing the death rate from cancer. An early diagnosis is enabled by the development of various cancer markers and improved detection capability to sense extremely low concentrations of cancer markers. Nanoscale structured sensors contribute to improving the detection sensitivity noticeably because the increased surface-to-volume ratio by the miniaturization plays a key role in sensing biomarkers. Among these nanoscale sensors, silicon-based nanowires have many advantages in terms of low-cost fabrication, and chip-level integration, each of which is crucial in point-of-care testing (POCT). More to the point, silicon-based technology and the subsequent development in information technology through miniaturization have progressed remarkably over the past four decades. Therefore, it would be a great advantage to fully utilize the matured silicon technology in this area. Moreover, electrical detection, which does not require a labeling process, is much more practical for mobile or portable sensor systems. In the electronic sensor system, the direct electrical detection of cancer markers is feasible, as is keeping track of the changes in the conductance of the nanowires.

[1]Department of Electrical Engineering, KAIST, 335 Gwahangno, Yuseong-gu, Daejeon 305-701, Republic of Korea.
[a]E-mail: ykchoi@ee.kaist.ac.kr
[b]E-mail: chkim@nobelab.kaist.ac.kr
*Corresponding author

List of abbreviations after the text.

In this chapter, we discuss a silicon nanowire biosensor for cancer marker detection. The basic structure and the fabrication method of the silicon nanowire biosensor are described. Its operating principle is also explained in detail. Several strategies for achieving high sensitivity are discussed with a focus on its structural parameters, such as the nanowire size, as well as the environmental conditions, such as the distance of the biomolecules to the nanowire surface and the ionic concentration. Recent results from silicon nanowire biosensors to detect DNA and RNA, which can express the characteristics of cancers, are summarized. A direct detection method of proteins, which are relevant to cancer markers, is covered as well.

INTRODUCTION

Tacitly, the traditional trend in health care, concentrating on the treatment of diseases, has been slowly replaced by early diagnosis to prevent disease. In order to keep step with the trend, the need for high-performance biosensors has attracted attention as a viable tool in healthcare systems. One of the most essential features for a high-performance biosensor is high sensitivity. Nanotechnology, which has advanced rapidly, can be a powerful tool for improving the sensitivity of biosensors through maximization of the surface-to-volume ratio (SVR), allowing a small amount of change by biomolecules placed onto their surfaces to be monitored. In general, the limit of detection (LOD) of a biosensor is mainly limited by the dissociation constant (K_d), which is related to the thermodynamics of the affinity reaction. In the case of an antibody-antigen reaction for protein detection, the K_d value is $10^{-8} \sim 10^{-12}$ M; it is 10^{-15} M for the streptavidin-biotin reaction, which is known as the strongest binding affinity in nature (Bayer and Wilchek 1990). As a result, $10^{-9} \sim 10^{-14}$ M represents the lowest LOD range that can be acquired from a conventional biosensor. Therefore, in order to attain improved sensitivity, amplification methods such as the polymerase chain reaction (PCR) method are necessary. However, such an amplification method requires a labeling process, which inevitably involves time-consuming labor and pretreatment steps, which in turn demand skilled operators and specialized expensive equipment. In addition, these methods are associated with constraints in terms of real-time detection and result in unreliable data owing to the loss of samples during the manipulation steps. Recently, biosensor building blocks with a range of 1 to 100 nm in size were developed with the aid of nanotechnology. The nanoscale building blocks provide a size-matched interface between biomolecules and the biosensor system because the size of the building block is comparable to the size of the biomolecule, such as DNA, protein, and virus, which can cause disease (Fig. 9.1). Moreover, these building blocks show high sensitivity without extra amplification

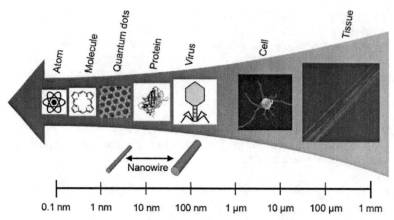

Figure 9.1. Size of the molecules and the nanostructures.

steps due to the high SVR, which is an inherent property of the nanoscale structure. Cantilever, quantum dot or nanoparticle (0-dimension), nanobelts (2-dimension), nanogaps (>2-dimension), nanotube (1-dimension), and nanowire (1-dimension)-based biosensors are typical biosensors that utilize such nanostructures. Among them, cantilever and quantum dot biosensors or those based on nanoparticle show extremely high sensitivity, selectivity, and a short response time. However, the requirement of massive and expensive equipment for their proper operation hinders these biosensors from being applied to chip-based biosensors. On the other hand, field effect transistor (FET)-based biosensors, such as nanotubes, nanobelts, nanogaps, and nanowires, do not require this type of equipment. Hence, they are proper candidates for application to chip-based biosensors (Patolsky et al. 2006a; Curreli et al. 2008). FET-based biosensors respond to the charges arising from target molecules and therefore allow label-free detection without pre- or post-treatments which are a risk sacrificing time, cost, and sample loss. They exhibit sufficiently high sensitivity (~ fM) to detect disease markers despite the fact that their sensitivities are lower than the sensitivity levels of the cantilever and quantum dot-based biosensors. One of the advantages of electrical biosensors is free of a transducer, which converts one signal to another type of signal because both the input and output signals are composed of electrical signals. For example, optical, chemical, mechanical, or biological signals have to be transformed to electrical signals, which can be directly displayed in an electronic terminal device for non-electrical biosensors. This advantage of the FET-based biosensors makes them promising candidates for chip-based point-of-care testing (POCT) systems. Among the FET-based biosensors, silicon nanowire (SiNW) has attracted a considerable amount of attention due to its simple fabrication, integration, and well-understood underlying physics by virtue of the matured silicon technology. Thus, in this chapter, SiNW biosensors are primarily discussed in depth.

The first report of a FET-based biosensor was a planar device termed ion-sensitive field effect transistor (ISFET) or chemical field effect transistor (CHEMFET), in the 1970s (Bergveld 2003). The ISFET comprised of a channel exposed to liquid and a liquid gate including target molecules. Detection of the target molecule was achieved by monitoring the change in the electrical conductivity of the channel, which stemmed from the intrinsic charges of the target molecules. ISFET was a novel attempt to utilize a FET as a biosensor. However, the sensitivity previously expected from the downscaling of the sensor size was not satisfactory due to the limited SVR from the bulky structure (3-dimension) and the unstable parameters affected by the temperature and illuminated light. Alternatively, the optics-based biosensor, which relies on fluorescence detection, entered the mainstream and led to the advancement of biosensors. This trend was reversed in the 2000s. Research into SiNW biosensors is in the spotlight due to the advances in nanofabrication technology. With the aid of nanotechnology, an extremely scaled nanowire with a high SVR was created, showing an improvement in the sensitivity level compared to the ISFET. The advanced silicon process technology enabled the fabrication of a nanowire up to the sub-10 nm range with good pattern fidelity and reproducibility. The nanowire can be made of Si, Ge, or metal oxide (e.g. ZnO, In_2O_3, or SnO_2). However, SiNW has been the most widely used, as it offers a reliable and reproducible fabrication method. An operational principle of the SiNW biosensor is the same as that of the ISFET. Charged target molecules result in a change of the conductance in the SiNW through a change of the flowing current. Thus, the conductance or current can be a type of sensing metric. Although the working principles are the same, the SiNW biosensor shows extremely high sensitivity compared to the ISFET. This is easily understood by the fact that the SiNW is composed of a one-dimensional structure; hence, it inherently has a high SVR. In contrast, it should be recalled that the ISFET is comprised of a three-dimensional bulky structure. With the use of the SiNW-based biosensor, the detection of various biomolecules, such as DNA, protein, virus, and single cells, was recently reported. In an extension of these previous works, multiplexed detection techniques were also developed. Multiplexed detection with high selectivity is crucial to avoid a false-positive or false-negative results, as many biomolecules are related to one specific type of cancer. In other words, similar types of biomolecules should be selectively detected for a more careful diagnosis. Lastly, a detection method for cancer markers, based on the SiNW, will be discussed.

DEVICE STRUCTURE AND OPERATIONAL PRINCIPLES

Device Structure and Fabrication Method

A typical SiNW biosensor is composed of a SiNW channel, read-out pads, and a back gate under the gate dielectric layer (Fig. 9.2A). The nanowire channel is the sensing region, and read-out pads connected by the channel are the output region that extracts the sensing signals. A certain fixed bias applied to the gate induces homogeneous and uniform carrier density across the SiNW; hence, the conductivity of the SiNW is constant. When biomolecules are immobilized on the SiNW surface, the intrinsic charges from the molecules lead to a change of the carrier density, thus causing the conductance of the SiNW to change.

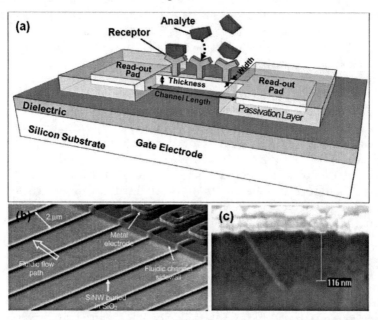

Figure 9.2. **Structure of a SiNW biosensor. (A)** Schematic of a SiNW biosensor and its operational principle. A sensing channel is located between the read-out pads and a back gate is underneath the channel. Combined target molecules to receptors affect the electrical properties of the channel. **(B)** Uniform and well aligned SiNW biosensors fabricated by a top-down method and **(C)** non-uniform SiNW biosensor fabricated by a bottom-up method. (b) Reprinted and/or adapted with permission from Gao et al. 2007 (Copyright 2007 American Chemical Society).

The SiNW can be patterned by either a top-down or a bottom-up method for biosensor applications. In the bottom-up method, SiNWs are grown using the vapor-liquid-solid (VLS) technique (Wagner and Ellis 1964) then spread on a substrate where other peripheral circuits have been patterned. Even though a nanoscale-sized pattern beyond the lithographic limit can be achieved by the bottom-up method, difficulties in aligning and non-identical property (Fig. 9.2C) due to different orientation become a serious concern compared to the top-down method. The top-down method employs a conventional silicon process, and a silicon-on-insulator (SOI) wafer is typically used as a substrate (Li et al. 2005). An SOI wafer consists of three layers: top silicon working as a sensing domain, buried oxide acting as a gate dielectric, and bottom silicon serving as a back gate. The top silicon was initially reduced in thickness down to the desired nanowire height by iterative oxidation and etching process known as a body thinning step. The reduced top silicon was then doped with boron or phosphorus according to the desired SiNW type (boron for a p-type channel and phosphorus for an n-type channel) with the aid of ion implantation. After annealing for dopant activation, SiNW patterns were delineated using electron-beam (simply e-beam) lithography followed by dry etching to remove the top silicon except in the device region. Additional implantation with the same dopants but with a high dose is applied for the read-out pads in order to reduce the contact resistance. Alternatively, metal is directly deposited on the read-out pads. Except for the sensing domain, all other areas should be passivated in order to prevent parasitic current flow, electrophoresis, and work function change of the read-out pads due to the nonspecific binding of the target molecules. Major advantages of the top-down method include excellent controllability for the positioning of the SiNWs and its chip-level integration capability. All SiNWs fabricated by the top-down method have the same crystal orientation and are well aligned at the designed position (Fig. 9.2B). These properties reduce the process-induced variability and thereby minimize the statistical fluctuation of the device characteristics. Perfectly controlled widths and lengths can also be achieved by the top-down method; these are important parameters for improving the sensitivity. However, the high cost and low throughput due to e-beam lithography for tight control of the width and length are disadvantages of the top-down method. These problems are solved by the adoption of spacer lithography. Choi et al. developed a spacer lithography technique which produced a nanowire with a width smaller than 10 nm through optical lithography (Choi et al. 2003). However, biosensors using this technique have yet to be reported.

Operational Principle and Sensing Metrics

The most important sensing component in the SiNW biosensor is the nanoscale channel. The conductance of the SiNW is determined by the majority carrier density (e.g. electrons for the n-type and holes for the p-type SiNW). The conductance can be extracted from the measured current flow via the channel. The majority carrier density is affected by external charges when charged molecules are immobilized on the SiNW surface; thus, the conductance is changed according to the polarity and density of the external charges, and the channel polarity of the SiNW. Representative structural parameters affecting the conductance are the width and doping concentration of the SiNW, and the environmental parameters are the distance of the molecules to the SiNW surface and the ionic strength. The width of the SiNW is the most important structural parameter for the maximization of the sensitivity (Li et al. 2005; Nair and Alam 2007). The thickness of the depleted or accumulated layer induced by the external charges is a few nanometers; however, the bulk region remains unchanged. The conductance change originates mainly from the depletion or accumulation layer rather than from the unchanged bulk region. Thus, the higher ratio of the depletion or accumulation layer to the bulk region induces a large conductance difference, thereby assuring higher sensitivity. This explains why many researchers are interested in the SVR and why the one-dimensional SiNW is a good candidate for biosensors. The depletion or accumulation thickness can be controlled by the doping concentration of the SiNW. A decreased doping concentration creates a thickened depletion or accumulation layer; thus, a low doping concentration is preferred for the high sensitivity of a biosensor (Nair and Alam 2007).

The properties of biomolecules, such as charge density and bioaffinity, are significantly influenced by the surrounding environment. Tight control of these properties guarantees stable biosensor performance. Phosphate-buffered silane (PBS) is the most widely used buffer solution to preserve these properties, as it has a pH and electrolyte concentration similar to those of a physiological solution. However, the ionic strength generated by the electrolyte creates an electrostatic screening effect (Nair and Alam 2008). The electrostatic screening effect means that counter ions against the target molecule in the solution neutralize the charge of the target molecules; hence, the sensitivity of the biosensors is degraded by the electrostatic screening effect. In order to explain the electrostatic screening effect, the Debye length (λ_D) should be understood. λ_D is defined as the maximum distance in which the charge of the target molecule can affect the characteristics of the SiNW over the electrostatic screening effect. Thus, the charges existing out of λ_D from the SiNW surface play no role in the operation of the biosensor. In the case of serum, λ_D is ~0.7 nm, which is much smaller than the range of 10~15 nm for an antibody or 5~10 nm for a protein. Thus far, charges in the range of 0.7 nm from the SiNW surface can contribute to influencing a change in the conductance. In this sense, it is difficult to expect high sensitivity. In order to increase the sensitivity, a reduction of the electrolyte concentration is required. Responses according to the screening effect and λ_D were investigated by Stern et al. via the biotin-streptavidin binding. This exploitation was carried out at constant concentration of streptavidin under various concentrations of PBS (Stern et al. 2007b). The experiment was valid as it is well known that the K_d value of the streptavidin-biotin reaction is not affected by changes in the surrounding environment. In their report, the conductance change of a p-type SiNW was measured for different PBS concentrations. The conductance of the SiNW was increased by more than 20% after the addition of 10 nM of streptavidin in a 0.01×PBS (λ_D=7.3 nm) solution compared to the initial state i.e. only 0.01×PBS was added to the SiNWs (Figs. 9.3A and B). This indicates that the additional negative charges in the enlarged λ_D range effectively changed the conductance. When the same concentration of streptavidin in a 0.1×PBS (λ_D=2.3 nm) solution was added to the SiNWs, a conductance increment of only ~10% was observed. This conductance reduction was due to the strengthened electrostatic screening effect by the decreased value of λ_D for the increased concentration of the buffer solution. Finally, a 10-fold increased 1×PBS (λ_D=0.7 nm) solution with the same concentration of streptavidin was applied to the SiNWs. The conductance was nearly identical to the initial conductance due to the very short λ_D. From this result, they attempted to reduce the generation of a false-positive outcome. When λ_D is shorter than the thickness of the target molecules, the sensitivity is reduced. However, when λ_D is longer than the thickness of target molecules, unbound target molecules or other molecules in the solution can affect the SiNW conductance. Hence, an unwanted false-positive or false-negative result may occur. However, they successfully demonstrated that the response of SiNWs for deoxyribonucleic acid (DNA) detection arose not from the unbounded DNA in the 0.05×PBS but from the immobilized DNA (Figs. 9.3C and D).

Another notable experiment regarding λ_D and the electrostatic screening effect was carried out by Zhang et al. (Zhang et al. 2008). They demonstrated the electrostatic screening effect by controlling the distance between the target molecules and the SiNW surface in buffer solution with the same concentrations, whereas Stern et al. changed the concentration of the buffer solution with the same concentration of the target molecules. In their study, a probe peptide nucleic acid (PNA) and target DNA were used to control the distance between the target DNA and the SiNW surface. Six target DNAs with the same length but different sequences were synthesized in order to make different binding sites on the probe DNA. The different sequences of DNA left three-mismatched base pairs near the SiNW surface, which created a distance of 1.02 nm from the surface (Fig. 9.4A). The conductance according to the distance of the target DNAs decreased monotonously as the distance increased (Fig. 9.4B). These results confirm that the sensitivity of the SiNW biosensor is significantly affected

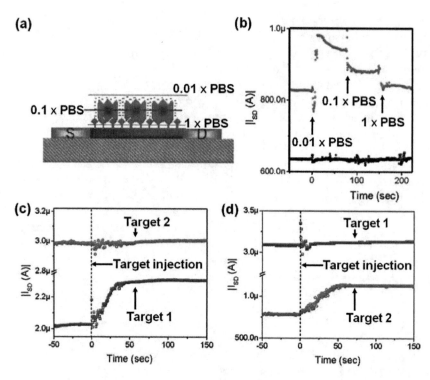

Figure 9.3. Electrolyte concentration effect on sensitivity. (A) Concept of Debye length change due to different concentrations of buffer solution. Higher concentration of buffer solution makes the shorter Debye length. **(B)** Real-time detection of streptavidin dissolved in different concentrations of buffer solution. The response was reduced for the same concentration of the streptavidin resolved in a high concentration of buffer solution. Responses on mixture of two different target DNA (target 1 and target 2) injection to **(C)** the modified NW by the probe DNA, which is matched to target 1 and **(D)** the modified NW by the probe DNA, which is matched to target 2. The target DNA in 0.05×PBS (λ_D=3.3 nm) produced no signals from non-complementary target DNA. **(A)-(D)** Reprinted and/or adapted with permission from Stern et al. 2007b (Copyright 2007 American Chemical Society).

by the target molecule's position, whether it is in the λ_D or out of the λ_D. As discussed earlier, a low electrolyte concentration leads to higher sensitivity. However, electrolyte concentrations lower than a certain critical value, as determined by the target biomolecules, are not desirable because a low electrolyte concentration degrades the bioaffinity of the biomolecules to the receptor. In addition, the charge density and polarity are also changed by the condition of the electrolyte solution. In order to increase the sensitivity in a high concentration electrolyte solution, the target molecules should be located at the SiNW surface as close as possible. Thus, the design of a linker and receptor is also an important issue.

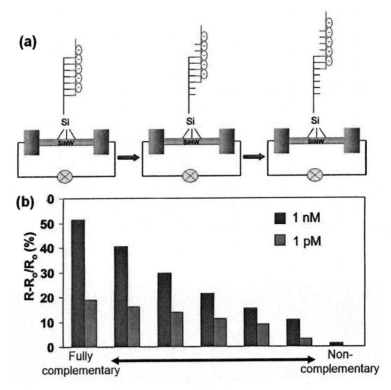

Figure 9.4. Charge layer position effect on sensitivity. (A) Schematic of the different positions of the charge layer formation. With the different target DNA sequences to the same probe PNA sequence, the charge layers are receded from the SiNW by a 3-base pair distance. **(B)** Resistance change according to the charge layer position. Closer charge layer to the SiNW (fully complementary) showed higher resistance change compared to the distanced one (non-complementary). **(A)** and **(B)** Reprinted and/or adapted with permission from Zhang et al. 2008 (Copyright 2008 American Chemical Society).

CANCER-RELATED BIOMOLECULE DETECTION

Detection of DNA

It is well known that some specific sequences of DNA cause cancer. Hence, the detection of a specific sequence of DNA is very important for the diagnosis of some types of cancer. DNA is one of the strongest negatively charged biomolecules due to its phosphate backbone; thus, the SiNW conductance is significantly changed by DNA immobilization or hybridization. Single-stranded DNAs are widely used as receptors to detect the hybridization of target DNA. However, the electrostatic repulsive force originating from the negative charges prevents the hybridization process.

To increase the hybridization efficiency, achieve high sensitivity, and reduce the response time, a high concentration of the electrolyte solution is used. In this highly concentrated electrolyte solution, positive ions neutralize the negative charges in the DNA and the hybridization efficiency is improved due to the reduced electrostatic repulsive force. However, as mentioned earlier, the short λ_D in the highly concentrated electrolyte solution diminishes the sensitivity of the device. The utilization of PNA with a specific binding property to complementary DNA solves this problem (Briones et al. 2004). PNAs are uncharged molecules; therefore, the repulsive electric force no longer affects the hybridization process in an electrolyte solution with a low concentration. In addition, the structural stability and neutral backbone of the PNA lead to high sensitivity compared to the probe DNA (Gao et al. 2007). Gao et al. reported a resistance change when PNA was used as a probe receptor for DNA detection. In this study, a resistance change of 200% was observed after hybridization of the target DNA to the probe PNA, whereas the resistance change was only 14% in the control experiment which used the probe DNA (Fig. 9.5A). With the aid of probe PNA, various DNA sequences related to cancer or disease have been detected. Hahm et al. reported the detection of ΔF508 in the cystic fibrosis transmembrane conductance regulator (CFTR) gene (Hahm and Lieber 2004). The results exhibited an LOD of 10 fM with a relatively short response time of less than 10 sec (Fig. 9.5B). Zhang et al. also succeeded in recognizing miRNA extracted from HeLa cells which is related to uterine cervical cancer (Zhang et al. 2009). In this work, an LOD of 1 fM was attained (Fig. 9.5C) and the resistance change by miRNA hybridization with probe PNA was approximately 50%. However, this value was less than 15% in the hybridization case of the probe DNA and the target miRNA with 1 nM of miRNA (Fig. 9.5D). These results confirm that the uncharged probe PNA was a more attractive receptor for detecting DNA with high sensitivity compared to the charged probe DNA.

The highly sensitive detection of target DNA was achieved not only by probe PNA but also by probe DNA. Wu et al. reported the detection of serine/threonine-protein kinase B-Raf (BRAF) gene mutation with probe DNA; this finding is related to papillary thyroid cancer (Wu et al. 2009). The hybridization process was carried out in a 1×PBS solution to ensure a successful hybridization. Afterwards, the buffer solution was dried under a nitrogen ambient atmosphere. Thus, the charges of the target BRAF gene directly influenced the electrical characteristics of the SiNW through air regardless of the electrostatic screening effect. The measured parameter in this work was the threshold voltage. The threshold voltage shift due to the 10 nM value of the target BRAF gene was about 1V, and a femto-molar concentration of the LOD was achieved (Fig. 9.6A). Moreover, one- and five-base mismatched DNA samples with a concentration of 10 nM were

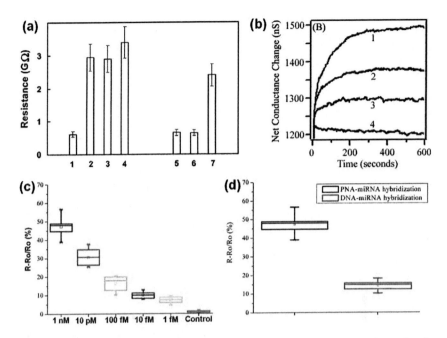

Figure 9.5. Improved sensitivity utilizing probe PNA. (A) Sensitivity comparison of probe PNA and DNA. Each number indicated the resistance measured from (1) initial SiNW, (2) probe DNA immobilization, (3) hybridized 1 nM of complementary target PNA on (2), (4) hybridized 1 nM of complementary target DNA on (2), (5) initial SiNW, (6) probe PNA immobilization, and (7) hybridized 1 nM of complementary target DNA on (6). Probe PNA showed higher resistance change after DNA hybridization. **(B)** Response of ΔF508 detection with probe PNA for the concentration of (1) 100 fM, (2) 30 fM, (3) 10 fM, and (4) 1 fM. Response of miRNA extracted from HeLa cell showed **(C)** 1 fM of LOD and **(D)** are achieved higher sensitivity utilizing the probe PNA compared to the probe DNA. (A) Reprinted and/or adapted with permission from Gao et al. 2007 (Copyright 2007 American Chemical Society) and **(B)** from Hahm and Lieber 2004 (Copyright 2004 American Chemical Society) **(C)** and **(D)** from Zhang et al. 2009 (Copyright 2008 Elsevier B.V.).

detected, and distinguishable threshold voltage shifts were observed (Fig. 9.6B). Measurement in air ambient to prevent the electrostatic screening effect is not a general method, but some groups reported similar results. Choi's group reported the detection result of an avian influenza antibody with a SiNW-based biosensor in air ambient (Ahn et al. 2010).

Although a low concentration of the buffer solution improved the hybridization efficiency and the sensitivity, these results could not be applied directly to undiluted serum samples. Bunimovich et al. demonstrated the detection of DNA in a buffer solution with a high concentration comparable to a physiological condition (Bunimovich et al. 2006). They used probe DNA as a receptor, but the formation of the probe DNA was different from that in other reports. The previously mentioned results used covalent bonding

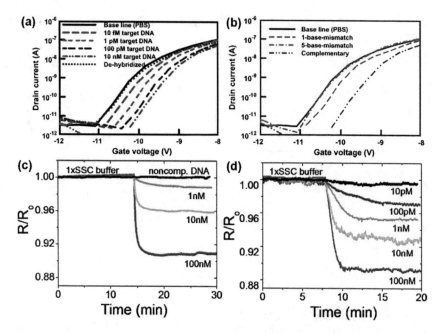

Figure 9.6. Highly sensitive DNA detection with DNA receptor. BRAF gene detection result **(A)** with femto-molar range LOD and **(B)** mismatched sequence detection for the 1- and 5-base-mismatched target BRAF gene. Both **(A)** and **(B)** showed high sensitivity and selectivity even though DNA was used as a receptor. DNA detection in 1×PBS **(C)** with the native oxide and **(D)** without the native oxide was demonstrated. Reduced distance of the DNA from the SiNW surface by removing the native oxide, improved the LOD down to 10 pM in buffer solution with high electrolyte concentration. **(A)** and **(B)** Reprinted and/or adapted with permission from Wu et al. 2009 (Copyright 2009 Elsevier B.V.) **(C)** and **(D)** from Bunimovich et al. 2006 (Copyright 2006 American Chemical Society).

to immobilize probe DNA or PNA on linkers; thus, the probe DNAs or PNAs were formed as a standing structure perpendicular to the SiNW surface. However, Bunimovich et al. used the physical binding method for the immobilization of the probe DNA. Negatively charged probe DNAs were physically adsorbed on a positively charged amine-terminated SiNW surface by electrostatic force; hence, the probe DNAs formed a stretched out structure on the SiNW surface. As a result, hybridized target DNAs also formed a stretched out structure and could be located in the λ_D length in spite of the high concentration of the buffer solution. In their experiments, they achieved an LOD value of 1 nM in an electrolyte concentration of 240 mM, which results in 0.7 nm for the λ_D value (Fig. 9.6C). In addition, improvement of two orders of magnitude in the LOD was demonstrated by removing native oxide from the SiNW surface (Fig. 9.6D).

One of the most important molecules related to cancer and DNA is telomerase. At the 3'-end of DNA, telomere (a repeat of the TTAGGG sequence) protects the information of the DNA. The length of the telomere is reduced after cell division. As a consequence, the cell vanishes as all telomeres disappear. The telomerase is a eukaryotic ribonucleoprotein complex; an activated telomerase prevents the reduction of the telomere by adding the repeated TTAGGG sequence to the telomere. Thus, the cell does not vanish and eventually becomes a cancer cell. Telomerase can be found in at least 80% of human cancers. Zheng et al. detected activated telomerase using SiNWs and probe DNA (Zheng et al. 2005). In order to test the activity of the telomerase extracted from a HeLa cell, the telomerase was injected into a p-type SiNW modified by probe DNA. Initially, binding of the telomerase on the probe DNA led to a decrement of the conductance because the charge polarity of the telomerase is positive at physiological pH levels. The conductance, which was initially decreased due to the telomerase, increased after the injection of deoxynucleotide triphosphates due to the added sequences at the end of the probe DNA synthesized by the telomerase. This result was observed in telomerase extracted from only 10 HeLa cells without any amplification.

Detection of Proteins

Protein is another important biomolecule related to cancer. Cancer cell causes the proliferation of certain proteins or raises the concentration of pre-existing proteins. In order to detect cancer-related proteins, researchers have usually used an antigen-antibody reaction. One of the most widely surveyed proteins is the prostate-specific antigen (PSA), which is related to prostate cancer. Zheng et al. detected PSA via an antigen-antibody reaction in a SiNW biosensor (Zheng et al. 2005). The reversible conductance change due to the injected PSA was linearly related to the concentration of the PSA, which provides a possibility for a quantitative analysis (Fig. 9.7A). The LOD value of the PSA detection was 2 fM in a diluted buffer solution, which corresponds to a λ_D value of 130 nm. The colorectal marker carcinoembryonic antigen (CEA) and the colon cancer marker mucin-1 were also detected by the same experimental configuration, with LOD values of approximately 0.5 fM. In that work, the mechanism of the SiNW biosensor was verified by utilizing an n- and p-type SiNW for the detection of negatively charged PSA. The increased conductance in the p-type SiNW and decreased conductance in the n-type SiNW were confirmed by the negatively charged PSA because the majority of carriers in each type of the SiNW accumulated or depleted according to the external charge polarity. A mixture of PSA and background serum proteins was used for the specificity test. The test showed high specificity of PSA detection with an LOD value of 26 fM against a concentration that was 12 orders higher in background serum proteins. Multiplexed detection was also noted. Three

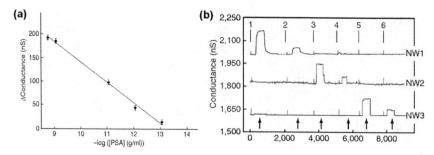

Figure 9.7. Multiplexed detection of PSA, CEA, and mucin-1. (A) Linear relation between the conductance change and the concentration of PSA. This result provides the possibility for a quantitative analysis. **(B)** Multiplexed detection of PSA, CEA, and mucin-1. Each antibody of PSA, CEA, and mucin-1 was immobilized on NW1, NW2, and NW3, respectively. (1) 0.9 ng/ml PSA, (2) 1.4 pg/ml PSA, (3) 0.2 ng/ml CEA, (4) 2 pg/ml CEA, (5) 0.5 ng/ml mucin-1, and (6) 5 pg/ml mucin-1 were sequentially injected. Injection of buffer solution to wash out the previously injected analyte was subsequently carried out after each analyte injection step (denoted by the black arrow points). The conductance change occurred only when the specific binding was made between the immobilized antibody on the NW and a targeted antigen in the injected solution. **(A)** and **(B)** Reprinted and/or adapted with permission from Zheng et al. 2005 (Copyright 2005 Nature Publishing Group).

independent devices modified by the antibodies of PSA, CEA, and mucin-1 were prepared for the multiplexed detection and a mixture of PSA, CEA, and mucin-1 was then injected into the devices. A response to the mixture was observed in only the device that matched to a specific target (Fig. 9.7B). In that work, high sensitivity was achieved by a buffer solution with a low concentration. Apparently, a decrement in the sensitivity is unavoidable with a highly concentrated buffer solution. Stern et al. achieved an LOD value of 100 fM for immunoglobulin G (IgG) and immunoglobulin A (IgA) detection in a highly concentrated buffer solution close to physiological serum conditions (Stern et al. 2007a). The obtained LOD is poorer than that in a buffer solution with a low concentration; however, this represents a greatly improved value compared to the values noted in previous reports. This low LOD value was achieved by removing the native oxide and employing the aforementioned chamber-type microfluidics.

Kim et al. reported another result of PSA detection (Kim et al. 2007) with n-type SiNW. The measured LOD was in the atto-molar concentration range, which is the highest sensitivity reported to date (Fig. 9.8). This extremely high level of sensitivity was achieved through an optimization of the initial conductance to less than 500 nS. The low conductance was achieved through carefully controlled doping concentration, width, and length. Real-time detection of PSA was carried out for different pH values of the solution. The selected pH values were 7.8 and 6.0, where the isoelectric point (pI) of PSA is 6.9. Because the pI value is smaller than 7.8 and larger than 6.0,

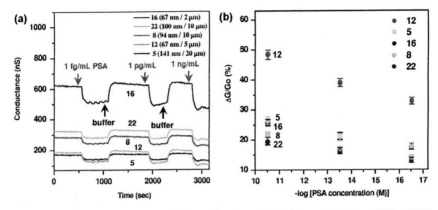

Figure 9.8. Ultrahigh sensitivity for PSA detection. (A) Real-time detection of PSA. SiNW of various dimensions creates a different response and sensitivity. **(B)** The acquired LOD was approximately in an atto-molar range, which is the lowest LOD reported to date. **(A)** and **(B)** Reprinted and/or adapted with permission from Kim et al. 2007 (Copyright 2007 American Institute of Physics).

the PSA creates negative charges and positive charges in the solutions with pH value of 7.8 and 6.0, respectively. Thus, the conductance of the n-type SiNW is decreased in the solution with a pH of 7.8 and increased in the solution with a pH of 6.0. This is consistent with the mechanism of the SiNW biosensor.

Applications

The introduced SiNW is applicable to various areas of health care and disease diagnoses, especially to a portable biosensor, POCT systems, and drug discovery systems. A SiNW biosensor fabricated by a conventional silicon process is suitable for use as a portable biosensor due to its small size. Peripheral control and signal processing circuits can be monolithically fabricated with a SiNW biosensor; hence, this co-integrated chip can provide preliminary health information prior to a visit to a hospital. Construction of a POCT system is possible through label-free and real-time detection. SiNW-based biosensors can also be adapted for use with drug discovery research. In the drug discovery process, numerous chemicals or biomolecules are typically tested and screened with high throughput. To speed up the procedure, multiplexed detection and automatic data processing are necessary. This type of automatic data processing can be achieved in a chip-based analysis along with label-free electrical detection. For these reasons, the SiNW-based biosensor has attracted continuous attention from various fields.

KEY FACTS

Electrical detection: Electrical detection refers to when the output from a biosensor is an electrical signal. The type of signals created by the receptor can be colored, fluorescent, mechanical, massive, or electrical signal. Except for the electrical signal, all other signals should be converted to an electrical signal through the transducer for a chip-based sensor kit. Thus, electrical detection by a biosensor is attractive for a small portable device that can be embedded into a smart phone due to the absence of a transducer.

Label-free detection: The time-consuming labeling step is difficult for non-skilled personnel, requires expensive equipment and difficult labor, and results in a loss of samples and contamination. Hence, the label-free detection method is essential in various fields, such as those that use portable biosensors and POCT systems, due to the simple manipulation of the samples and the reduced sensing step accompanied with fast detection.

DEFINITIONS

- *Dopant:* The species introduced in a semiconductor substrate to change the physical, chemical, or electrical properties (e.g. electron-rich or hole-rich in the semiconductor) of the solid.
- *FET:* Field effect transistor. The device whose operation is controlled by an electric field by gate bias.
- *Implantation (or Ion implantation):* A process of introducing dopants into a semiconductor by ion acceleration under an electrical field. They can also be impacted into another solid with an arbitrary angle.
- *LOD:* Limit of detection. The lowest analyte concentration which can be detected by a particular biosensor.
- *PCR:* Polymerase chain reaction. An amplification method that produces millions of copies of a target DNA or RNA.
- *pI value:* Isoelectric point. A certain pH value at which biomolecules show an electrically neutral property. The biomolecules show a negatively charged property when the pH value of the surrounding solution is higher than the pI value. However, they show a positively charged property when the pH value of the surrounding solution is lower than the pI value.
- *POCT:* Point-of-care testing. Diagnosis of a disease in a place where the patient is.
- *Response time:* Required time to obtain a stable output signal from an injection of target analytes.

- *Sensitivity*: The ability to detect a low concentration of the targeted analytes. It is expressed in terms of the LOD.
- *Specificity (or Selectivity)*: The ability to detect targeted analytes from a solution mixed with other biomolecules selectively.

SUMMARY

- Compared to the bottom-up method, the top-down method offers identical and well-aligned SiNWs with peripheral circuits monolithically.
- Biomolecules charged by the same polarity to majority carriers lowered the conductance of SiNW while those charged by the opposite polarity to the majority carriers increased the conductance of SiNW.
- A narrow width and lower doping concentration are desirable for high sensitivity.
- Highly concentrated buffer solution preserved the charge density and bioaffinity of the biomolecules; however, this also degraded the device sensitivity due to the electrostatic screening effect caused by the ionic strength.
- The CFTR gene and miRNA extracted from a HeLa cell were detected in a buffer solution with a low concentration at a high level of sensitivity.
- The activity of telomerase, an enzyme which is closely related to cancer, was also detected using a probe DNA platform on the SiNWs.
- An atto-molar LOD value was achieved for the detection of PSA after controlling the structural parameters, and immediate multiplexed detection was effectively carried out for PSA, CEA, and mucin-1 protein.

ACKNOWLEDGMENT

We thank J.-H. Ahn and J.-Y. Kim for their help in preparing the manuscript. This work was supported in part by the National Research and Development Program under Grant 2010-0002108 for the development of biomedical function monitoring biosensors and in part by the National Research Foundation of Korea funded by Korean government under Grant 2010-0018931.

ABBREVIATIONS

BRAF	:	Serine/threonine-protein kinase B-Raf
CEA	:	Carcinoembryonic antigen
CFTR	:	Cystic fibrosis transmembrane conductance regulator
CHEMFET	:	Chemical field effect transistor
DNA	:	Deoxyribonucleic acid
K_d	:	Dissociation constant
λ_D	:	Debye length
FET	:	Field effect transistor
IgA	:	Immunoglobulin A
IgG	:	Immunoglobulin G
ISFET	:	Ion-sensitive field effect transistor
LOD	:	Limit of detection
PBS	:	Phosphate-buffered saline
PCR	:	Polymerase chain reaction
pI	:	Isoelectric point
PNA	:	Peptide Nucleic Acid
POCT	:	Point-of-care testing
PSA	:	Prostate-specific antigen
RNA	:	Ribonucleic acid
SiNW	:	Silicon nanowire
SOI	:	Silicon-on-insulator
SVR	:	Surface-to-volume ratio
VLS	:	Vapor-liquid-solid

REFERENCES

Ahn J-H, S-J Choi, J-W Han, TJ Park, SY Lee and Y-K Choi. 2010. Double-gate nanowire field effect transistor for biosensor. Nano Lett 10: 2934–2938.

Bayer EA and M Wilchek. 1990. Biotin-binding proteins: Overview and prospects. Methods Enzymol 184: 49–51.

Bergveld P. 2003. Thirty years of ISFETOLOGY. What happened in the past 30 years and what may happen in the next 30 years. Sens. Actuators, B 88: 1–20.

Briones C, E Mateo-Mariti, C Gomez-Navarro, V Parro, E Roman and JA Martin-Gago. 2004. Ordered self-assembled monolayers of peptide nucleic acids with DNA recognition capability. Phys Rev Lett 90: 208103.

Bunimovich YL, YS Shin, W-S Yeo, M Amori, G Kwong and JR Heath. 2006. Quantitative real-time measurements of DNA hybridization with alkylated nonoxidized silicon nanowires in electrolyte solution. J Am Chem Soc 128: 16323–16331.

Choi Y-K, J Grunes, J Boker and GA Somorjai. 2003. Fabrication of sub-10-nm silicon nanowire arrays by size reduction lithography. J Phys Chem B 107: 3340–3343.

Curreli M, R Zhang, FN Ishikawa, H-K Chang, RJ Cote, C Zhou and ME Thompson. 2008. Real-time, label-free detection of biological entities using nanowire-based FETs. IEEE Trans. IEEE Trans. Nanotechnol 7: 651–667.

Gao Z, A Agarwal, AD Trigg, N Singh, C Fang, C-H Tung, Y Fan, KD Buddharaju and J Kong. 2007. Silicon nanowire arrays for label-free detection of DNA. Anal Chem 79: 3291–3297.

Hahm J-I and CM Lieber. 2004. Direct ultrasensitive electrical detection of DNA and DNA sequence variations using nanowire nanosensors. Nano Lett 4: 51–54.

Kim A, CS Ah, HY Yu, J-H Yang, I-B Baek, C-G Ahn, CW Park and MS Jun. 2007. Ultrasensitive, label-free, and real-time immunodetection using silicon field-effect transistors. Appl Phys Lett 91: 103901.

Li Z, B Rajendran, TI Kamins, X Li, Y Chen and RS Williams. 2005. Silicon nanowires for sequence-specific DNA sensing: device fabrication and simulation. Appl Phys A: Mater Sci Process 80: 1257–1263.

Nair PR and MA Alam. 2007. Design considerations of silicon nanowire biosensor. IEEE Trans. Electron Devices 54: 3400–3408.

Nair PR and MA Alam. 2008. Screening-limited response of nanobiosensors. Nano Lett 8: 1281–1285.

Patolsky F, G Zheng and CM Lieber. 2006a. Nanowire sensors for medicine and the life sciences. Nanomedicine 1: 51–65.

Stern E, JF Klemic, DA Routenberg, PN Wyrembak, DB Turner-Evans, AD Hamiton, DA LaVan, TM Fahmy and MA Reed. 2007a. Label-free immunedetection with CMOS-compatible semiconducting nanowires. Nature 445: 519–522.

Stern E, R Wagner, FJ Sigworth, R Breaker, TM Fahmy and MA Reed. 2007b. Importance of the Debye screening length on nanowire field effect transistor. Nano Lett 7: 3405–3409.

Wagner RS and WC Ellis. 1964. Vapor-liquid-solid mechanism of single crystal growth. Appl Phys Lett 4: 89–90.

Wu C-C, F-H Ko, Y-S Yang, D-L Hsia, B-S Lee and T-S Su. 2009. Label-free biosensing of a gene mutation using a silicon nanowire field-effect transistor. Biosens Bioelectron 25: 820–825.

Zhang G-J, G Zhang, JH Chua, R-E Chee, EH Wong, A Agarwal, KD Buddharaju, N Singh, Z Gao and N Balasubramanian. 2008. DAN sensing by silicon nanowire: Charge layer distance dependence. Nano Lett 8: 1066–1070.

Zhang G-J, JH Chua, R-E Chee, A Agarwal and SM Wong. 2009. Label-free direct detection of MiRNAs with silicon nanowire biosensors. Biosens Bioelectron 24: 2504–2508.

Zheng G, F Patolsky, Y Cui, WU Wang and CM Lieber. 2005. Multiplexed electrical detection of cancer markers with nanowire sensor arrays. Nat Biotechnol 23: 1294–1301.

SECTION 2: BLOOD, MOLECULES AND CELLS

10

DNA-electrochemical Biosensors and Oxidative Damage to DNA: Application to Cancer

Victor Constantin Diculescu[2] and Ana Maria Oliveira Brett[1,*]

ABSTRACT

In recent years increased attention has been focused on the ways in which endogenous and exogenous stimuli interact with DNA, with the goal of understanding the toxic as well as chemotherapeutic effects of many molecules. The reactions with chemicals cause changes in the structure of DNA and the base sequence leading to perturbations in DNA replication and consequently to different diseases especially cancer. Thus, it is very important to explain the factors that determine affinity and selectivity in binding molecules to DNA, identify these chemicals and ascertain their potency so that human exposure to them can be minimized.

[1]Departamento de Química, Faculdade de Ciências e Tecnologia, Universidade de Coimbra, 3004-535 Coimbra, Portugal; E-mail: brett@ci.uc.pt
[2]Instituto Pedro Nunes, Laboratório de Electroanálise e Corrosão, Rua Pedro Nunes, 3030-199 Coimbra, Portugal; E-mail: victorcd@ipn.pt
*Corresponding author

List of abbreviations after the text.

The need for analyzing gene sequences, oxidative damage to DNA and the understanding of DNA interactions with molecules or ions led to the development of DNA- biosensors. Electrochemical techniques have the advantage of a rapid response time, being quantitative, sensitive, suitable for automation, cost effective, disposable, enabling *in situ* generation of short-lived radical intermediates and the detection of their interaction with DNA. The DNA-modified electrode is a very good model for simulating the nucleic acid interaction with cell membranes, potential environmental carcinogenic compounds and to clarify the mechanisms of action of drugs used as chemotherapeutic agents, without using animal tests. How the electrochemical method can explain the mechanism of interaction between different compounds and DNA is briefly described. The comprehensive descriptions of research on DNA and DNA biosensing capabilities will show the great possibilities of using electrochemical transduction in DNA diagnostics.

INTRODUCTION

The recent advance in molecular genetics allowed understanding the molecular mechanisms involved in the neoplasic transformations (Hanahan and Weinberg 2000). Cancer arises through a number of biochemical transformations (Hartwell and Kastan 1994) that induce the formation of cells with a set of particular properties such as unlimited proliferation potential and resistance to anti-proliferative and apoptotic signals (Luo et al. 2009).

The complex series of cellular changes participating in cancer development are mediated by a diversity of endogenous and exogenous stimuli (Evans et al. 2004). One type of endogenous damage arises from intermediates of oxygen reduction, the reactive oxygen species (ROS). Endogenous ROS are produced as a result of various metabolic processes and biochemical reactions (Grivennikov et al. 2010). The cell can protect itself from ROS using different mechanisms that involve repairing enzymes and/or antioxidants (Jackson and Loeb 2001). Under normal physiological conditions a balance is maintained between the endogenous ROS and the elimination of the damage produced. However, when an imbalance occurs, biological molecules such as DNA may undergo oxidative damage, a process involved in the pathogenesis of many diseases (Evans et al. 2004; Cooke et al. 2003). It is now generally accepted that the main reason for the development of cancer is the genetic disorder produced by DNA damage after its interaction with a variety of compounds.

Besides ROS, several other compounds found in cellular environment such as metal ions and drugs as well as the ionizing radiation involve interactions with DNA (Fojta 2005; Palecek 2009). These interactions may lead to chemical reactions that can cause mutations in DNA leading to perturbation in its replications and consequently malfunctioning and cellular death. Thus, it is very important to explain the factors that determine the affinity and selectivity in binding molecules to DNA since a qualitative understanding of the reasons that determine selection of DNA reaction sites is useful in designing sequence-specific DNA binding molecules for application in chemotherapy and in explaining the mechanism of action of anti-neoplasic drugs.

The need for analyzing gene sequences, oxidative damage to DNA and the understanding of DNA interactions with molecules or ions led to the development of DNA-biosensors (Wang 2006). Optical, piezoelectric, surface acoustic wave and electrochemical methods have been applied for the transductions of the signals that occur at the surface of a DNA-biosensor (Soper et al. 2006).

When compared with the other transducers, the electrochemical transduction is dynamic and the electrode provides a tuneable charged reagent as well as a detector of all surface phenomena, which greatly enhance the biosensing capabilities. Due to the existing resemblance between electrochemical and biological reactions it can be assumed that the oxidation mechanisms taking place at the electrode and in the body share similar principles (Rauf et al. 2005).

To design DNA-based biosensors it is essential to understand the structure and the electrochemical DNA properties. Also, the performance of the DNA biosensor and the electrochemical response are dictated by the DNA immobilization procedure. Therefore, a full understanding of the surface morphology of the DNA-electrochemical biosensor is necessary to guarantee the correct interpretation of the experimental results.

DNA STRUCTURE

The deoxyribonucleic acid (DNA) is formed by two antiparallel polynucleotide strands running in opposite directions. Each strand is formed by monomer units called nucleotides. Each nucleotide is formed by a phosphate group, a sugar and heterocyclic base. The alternating phosphate and sugar groups in one strand provide the continuity of the polymer performing a structural role and represent the DNA backbone. The genetic information is coded by the purine bases, adenine (A) and guanine (G), and the pyrimidine bases, cytosine (C) and thymine (T), as a function of their consecutive order in the strand, Fig. 10.1.

The two strands of a DNA molecule are held together by hydrogen bonds between complementary bases: two between adenine and thymine and three between guanine and cytosine, Fig. 10.1. The hydrogen bonds between purines and pyrimidines together with base stacking and electrostatic interactions between negative charged phosphate groups stabilize the DNA double helix structure (double stranded or dsDNA) in which both strands

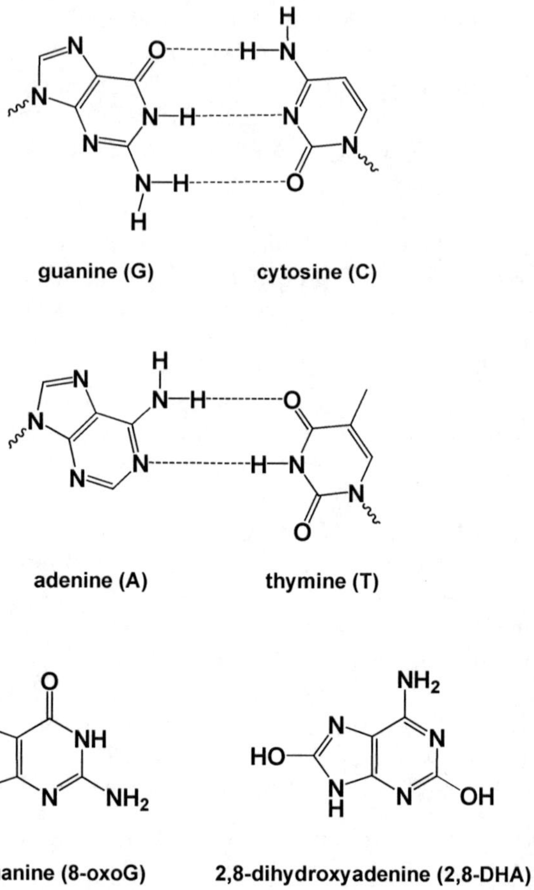

Figure 10.1. Chemical structures of DNA bases. Chemical structures of: DNA bases guanine, adenine, cytosine, thymine and the formation of hydrogen bonds between complementary bases; and biomarkers for DNA damage 8-oxoguanine and 2,8-dihydroxyadenine.

run along a common axis. The bases are oriented perpendicular to this axis and stacked inside the helix whereas the sugar-phosphate backbone is accessible to the surrounding environment. The specificity of the base pairing is the most important aspect of the DNA double helix since one strand of the DNA is the complement of the other.

Under conditions of extremes of pH or of heat, dsDNA denaturation occurs and its physical properties in solution change although no covalent bonds are broken: only the unwinding and separation of the double helical DNA structure occurs. The hydrogen bonds between the complementary bases on opposite strands are broke and the double-helix structure of dsDNA is disrupted into the two complementary strands forming the so called single-stranded DNA (ssDNA).

ELECTROCHEMISTRY OF DNA

The electrochemical behaviour of DNA and its components at different types of electrodes have been investigated for a number of years. At mercury electrodes (Fojta 2005; Palecek 2009), adenine and cytosine residues as well as guanine residues in a polynucleotide chain are reducible. However, the use of mercury electrodes is limited to the negative potential range and the information obtained allowed conclusions only about reduction. Moreover, because of the toxicity of mercury, the popularity of mercury electrodes has recently considerably declined. Thus, the use of solid electrodes in general, and carbon in particular, expanded in recent years (Oliveira Brett et al. 2004b).

All DNA bases, purines: guanine and adenine and pyrimidines: cytosine and thymine can be electrochemically oxidized at carbon electrodes, Fig. 10.2 (Oliveira Brett et al. 2004b). The purines are oxidized at lower potentials than the pyrimidines where oxidation occurs near the potential corresponding to oxygen evolution and consequently are more difficult to detect. Also, the electrochemical oxidation of nucleotides of all DNA bases has been studied and the results showed that for all bases the corresponding nucleotides are oxidized at potential approximately 200 mV more positive than the base. For these reasons, the electrochemical detection of DNA has been based on the appearance of purine bases oxidation peaks.

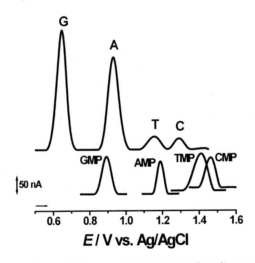

Figure 10.2. Electrochemical oxidation of all DNA bases. Base line corrected differential pulse voltammograms obtained for a 20 μM equimolar mixture of guanine **(G)** adenine **(A)** thymine **(T)** and cytosine **(C)** 20 μM guanosine-monophosphate (GMP), 20 μM adenosine-monophosphate (AMP), 500 μM thymidine-monophosphate (TMP) and 500 μM cytidine-monophosphate (CMP) in pH 7.4 0.1 M phosphate supporting electrolyte. [Adapted from (Oliveira Brett et al. 2004b) with permission.]

Electrochemical oxidation of DNA samples has been extensively studied with a glassy carbon electrode (Oliveira and Oliveira Brett 2010) and showed that only the oxidation of purines residues in the polynucleotide chain can be observed and gives rise to two well separated oxidation peaks, Fig. 10.3. Using differential pulse voltammetry (DPV), the less positive peak corresponds to the oxidation of guanine residues and the peak at more positive potentials is due to the oxidation of adenine residues. Large differences in the currents obtained for dsDNA and ssDNA were observed. The greater difficulty for the transition of electrons from the inside of the rigid helix of dsDNA to the electrode surface than from the flexible ssDNA, where guanine and adenine residues can reach the surface, leads to much higher peak currents for ssDNA. Thus, the oxidation currents of guanine and adenine residues in DNA can be used to probe individual A–T and G–C pairs in dsDNA.

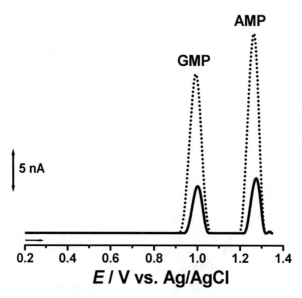

Figure 10.3. Electrochemical oxidation of DNA samples. Base line corrected differential pulse voltammograms obtained with the GCE in solutions of 60 µg ml⁻¹ (•••) ssDNA and (—) dsDNA in pH 4.5 0.1 M acetate buffer. [unpublished results.]

ADSORPTION OF DNA AT ELECTRODE SURFACE

When natural or synthetic DNA molecules interact with electrode surfaces adsorption occurs. The knowledge about the adsorption of nucleic acids onto the electrode surface leads to the development of DNA-modified electrodes, also called DNA-electrochemical biosensors (Oliveira Brett et al. 2006).

The development of an electrochemical biosensor consists in the immobilization of biological material on the sensor surface by controlling the potential applied to the electrode (Oliveira Brett and Chiorcea Paquim 2005). The atomic force microscopy (AFM) results (Oliveira Brett and Chiorcea 2003a,b, 2005; Oliveira Brett et al. 2004a), Fig. 10.4, have already shown the importance of morphological characterization of biosensors surface for the understanding of the adsorption processes of biomolecules at the electrode surface and a correct evaluation of all parameters that could influence the response of the biosensor.

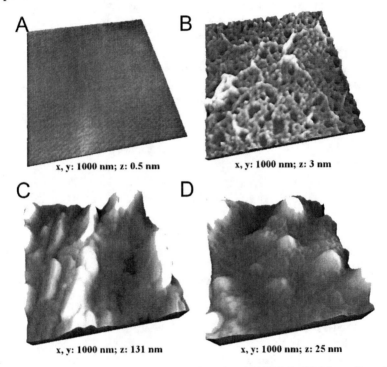

Figure 10.4. Adsorption of DNA at the electrode surface. MAC Mode AFM three-dimensional images in air of: **(A)** clean HOPG electrode; **(B)** thin film dsDNA-biosensor surface, prepared onto HOPG by 3 min free adsorption from 60 µg/mL dsDNA in pH 4.5 0.1 M acetate buffer; **(C)** multi-layer film dsDNA-biosensor, prepared onto HOPG by evaporation of three consecutive drops each containing 5 µL of 50 µg/mL dsDNA in pH 4.5 0.1 M acetate buffer; **(D)** thick film dsDNA-biosensor, prepared onto HOPG by evaporation from 37.5 mg/mL dsDNA in pH 4.5 0.1 M acetate buffer. [Adapted from (Oliveira Brett et al. 2007) with permission.]

The DNA properties, such as flexibility and DNA–drug interactions, are influenced by the adsorbed DNA structure (ssDNA or dsDNA), concentration, pH and supporting electrolyte (Oliveira Brett and Chiorcea 2003a, 2003b). A full understanding of the surface morphology of the DNA-electrochemical biosensor is necessary to guarantee the correct interpretation of the experimental results.

Highly oriented pyrolytic graphite (HOPG) and glassy carbon (GCE) electrodes are usually used as the immobilization material for the development of DNA-electrochemical biosensors. The interactions between DNA and the different carbon surfaces, the adsorption and the degree of surface coverage are very similar. However, HOPG surface is extremely smooth and atomically flat, Fig. 10.4A, and enables to study the topography changes when the sensor surface is modified with DNA, Fig. 10.4.

It has been shown that the coverage and the robustness of the DNA-biosensor are influenced by the DNA immobilization procedure on the electrode surface. It was possible to visualize directly, Fig. 10.4, the surface characteristics of dsDNA films prepared on a HOPG electrode using ex situ MAC mode AFM; different immobilization methodologies lead to structural changes on the DNA biosensor surface and consequently different sensor response. Images of HOPG electrode modified by thin or thick films of dsDNA showed that the thin films forms a network structure, Fig. 10.4B, with holes that expose the electrode surface. On the other hand, the thick films of dsDNA, Figs. 10.4C and 10.4D, completely cover the electrode surface with a multilayer film having a rough morphology.

ELECTROCHEMICAL DNA BIOSENSOR

DNA-electrochemical biosensors enable the study of the interaction of DNA immobilized on the electrode surface with analytes in solution. Interactions of the surface-confined DNA with the damaging agent are converted, via changes in the electrochemical properties of the DNA recognition layer, into measurable electric signals, Table 10.1.

The immobilization of the dsDNA probe on the electrode surface is usually done in pH 4.5 due to the better adsorption of DNA on the carbon surface, leading to an enhanced electrochemical response. There are different procedures that can be followed in the DNA-electrochemical biosensor construction.

1. *Thin-Layer dsDNA Biosensor*: prepared by immersing the GCE surface in a 60 μg mL^{-1} dsDNA solution at + 0.30 V applied potential during 10 min, Fig. 10.4B.
2. *Multi-Layer dsDNA Biosensor*: prepared by successively covering the GCE surface with three drops of 5 μL each of 50 μg mL^{-1} dsDNA solution. After placing each drop on the electrode surface the biosensor is dried under a flux of N$_2$, Fig. 10.4C.
3. *Thick-Layer dsDNA Biosensor*: prepared by covering the GCE surface with 10 μL of 35 mg mL^{-1} dsDNA solution and allowing it to dry in normal atmosphere, Fig. 10.4D.

Table 10.1. Key facts of electrochemical DNA biosensor. Key facts on electrochemistry, working principle, its application in DNA biosensor technology and the advantages when compared with other techniques.

1. Electrochemistry involves chemical phenomena associated with the charge transfer.
2. Three electrodes are immersed into an electrochemical cell that contains a conductive solution. Applying different potentials, the electrodes may act as a sink or source of electrons such as the electric charge is transferred between them and the compound.
3. The potential (E) applied to the electrode is varied in a controlled manner and the current (I) registered. The I vs. E curve is the recorded voltammograms.
4. The steps involved during the study of electrochemical detection of oxidative DNA damage by a compound are:
    - Immobilization of DNA at the electrode surface;
    - the incubation of the biosensor in the compound-containing solution for a given period of time;
    - the transduction of the electroanalytical detection of DNA damage by DPV in buffer.
5. The *in situ* generation of metabolites is achieved when during the incubation phase a potential is applied to the biosensor surface causing the compound to undergo redox reactions leading to the formation of reactive redox products .
6. Damage to DNA is electrochemically recognized by changes into purine bases oxidation signals and/or occurrence of new oxidation peaks.

The existence of pores in the thin dsDNA layer, Fig. 10.4B, leaving areas of the HOPG surface uncovered can cause misleading results. The drug molecules from the bulk solution will diffuse and adsorb non-specifically on the electrode's uncovered regions. If the drugs are electroactive, this leads to two different contributions to the electrochemical signal, one from the simple adsorbed drug and the other due to the damage caused to immobilized DNA, being difficult to distinguish between them.

A complete coverage of the electrode surface is obtained using the multi-layer and thick dsDNA films, Figs. 10.4C and 10.4D. The DNA-electrode surface interactions are stronger and these DNA films are more stable. The big advantage of these dsDNA biosensors is that the surface is completely covered and consequently the undesired binding of molecules to the electrode surface is not possible.

BIOMARKERS FOR DNA-DAMAGE

Hazard compounds such as drugs and carcinogens interact with DNA causing irreversible damage. Numerous DNA damage products are formed due to bases and sugar modifications, covalent crosslinks, single and double stranded breaks (Fojta 2005). However, most research interest has focused on nucleobase modifications.

Some DNA adducts are monitored as specific biomarkers of exposure of organisms to different genotoxic agents Among them, several mutagenic products such as 8-oxoguanine (8-oxoG), 2,8-dihydroxyadenine (2,8-DHA),

5-formiluracil, 5-hydroxycitosine e 5,6-dihydroxythymine may be produced upon exposure of DNA to free radicals or ionizing radiation (Evans et al. 2004).

The oxidation products of guanine, 8-oxoG, and adenine, 2,8-DHA, Fig. 10.1, are the most commonly measured products of DNA oxidative damage. The *in vivo* formation of 8-oxoG is highly mutagenic since it pairs more easily with A, and, if not repaired by enzymes, may lead to substitution of C by A in the complementary strands which in turn leads to the substitution of G by T after DNA replication.

The electroactivity of 8-oxoG (Oliveira Brett et al. 2000) and of 2,8-DHA (Diculescu et al. 2007) was investigated and their oxidation peaks were chosen to monitor DNA oxidative damage since the oxidation potentials are lower and well-separated from the oxidation potentials of the respective bases.

DNA BIOSENSORS FOR THE *IN SITU* DETECTION OF OXIDATIVE DNA DAMAGE

Molecules and ions interact with DNA in three significant ways: electrostatic, groove-binding and intercalation (Rauf et al. 2005). These interactions can cause changes in the structure of DNA and the base sequence leading to perturbation of DNA replication. How the electrochemical method can explain the mechanism of interaction between different compounds or ionizing radiation and DNA is illustrated briefly in the following examples.

Metals and Metal Complexes

Metals

Although certain metals are essential to living systems, being required for enzymatic reactions or other physiological processes, others are highly toxic involving an increased risk of various cancers and adverse health effects.

The evaluation of the interaction of divalent cations, Pb, Cd, Ni and Pd, with dsDNA, was studied by AFM and DPV (Chiorcea-Paquim et al. 2009). The electrochemical behaviour of these metal–DNA complexes was related to the different adsorption patterns and conformational changes obtained by the AFM images. The dsDNA interaction was specific with each metal cation, inducing structural changes in the DNA structure, local denaturation of the double helix, and oxidative damage. For cadmium and nickel, oxidative damage to DNA was observed for the concentrations studied and the formation of 8-oxoG and 2,8-DHA was electrochemically detected.

Palladium interaction with dsDNA induced condensation of the dsDNA secondary structure, which led to the aggregation of helixes forming very compact and thick filaments. The voltammetric data for the palladium–DNA complex showed a sharp decrease of the guanine and adenine oxidation peak currents, consistent with the DNA condensation, but no DNA oxidative damage was detected for the range of concentrations used.

Metal Complexes

The development of new chemotherapeutic agents led to the synthesis of polynuclear metal complexes, a new class of third generation anticancer agents with specific chemical and biological properties designed as alternatives to first-generation agents.

The interaction of dsDNA with two polynuclear Pd(II) chelates with the biogenic polyamines spermidine (Spd) and spermine (Spm), Pd(II)-Spd and Pd(II)-Spm, as well as with the free ligands Spd and Spm, was studied using AFM, voltammetry and gel electrophoresis (Corduneanu et al. 2010). The interaction of Spd and Spm with DNA occurred even for a low concentration of polyamines and caused no oxidative damage to DNA. The Pd(II)-Spd and Pd(II)-Spm complexes were found to induce greater morphological changes in the dsDNA conformation, when compared with their ligands. The interaction induced distortion and local denaturation of the DNA structure with release of some guanine bases that were electrochemically detected. The DNA strands partially opened give rise to palladium intra- and interstrand cross-links, leading to the formation of DNA adducts and aggregates.

Reactive Oxygen (ROS) and Nitrogen (RNS) Species

Quercetin

Quercetin, a major flavonoid in the human diet, acts as a pro-oxidant under certain circumstances (Oliveira Brett and Diculescu 2004c). The formation of quercetin radicals via auto-oxidation of the catechol ring leads to the generation of superoxide radicals that can promote oxidative damage to DNA.

Quercetin interaction with dsDNA was investigated using a dsDNA biosensor in order to evaluate the occurrence of DNA damage caused by oxidized quercetin. The dsDNA biosensor was incubated in a solution of quercetin and the DPV recorded in buffer showed the quercetin peak followed by small peaks of guanine and adenine residues, Fig. 10.5. When a potential of + 0.40 V was applied to a DNA-electrochemical biosensor, previously incubated in quercetin, the quercetin molecules bound to DNA were oxidized

A

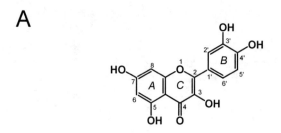

B

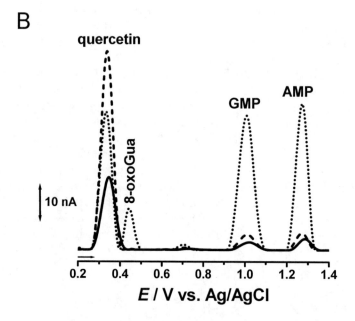

Figure 10.5. *In Situ* **detection of quercetin-DNA interaction. (A)** Chemical structure of quercetin; **(B)** Base line corrected differential pulse voltammograms in pH 4.3 0.1 M acetate buffer obtained with a multi-layer dsDNA biosensor incubated for 10 min in: 100 µM quercetin (- - -) before and after applying + 0.40 V for 300 s (—) with and (•••) without bubbling N_2 in the solution. [Adapted from (Oliveira Brett and Diculescu 2004c) with permission.]

leading to formation of ROS. The radicals formed damaged the dsDNA and this process was detected by the occurrence of high oxidation peaks of GMP and AMP, Fig. 10.5. Moreover, the DPV obtained in these conditions showed a peak at + 0.45 V, confirming the formation of 8-oxoG.

To prove the involvement of ROS in the process of DNA damage during quercetin oxidation, experiments were carried out after removal of O_2 from the solution which impeded the formation of ROS. In these conditions, the DPV, Fig. 10.5, showed only small oxidation peaks of DNA and no 8-oxodG proving that no damage had occurred in the absence of ROS.

Nitric Oxide

Recently, DNA damage due to RNS has become an interesting subject since high nitric oxide (NO) concentration in cells was reported to produce genotoxic effects.

The dsDNA biosensor was used to study the interaction between DNA and RNS released by a NO-releasing compound, diethylenetriamine/nitric oxide (DETA/NO) (Diculescu et al. 2005a). The DP voltammograms obtained after incubation of the biosensor in DETA/NO showed small DNA oxidation peaks proving that no damage occurred. When a potential of –0.60 V is applied during the incubation procedure, O_2 is reduced and $O_2^{-\bullet}$ radicals produced at the electrode surface reacted with the NO molecules giving rise to peroxynitrite ($ONOO^-$) that damage DNA. The voltammograms obtained in these conditions, Fig. 10.6, showed two large oxidation peaks for GMP and AMP corresponding to the structural modifications of the

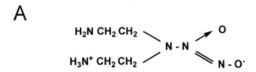

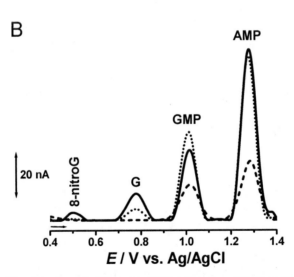

Figure 10.6. *In Situ* **detection of nitric oxide-DNA interaction. (A)** Chemical structure of DETA/NO. **B)** Base line corrected differential pulse voltammograms obtain in pH 4.5 0.1 M acetate buffer with a dsDNA-biosensor previously incubated in 1.5 mM DETA: (‒ ‒ ‒) during 5 min, or at –0.60 V during (•••) 2 and (—) 3 min. [Adapted from (Diculescu et al. 2005a) with permission.]

dsDNA double helix. The peak at E_{pa} = + 0.77 V showed that some guanine bases were released during peroxynitrite interaction with DNA. Also, a new peak is observed at E_{pa} = + 0.49 V, Fig. 10.6, due to oxidative damage to immobilized DNA after interaction with peroxynitrite. This peak is due to the formation of 8-nitroguanine, a highly mutagenic product.

DRUGS

Adriamycin

The ability of antitumour antibiotics to intercalate between the DNA base-pairs has the advantage of bringing the toxic species (the free radicals) into proximity with the target. The antitumour antibiotic adriamycin generates ROS which have the potential to damage DNA.

Electrochemical *in situ* sensing of DNA damage caused by reduced adriamycin intercalated into DNA was investigated using the dsDNA biosensor (Oliveira Brett et al. 2002). The voltammograms obtained with a thin-layer DNA biosensor incubated in an adriamycin solution, Fig. 10.7, have shown adriamycin oxidation peak at +0.50 V and a small oxidation peak of guanine residues. In order to reduce adriamycin molecules intercalated in DNA, a potential of - 0.60 V was applied to a new biosensor previously incubated in adriamycin. A high oxidation peak for guanine occurred at +0.84 V showing structural modifications of the dsDNA, and the oxidation peak of 8-oxoG appeared at +0.38 V, Fig. 10.7. These results correspond to the direct oxidative damage to DNA caused by adriamycin which occurs through the formation of the semiquinone radical intercalated in the double helix that oxidizes the guanine residues and generates 8-oxoG: In this mechanism adriamycin radicals are able to directly cause oxidative damage to DNA and ROS were not directly involved in the genomic mutagenic lesions.

Imatinib Mesilate

Imatinib mesilate is a relatively small molecule with activity against the *BCR-ABL* tyrosine kinase, a protein expressed by all patients with chronic myelogenous leukemia (CML) but also may involve DNA damage in the cells expressing this protein.

The interaction of DNA with the antileukemia drug imatinib was investigated in bulk solution and at a dsDNA biosensor using DPV (Diculescu et al. 2006). It was found that imatinib binds to dsDNA and this interaction leads to modifications in the dsDNA structure, electrochemically recognized through changes of the anodic oxidation peaks of guanine and adenine bases, Fig. 10.8. When a multi-layer dsDNA-biosensor was

A

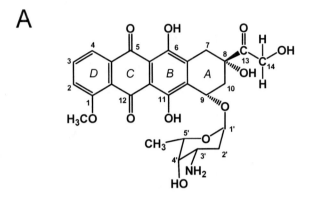

B

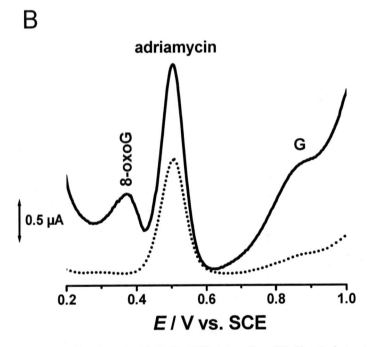

Figure 10.7. *In Situ* detection of adriamycin-DNA interaction. **(A)** Chemical structure of adriamycin. **(B)** Base line subtracted differential pulse voltammograms obtained with the dsDNA biosensor in pH 4.5 0.1 M acetate buffer after being immersed in a 5 μM adriamycin solution during 3 min and rinsed with water before the experiment in buffer: (•••) without applied potential; (—) applying a potential of –0.6 V during 60 s. [Adapted from (Oliveira Brett et al. 2002) with permission.]

incubated in an imatinib solution and a conditioning potential of + 0.90 V was applied, the imatinib molecules attached to the dsDNA film were oxidized leading to the formation of imatinib oxidation product, the peak at + 0.32 V,

Fig. 10.8, and a new small peak at + 0.45 V showed that oxidative DNA damage have occurred, Fig. 10.8. Using polyhomonucleotides of known sequence, poly[G] and poly[A] has proved that the interaction between imatinib and DNA takes place at adenine enriched segments and the peak + 0.45 V was due to 2,8-DHA formation. This interaction mechanism was proposed and the formation of 2,8-DHA explained (Diculescu et al. 2006).

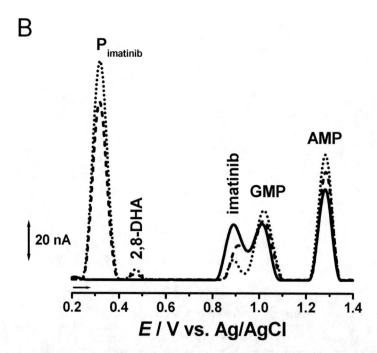

Figure 10.8. *In Situ* **detection of imatinib-DNA interaction. (A)** Chemical structure of imatinib. **B)** Base line corrected differential pulse voltammograms obtained with the dsDNA biosensor in pH 4.5 0.1 M acetate buffer after incubation for 2 min with 5 μM glivec (—) before and after application of + 0.90 V during (---) 1 and (•••) 2 min. [Adapted from (Diculescu et al. 2006a) with permission.]

Thalidomide

Thalidomide (TD) was originally developed as a sedative and anti-emetic drug to combat morning sickness during pregnancy. However, TD teratogenic side effects appeared in newborn children.

The interaction of TD with dsDNA was studied using AFM at HOPG, and DPV at GCE, (Oliveira et al. 2009). The AFM images show the formation of thin and incomplete TD–DNA network films with a number of embedded molecular aggregates and regions of uncovered HOPG. Both the TD–dsDNA aggregates and network thickness directly depended on the TD concentration and incubation time. In agreement, the voltammetric data showed that the modifications caused by TD to the DNA double helical structure are time-dependent. The DP voltammograms obtained after different incubation times showed four small well-defined oxidation peaks, Fig. 10.9. The two oxidation peaks of guanine and adenine residues were observed, although they showed a large decrease of the oxidation current due to the TD–DNA condensation, when compared with the results obtained from the control dsDNA solution. The oxidation peak found at + 0.45 V is attributed to 8-oxoGua and/or 2,8 oxoAde oxidation, and the peak observed at + 0.80 V is due to the oxidation of TD intercalated in the dsDNA.

Methotrexate

Methotrexate (MTX) is an antimetabolite of folic acid, that targets the enzyme dehydrofolate reductase which plays a supporting but essential role for the synthesis of thymine nucleotide. Also, it has been shown that the MTX treatment causes the accumulation of 8-oxoG in cells.

The *in situ* evaluation of dsDNA-methotrexate (MTX) interaction was investigated by voltammetry at a dsDNA biosensor and characterized by AFM. The AFM images have shown the reorganization of the DNA self-assembled network upon binding MTX and the formation of a more densely packed and slightly thicker MTX–dsDNA lattice with a large number of aggregates embedded into the network film. The intercalation of MTX between complementary base pairs of dsDNA led to the increase of purine oxidation peaks due to the unwinding of the dsDNA. The dsDNA-electrochemical biosensor and the polyhomopurinenucleotide single stranded sequences of guanine and adenine, poly[G] and poly[A]-electrochemical biosensors, were used to understand the mechanism of MTX-dsDNA interaction.

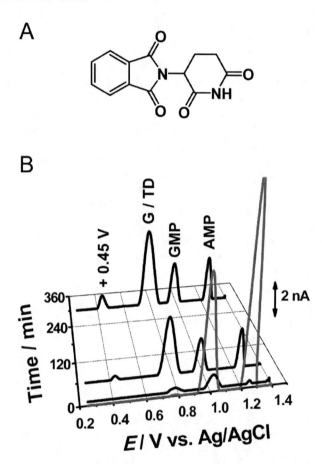

Figure 10.9. *In Situ* **detection of thalidomide-DNA interaction. (A)** Chemical structure of thalidomide. **(B)** Base line corrected DP voltammograms of (—) control 100 μg mL⁻¹ dsDNA and (—) incubated solutions in pH 4.5 0.1 M acetate buffer of 100 μg mL⁻¹ dsDNA with ~40 μM TD during 10 min, 1 hr and 5 hr. [Adapted from (Oliveira et al. 2009) with permission].

Ionizing Radiation

The application of ionizing radiation in cancer treatment as an alternative to surgery was recognized soon after the discovery of Xrays and has been used for several decades in curative treatments of cancerous tumours. In particular, γ-radiation has been used in radiotherapy and it is known that exposure gives rise to genomic instability.

Polyhomonucleotides, poly[G], poly[A], poly[T], and poly[C], and calf thymus ssDNA and dsDNA aqueous solutions previously exposed to γ radiation doses between 2 and 35 Gy, were studied by DPV using a GCE (Piedade et al. 2006). The generation of 8oxoG, 2,8-DHA,

5-formyluracil, base-free sites, and single- and double-stranded breaks in the γ-irradiated DNA samples was detected voltammetrically, Fig. 10.10, with the amount depending on the irradiation time. It was found that the current peaks obtained for 8-oxoG increase linearly with the radiation dose applied to the nucleic acid sample, and values between 8 and 446 of 8-oxoG per 10^6 guanines per Gy were obtained according to the nucleic acid sample (Piedade et al. 2006). The results showed that voltammetry can be used for monitoring and simultaneously characterizing different kinds of DNA damage caused by γ radiation exposure.

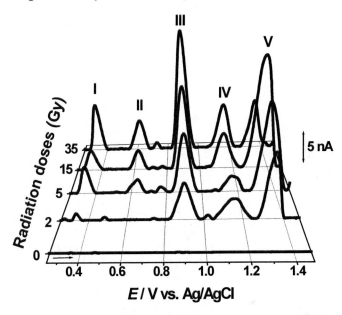

Figure 10.10. Detection of γ-radiation-DNA interaction. 3D plot of the baseline-corrected differential pulse voltammograms obtained in pH 7.4 0.1M phosphate buffer supporting electrolyte for 80 μg/mL dsDNA γ-irradiated between 0 and 35 Gy. Peak I – 8-oxoG; Peak II – free G and 2,8-DHA; Peak III – GMP and free A; Peak IV – AMP and free T; Peak V – free pyrimidines, 5-foUra and pyrimidine residues. [Adapted from (Piedade et al. 2006) with permission.]

APPLICATIONS TO OTHER AREAS OF HEALTH AND DISEASE

The aim of developing dsDNA-modified electrodes is to study the interaction of dsDNA immobilized on the electrode surface with analytes in solution and to use the biosensor to evaluate and to predict DNA interactions and damage by health hazardous compounds based on their ability to bind to nucleic acids. Other potential applications of DNA biosensors include molecular diagnostics, pharmacogenomics, drug screening, medical diagnosis, food analysis, bioterrorism and pollution or environmental monitoring.

The biosensors developed up to date are applied mostly for fundamental studies. The reason is that cancer development does not involve particular mutations and besides genome-related changes, other complex molecular alterations such as protein expression occur during the development of cancer cells. Therefore, there is an excess of biomarkers that can be analyzed for tumour classification in order to guide diagnosis. Despite considerable work in the biosensor field, there is still no general platform that can be ubiquitously applied to detect the amount of biomolecules in diverse clinical samples.

CONCLUSION

Electrochemical research on DNA is of great relevance to explain many biological mechanisms. The DNA-modified electrode is a very good model for simulating the nucleic acid interaction with cell membranes, potential environmental carcinogenic compounds and to clarify the mechanisms of action of drugs used as chemotherapeutic agents, without using animal tests.

The use of DNA-electrochemical biosensors for the understanding of DNA interactions with molecules or ions exploits the use of voltammetric techniques for *in situ* generation of reactive intermediates and is a complementary tool for the study of biomolecular interaction mechanisms. Additionally, the interpretation of electrochemical data can contribute to elucidation of the mechanism by which DNA is oxidatively damaged by such substances, in an approach to the real action scenario that occurs in the living cell.

The development of the DNA-electrochemical biosensor has opened wide perspectives using a particularly sensitive and selective method for the detection of specific interactions. The possibility of foreseeing the damage that these compounds cause to DNA integrity arises from the pre-concentration of either the starting materials or the redox reaction products on the DNA-biosensor surface, thus permitting the electrochemical probing of the presence of short-lived intermediates and of their damage to DNA.

DEFINITIONS

- *base pair*: two nucleotides inn DNA that are paired by hydrogen bonds—for example, G with C and A with T.

- *biomarker*: a compound used as an indicator of a biological state.
- *biosensor*: a device incorporating a biological sensing element connected to a transducer.
- *denaturation*: change in conformation of a nucleic acid caused by heating or by exposure to chemicals and usually resulting in loss of biological function.
- *differential pulse voltammetry*: a useful electrochemical technique since it allows low detection limits (10^{-8} M)
- *hydrogen bond*: A weak bond in which an atom shares an electron with a hydrogen atom; hydrogen bonds are important in the specificity of base pairing in nucleic acids.
- *in situ*: in place,
- *in vivo*: in a living cell or organism.
- *intercalation*: the insertion of planar aromatic ring systems of a compound between the base-pairs.
- *MAC mode AFM*: magnetic AC mode atomic force microscopy,
- *mutation*: chemical modification of any DNA base,
- *polyhomonucleotide*: single stranded DNA or RNA molecule that contains only one type of base.

SUMMARY

- In recent years increased attention has been focused on the ways in which molecules interact with DNA. Toxic compounds may induce oxidative DNA damage which is the main cause of cancer. The need for understanding the DNA interactions with molecules or ions and analyzing oxidative damage to DNA led to the development of DNA-biosensors. The electrochemical detection a particularly sensitive and selective method for the investigation of specific interactions.
- dsDNA consists of two antiparallel polynucleotide chains formed by monomeric nucleotide units containing four different nitrogen bases. The cellular genetic information is coded by the purine bases, adenine (A) and guanine (G), and the pyrimidine bases, cytosine (C) and thymine (T), as a function of their consecutive order in the chain. The two strands of nucleotides are twisted into a double helix, held together by two hydrogen bonds between the A·T and three between G·C bases of each strand.
- All DNA bases can be electrochemically oxidized at carbon electrodes. The purines (G and A) are oxidized at lower potentials than the pyrimidines (T and C). The electrochemical oxidation of DNA shows only the oxidation of purines residues. Large differences in the currents obtained for dsDNA and ssDNA were observed.

- The development of an electrochemical biosensor consists in the immobilization of biological material on the sensor surface by controlling the potential applied to the electrode. The performance, sensitivity and reliability of the DNA biosensor are dictated by the DNA immobilization procedure. A full understanding of the surface morphology of the DNA-electrochemical biosensor is necessary to guarantee the correct interpretation of the experimental results.
- The DNA biosensors enable the study of the interaction of DNA immobilized on the electrode surface with analytes in solution. Interactions of DNA with the damaging agent are converted, via changes in the electrochemical properties of the DNA recognition layer, into measurable electric signals. Several architectures are available but the choice of the best approach to be used depends on the drug and the time necessary to cause DNA damage.
- The oxidation product of guanine, 8-oxoG, and of adenine, 2,8-DHA, are considered the most commonly measured product of DNA oxidative damage. Both compounds are electroactive and their oxidation peaks were chosen to monitor DNA oxidative damage since the oxidation potentials are lower than the oxidation potentials of the respective bases.
- The electrochemical DNA biosensor enables the pre-concentration of compounds on the biosensor surface. Controlling the potential applied, the *in situ* electrochemical generation of radical intermediates is possible. Monitoring the changes of G and A oxidation peak currents or the appearance of new redox peaks such as 8-oxoG and 2,8-DHA it is possible to conclude about the damaging and potential toxic effect of different compounds such as: metal ions and metal complexes, reactive oxygen and nitrogen species, and drugs.
- Other potential applications of DNA biosensors include molecular diagnostics, pharmacogenomics, drug screening, medical diagnosis, food analysis, bioterrorism and pollution or environmental monitoring.

ACKNOWLEDGEMENTS

Financial support from Fundação para a Ciência e Tecnologia (FCT), Post-Doctoral Grant SFRH/BPD/36110/2007 (V.C. Diculescu), PTDC/QUI/098562/2008 and PTDC/SAU-BEB/104643/2008, POCI 2010 (co-financed by the European Community Fund FEDER), and CEMUC-R (Research Unit 285), is gratefully acknowledged.

ABBREVIATIONS

A	:	adenine
AFM	:	atomic force microscopy
AMP	:	adenosine-monophosphate
C	:	cytosine
CMP	:	cytidine-monophosphate
DETA/NO	:	diethylenetriamine/nitric oxide
DPV	:	differential pulse voltammtery
dsDNA	:	double stranded DNA
G	:	guanine
GMP	:	guanosine-monophosphate
GCE	:	glassy carbon electrode
HOPG	:	highly organized pyrolitic graphite
MTX	:	methotrexate
poly[A]	:	polyadenylic acid
poly[C]	:	polycytidylic acid
poly[G]	:	polyguanylic acid
poly[T]	:	polythymidylic acid
RNS	:	reactive nitrogen species
ROS	:	reactive oxygen species
Spd	:	spermidine
Spm	:	spermine
ssDNA	:	single stranded DNA
T	:	thymine
TD	:	thalidomide
TMP	:	thymidine-monophosphate
2,8-DHA	:	2,8-dihydroxyadenine
8-oxoG	:	8-oxoguanine

REFERENCES

Chiorcea-Paquim AM, O Corduneanu, SCB Oliveira, VC Diculescu and AM Oliveira Brett. 2009. Electrochemical and AFM Evaluation of Hazard Compounds-DNA Interaction. Electrochim. Acta 54: 1978–1985.

Cooke MS, MD Evans, M Dizdaroglu and J Lunec. 2003. Oxidative DNA damage: mechanisms, mutation, and disease. Faseb J 17: 1195–1214.

Corduneanu O, A.-M Chiorcea-Paquim, V Diculescu, SM Fiuza, MPM Marques and AM Oliveira-Brett. 2010. DNA Interaction with Palladium Chelates of Biogenic Polyamines Using Atomic Force Microscopy and Voltammetric Characterization. Anal Chem 82: 1245–1252.

Diculescu VC, RM Barbosa and AM Oliveira Brett. 2005a. *In Situ* Sensing of DNA Damage by a Nitric Oxide-Releasing Compound. Anal Lett 38: 2525–2540.

Diculescu VC, M Vivan and AM Oliveira Brett. 2006. Voltammetric Behavior of Antileukemia Drug Glivec. Part III—*In Situ* DNA Oxidative Damage by the Glivec Electrochemical Metabolite. Electroanal 18: 1963–1970.

Diculescu VC, JAP Piedade and AM Oliveira-Brett. 2007. Electrochemical behaviour of 2,8-dihydroxyadenine at a glassy carbon electrode. Bioelectrochem. 70: 141–146.

Evans MD, M Dizdaroglu and MS Cooke. 2004. Oxidative DNA damage and disease: induction, repair and significance. Mutat Res 567: 1–61.

Fojta M. Detecting DNA damage with electrodes. pp. 385–431. *In:* E. Paleček, F. Scheller and J. Wang. (eds.) 2005. Electrochemistry of Nucleic Acids and Proteins—Towards Electrochemical Sensors for Genomics and Proteomics. Elsevier, Amsterdam, The Netherlands.

Grivennikov SI, FR Greten and M Karin. 2010. Immunity, Inflammation, and Cancer. Cell 140: 883–899.

Hartwell LH and MB Kastan. 1994. Cell cycle control and cancer. Science. 266: 1821–1828.

Hanahan D and RA Weinberg. 2000. The Hallmarks of Cancer. Cell 100: 57–70.

Jackson AL and LA Loeb. 2001. The contribution of endogenous sources of DNA damage to the multiple mutations in cancer. Mutat Res Fund Mol M 477: 7–21.

Luo J, NL Solimini and S Elledge. 2009. Principles of cancer therapies: oncogene and non oncogene addiction. Cell 136: 823–837.

Oliveira Brett AM and A-M Chiorcea. 2003a. Atomic force microscopy of DNA immobilized onto a highly oriented pyrolytic graphite electrode surface. Langmuir 19: 3830–3839.

Oliveira Brett AM and A-M Chiorcea. 2003b. Effect of pH and applied potential on the adsorption of DNA on highly oriented pyrolytic graphite electrodes. Atomic force microscopy surface characterisation, Electrochem. Commun. 5: 178–183.

Oliveira Brett AM and A-M Chiorcea Paquim. 2004a. Atomic force microscopy characterization of an electrochemical DNA-biosensor, Bioelectrochem 63: 229–232.

Oliveira Brett AM, JAP Piedade, LA da Silva and VC Diculescu. 2004b. Electrochemical determination of all DNA bases. Anal Biochem 332: 321–329.

Oliveira-Brett AM and VC Diculescu. 2004c. Electrochemical study of quercetin-DNA interaction. Part II—*In situ* sensing with DNA-biosensor. Bioelectrochem. 64: 143–150.

Oliveira Brett AM and A-M Chiorcea Paquim. 2005. DNA imaged on a HOPG electrode surface by AFM with controlled potential, Bioelectrochem 66: 117–124.

Oliveira SCB and AM Oliveira Brett. 2010. DNA-Electrochemical Biosensors: AFM Surface Characterisation and Application to Detection of *In Situ* Oxidative Damage to DNA. Comb. Chem. High T Scr 13: 628–640.

Oliveira Brett AM, JAP Piedade and SHP Serrano. 2000. Electrochemical oxidation of 8-oxoguanine. Electroanal 13: 199–203.

Oliveira-Brett AM, M Vivan, IR Fernandes and JAP Piedade. 2002. Electrochemical detection of *in situ* adriamycin oxidative damage to DNA. Talanta 56: 959–970.

Oliveira-Brett AM, AM Chiorcea Paquim, VC Diculescu JAP Piedade. 2006. Electrochemistry of nanoscale DNA surface films on carbon. Med Eng Phys 28: 963–970.

Oliveira SCB, AM Chiorcea-Paquim, SM Ribeiro, ATP Melo, M Vivan and AM Oliveira-Brett. 2009. *In situ* electrochemical and AFM study of thalidomide–DNA interaction. Bioelectrochem 76: 201–207.

Palecek E. 2009. Fifty years of nucleic acids electrochemistry. Electroanal 21: 239–251.

Piedade JAP, PSC Oliveira, MC Lopes and AM Oliveira-Brett. 2006. Voltammetric determination of γ radiation-induced DNA damage. Anal Biochem 355: 39–49.

Rauf S, JJ Gooding, K Akhtar, MA Ghauri, M Rahman, MA Anwar and AM Khalid. 2005. Electrochemical approach of anticancer drugs–DNA interaction. J Pharmaceut Biomed 37: 205–217.

Soper SA, K Brown, A Ellington, B Frazier, G Garcia-Manero, V Gau, SI Gutman, DF Hayes, B Korte, JL Landers, D Larson, F Ligler, A Majumdar, M Mascini, M Nolte, Z Rosenzweig, J Wang and D Wilson. 2006. Point-of-care biosensor systems for cancer diagnostics/prognostics. Biosens Bioelectron 21: 1932–1942.

Wang J. 2006. Electrochemical biosensors: Towards point-of-care cancer diagnostics. Biosens Bioelectron 21: 1887–1892.

11

Asparaginase-based Asparagine Biosensors and Their Application to Leukemia

Neelam Verma[1,a,*] and Kuldeep Kumar[1,b]

ABSTRACT

The uncontrolled abnormal cell growth and development process leads to cancer formation. Leukemia is a blood forming cells cancer in the bone marrow. Acute lymphocytic leukemia accounts for 75% of all cases of childhood leukemia, and is a malignant proliferation of lymphoid cells that is blocked at an early stage of differentiation. This disease generally occurs in children between the ages of 2 and 5 yr. Chemotherapy treatment in ALL includes multi drug, the combination of prednisone, vincristine and L-asparagines. L-asparagine is an essential amino acid required for the growth of tumor cells whereas growth of normal cells is independent of its requirement. Normal tissues mainly synthesize L-asparagine in sufficient amounts for their metabolic needs with their own enzyme machinery asparagine synthetase but malignant cells require an external source of L-asparagine for growth and multiplications. Hence monitoring of asparagines levels in ALL patients is desirable. Quantitative plasma amino acid values in leukemic blood are determined by spectrophotometric methods and paper chromatography methods. Biosensors can be an alternative promising

[1]Biosensor Technology Lab, Department of Biotechnology, Punjabi University, Patiala-147002, India.
[a]E-mail: neelam_verma2@rediffmail.com
[b]E-mail: kuldeepbio@rediffmail.com
*Corresponding author

List of abbreviations after the text.

technology to detect L-asparagine in physiological fluids at levels as low as nanolevels. Asparagine biosensor based on L-asparaginase obtained from *Erwinia caratovora* and a novel, diagnostic *E. coli* K-12 Asparaginase based Asparagine biosensor for monitoring asparagines levels in leukemia have been highlighted. Various immobilization strategies have been applied to improve the stability of the biocomponent.

INTRODUCTION

The uncontrolled abnormal cell growth and development process leads to cancer formation. Leukemia is a blood forming cells cancer in the bone marrow. There are four main types of leukemia.1. Acute lymphocytic leukemia (ALL), 2. Acute myeolocytic leukemia (AML), 3. Chronic lymphocytic leukemia (CLL), and 4. Chronic myeolocytic leukemia (CML). ALL is more common in children, and the others AML, CLL and CML are more prevalent in adults. (www.emedicinehealth.com). Acute lymphocytic leukemia accounts for 75% of all cases of childhood leukemia, is a malignant proliferation of lymphoid cells that is blocked at an early stage of differentiation. Both qualitative and quantitative changes in blood proteins and amino acid nitrogen levels have been observed in patients with leukemia (Kelley and Waismen 1957).

Chemotherapy treatment in ALL includes multi drug, the combination of prednisone, vincristine, and L-asparagine (Rizzari et al. 2006).

A prerequisite for making an effective medication for the treatment of cancer is that some fundamental difference between normal cells and cancer cells must be defined. The chemotherapeutic agent must exploit this cellular difference in such a way that normal cells are spared and only cancer cells are injured. L-asparagine is an essential amino acid required (Conter et al. 2004) for the growth of tumor cells where as growth of normal cells is independent of its requirement. Normal tissues mainly synthesize L-asparagine in amounts sufficient for their metabolic needs with their own enzyme asparagine synthetase but malignant cells require an external source of L-asparagine for growth and multiplication. In the presence of L-asparaginase, the tumor cells are deprived of an important growth factor and cannot survive. When L-asparaginase destroys asparagines, ammonia is the by product. In patients with compromised liver function, the transient high levels of ammonia in the blood could pose a toxic effect. Liver disease does not omit the use of L-asparaginase but it is desirable to watch symptoms referable to liver disease, generally neurologic abnormalities/ hepatic encephalopathy (Savitri and Wamik 2003).

L-asparaginase is used in combination as a drug to suppress the cancer cells growth. The present chapter deals with various approaches for selection of source, purification and immobilization of asparaginase or whole cells for the construction of biosensors for monitoring asparagines levels in leukemic and normal healthy subjects blood samples.

Leukemia

Acute lymphocytic leukemia accounts for 75% of all cases of childhood leukemia, is a malignant proliferation of lymphoid cells that is blocked at an early stage of differentiation. Chemotherapy treatment in ALL includes multi drug, the combination of prednisone, vincristine, and L-Asparagine (Rizzari et al. 2006).

A prerequisite for making an effective medication for the treatment of cancer is that some fundamental difference between normal cells and cancer cells must be defined. The chemotherapeutic drug must exploit this cellular difference in such a way that normal cells are spared and only cancer cells are injured. L-Asparaginase exploits the unusual high requirement tumor cells have for the amino acid asparagine.

L-asparagine is an essential amino acid required (Conter et al. 2004) for the growth of tumor cells where as growth of normal cells is independent of its requirement. Mostly normal tissues synthesize L-asparagine in amounts sufficient for their metabolic needs with their own enzyme asparagine synthetase but malignant cells require an external source of L-asparagine for growth and multiplications. In the presence of L-asparaginase, the tumor cells are deprived of an important growth factor and cannot survive. When L-asparaginase destroys asparagines, ammonia is the by product. In patients with compromised liver function, the transient high levels of ammonia in the blood could pose a toxic effect. Liver disease does not omit the use of L-asparaginase but it is desirable to watch symptoms referable to liver disease, generally neurologic abnormalities/ hepatic encephalopathy (Savitri and Wamik 2003).

Conventional Methods to Detect Asparagines Levels

Quantitative plasma amino acid values in leukemic blood were determined by the spectrophotometric method and paper chromatography method and a comparison was made between normal and leukemic patients (Kelley and Waisman 1957). A specific quantitative colorimetric assay for L-asparagine by mixing it with dilute ethanolic ninhydrin solution and noting its absorbance at 34–350 nm has been reported by Sheng et al. 1993. Selective measurement of glutamine and asparagines in aqueous media by near-infrared spectroscopy is described by Zhou et al. 1996. Flow injection analysis systems with spectrophotometric and potentiometric detection of L-Asparaginase has been described by Stein et al. 1996. *E.coli* asparaginase was given intramuscularly three times weekly for six and nine doses respectively as part of multi agent induction chemotherapy and CSF asparagines levels were monitored before, during and after asparaginase dosing by high-performance liquid chromatography (Woo et al. 1999). A method was developed for the detection of asparagine deamidation and aspartate isomerization by MALDI/TOF-Mass Spectrometry (Kameoka et al. 2003). DIONEX, 2007 has developed 3D amperometry for carbohydrate and amino acid analysis.

Asparagine Biosensor

Biosensors are attracting the attention of many investigators in the field of analytical biotechnology. Biosensor is an analytical tool or system consisting of an immobilized material in intimate contact or close proximity or coupled with a suitable transducer that converts the biological signal in quantifiable electrical signal. Conventional methods although are highly precise but suffer from the disadvantage of high cost, trained personnel requirement and are mostly laboratory bound. Biosensors are specific and can present distinct advantages in certain cases. A typical biosensor consists of two parts: immobilized biological component and transducer. The biological component may be enzymes, whole cells (bacteria, algae, fungi, yeast, animal or plant), organelles, tissues, receptors, antibodies, nucleic acids etc. The specificity of the enzyme is the main reason for use of enzymes for construction of the biosensor. Various immobilization procedures have been used in biosensor construction. In general the choice of procedure depends on the nature of the biological element, the type of transducer used, the physic-chemical properties of the analyte and the operating conditions in which the biosensor is to function. Monitoring of asparagines levels in ALL patients is desirable. Hence biosensor development can be important to detect asparagines levels in nano molar levels. For the construction of biosensors the following two requirements are to be fulfilled.

1.   Characterization of bioassay principle
2.   Bioassay Principle to be Compatible with the Transducer

L-asparaginase—An enzyme used as a biocomponent for construction of asparagine biosensor

L-asparaginase is an enzyme widely used on the clinical level as an antitumor agent for the treatment of acute lymphoblastic leukemia and lymphosarcoma. It is a relatively wide spread enzyme found in many animal tissues, microbes and plants and in the serum of certain rodents but not in man. The microbes are an excellent and the most preferred source of L-asparaginase as these can be cultured easily, extraction and purification of the enzyme from them is convenient, facilitating its large-scale production.

Source of L-asparaginase

Wide range of bacteria, fungi, yeast, algae and plants are very efficient producers of L-asparaginase. L-asparaginase from gram positive bacteria has received little attention. Broome 1961 showed that it was the enzyme L-asparaginase in the serum of guinea pig that had the antitumor factor. However the commercial production of L-asparaginase appeared feasible only after Mashburn and Wriston 1964 showed that L-asparaginase from *E. coli* also inhibited tumors in mice. There are two asparaginases from *E. coli* (EC-1 and EC-2) only one (EC-2) possesses anti lymphoma activity, being the most extensively studied. This isozyme differs from EC-1 by its broad pH activity profile and its higher substrate affinity. The important microbial source for L-asparaginase include *E. coli* (Cedar and Schwartz 1967), *Pseudomonas flourescenes* (Mardashev et al. 1975), luminous bacteria (Ramaih and Chanramohan 1992), *Entrobacter aerogenes* (Mukherjee et al. 2000), *Thermus thermophilus* (Prista and Kyriakidis 2001), *E. coli* (Zaho and Yu 2001), *Erwinina* sp. (Borkotaky and Bezbaruah 2002), *Bacillus subtilis* (Fisher and Wray 2002) *Aspergillus tumarii* and *Aspergilus terreus* (Sarquis et al. 2004), marine *actinomycetes* (Dhevagi and Poorani 2006), *Helicobacter pylori* (Dhavala et al. 2008), *Erwinia corotovora* (Mohsen and Youssri 2008), *E.coli* (Ghasemi et al. 2008), *Serratia marcescens* (Venil et al. 2009), *Enterbacter aerogenes* (Baskar et al. 2009), and *Bacillus cereus* (Sunitha et al. 2010). *Pectobacterium corotovorum* (Kumar et al. 2010), and *Bipolaris* sp. BR438 (Lapmak et al. 2010).

Purification and characterization of L-asparaginase

Extracellular L-asparaginase from candida utilis is partially purified by acetone and by column chromatography on DEAE, sephadex A-50 and sephadex G-200. Metal ions, -SH inhibitors, and chelating agents did not show any inhibition or activation of the enzyme (Sakamoto et al. 1977). Purification and characterization of two forms of L-asparaginase, L-asparaginase-I and L-asparaginase II obtained from *Sphagnum fallax* has been carried out by anion exchange chromatography by Heeschen et al. 1996. It was observed that pH optimum of enzyme is 8.2 and its molecular weight is 126,000 D. It has characteristics that are intermediate between those from higher plants and those from microorganisms. L-asparaginase from *Thermus thermophilus* has a dual L-asparaginase kinase activity. Is has been purified and its apparent molecular mass by SDS-PAGE is found to be 33 KDa by Prista and Kyriakidis 2001. Purification of the enzyme from *P. aeruginosa* by sephadex G-100 gel filtration and SDS-PAGE analysis of the protein has been performed by Bessoumy et al. 2004. The actinomycetes strain LA-29 isolated from the gut contents of fish, *Mugil cephalus* of the Veller estuary showed excellent asparaginase activity. The enzyme purification fold and final recovery of protein is 18 and 1.9% respectively which exhibited an activity of 13.57 IU/mg protein. The partially purified L-asparaginase inhibited the growth of leukemia cells in male Wister rats (Kumar et al. 2007).

Immobilization of L-Asparaginase

L-asparaginase from *Escheichia coli* has been immobilized by entrapment in a gel based on poly (2-hydroxyethyl methacrylate) with an activity 730 IU/g of dry gel. The apparent Michaelis constant for these gels was similar to that of the free enzyme. At 37°C the immobilized enzyme has a half life more than 40 d (Driscoll et al. 1975). In polyacrylamide the L-asparaginase properties from *E. coli* have been investigated: stability, pH dependence, heat stability and Km. It has been shown that the enzyme in gel has better stability than the native enzyme (Vinogrdova et al. 1977). Galev et al. 1981 immobilized bacterial L-asparaginase on polyacrylamide gel, which exhibited higher stability to denaturation and to the effect of a proteolytic enzyme. The immobilized enzyme has an apparent Km value 200-fold higher as compared with the free L-asparaginase. Edman et al. 1983 immobilized L-asparaginase under aseptic conditions in spherical microparticles of of polyacrylamide. To avoid direct contact between blood and enzyme, L-asparaginase was immobilized in microparticles on the outer surface of the capillary fibers of a hemofilter. The hemofilters were found to be very efficient in the transformation of L-asparagine to L-aspartic acid, *in vitro* as well as *in vivo* Gombotz and Hoffman 1985 immobilized L-asparaginase onto the porous polypropylene hollow fibers of a plasma filter. Immobilized enzymes have found applications as industrial, clinical and analytical biotools, because of their advantages over the free enzyme. The co-immobilized derivatives were utilized in extracorporeal devices to efficiently eliminate asparagines from the plasma (Minim and Filo 1994). The feasibility of the immobilization of *E. coli* L-asparaginase in to a hydrogel matrix mode of PEG and BSA has been demonstrated (Jean and Fortier 1996). After immobilization, a 200 fold increase in Km value was observed. At a physiological pH of 7.3, the immobilized enzyme retained high activity compared with only 43% for the native form. Enzyme immobilization by non covalent binding method of physical entrapment in gelatin and then coating a thin layer of it onto silicon surfaces has been studied (Subramanian et al. 1999). The effects of internal and external mass transfer systems on immobilized enzyme systems has been studied by Ladiwala et al. 2000, and Balco et al. 2001, stabilized L-asparaginase from *E. coli* via multisubunit covalent immobilization of the enzyme on to activated supports such as agarose-glutaraldehyde. Supports activated with different densities of reactive groups were used. L-asparaginase II from *E. coli* W3110 has been purified to homogeneity on DEAE-sepharose and immobilized in calcium alginate gelatin composites. The optimum pH for immobilized enzyme shifted from 7.5 to 8.5 (Youssef and Al-Omair 2008). The cell like hydrogel matrix has been prepared using carboxymethyl konjac glucomannan-chitosan nanocapsules for the immobilization of L-asparaginase. The immobilized enzyme has better stability and activity in contrast to the native enzyme (Wang et al. 2008). L-asparaginase is immobilized in hydrogel-magnetic nanoparticles using chitosan and hyaluronic acid (Teodor et al. 2008). The biocompatible hydrogel-magnetic nanoparticles have been prepared to entrap L-asparaginase for biomedical applications (Teodor et al. 2009). L-asparaginase of *Bacillus* sp. R36 is efficiently immobilized by covalent binding and characterized. Antitumor and antioxidant activities have also been investigated (Moharam et al. 2010).

Asparagine biosensors

L-asparaginase is used as an injectable drug and elimination of L-asparagine in blood involves the monitoring of L-asparagine in the blood of treated cancer patients (especially ALL patients) to avoid recurrence (Verma et al. 2007).

Biosensors can be a promising technology to monitor L-asparagine in physiological fluids at levels as low as nanolevels. Fraticelli and Meyerhoff 1983, developed an asparagines biosensor that could detect levels up to 10^{-5} M in human plasma samples through the use of *E. coli*. L-asparaginase in the soluble form, an online gas dialyzer for automated enzymatic analysis with potentiometer ammonia detection having an ammonia electrode incorporated in conjunction with a pre dialysis unit was used for the construction of the biosensor. In another study, an enzymatic method has been developed for the kinetic measurement of L-asparaginase activity and L-asparagine with an ammonia gas sensing electrode. The method is based upon the deamination of L-asparagine by L-asparaginase from *E. coli* resulting in the production of NH_3 (Tagami and Mastsuda 1990). Kim et al. 1995 have reported the use of garlic tissue electrode for the determination of L-asparagine where tissue cells were employed for conversion of L-asparagine into ammonia and ammonium gas electrode was used as a detector. Screen printed three electrode amperometric biosensors immobilizing L- and D-amino acid oxidase for the general purpose measurement of L- or D-amino acids has been described by Sarkar et al. 1999. A biosensor for asparagines has been described using a thermostable recombinant asparaginase from *Archaeoglobus fulgidus* which is cloned and expressed in *E. coli* as a fusion protein with a polyhistidine tail. After heat treatment to denature most of the native *E. coli* proteins, the enzyme has been purified by an immobilized metal ion affinity chromatography method. The activity of the enzyme was determined by monitoring the change in NH_3 concentration in solution. The enzyme has been immobilized and used with an ammonium selective electrode to develop a biosensor for L-asparagine (Wang et al. 2002). An automated kinetic enzymatic method for monitoring plasmatic L-asparaginase activity during therapy of acute lymphoblasic leukemia has been described by Orsonneau et al. 2004. The method is fast and easy to perform besides having better specificity and precision than the Nessler method. Tsurusawa et al. 2004, have demonstrated a highly sensitive enzyme coupling method to determine minimum levels of L-asparaginase activity necessary for maintaining asparagines depletion under L-asparaginase treatment in acute lymphoblastic leukemia. It was shown that asparagines levels are strongly correlated with plasma L-asparaginase activity even at low enzyme activities (50 IU/ml).

ASPARAGINE BIOSENSOR APPLICATION TO LEUKEMIA

Verma et al. 2007, developed a novel, diagnostic *E. coli* K-12 asparaginase based asparagine biosensor for monitoring asparagines levels in leukemia. Various immobilization techniques have been applied to improve the stability of the enzyme asparaginase. Response time studies have been performed for different immobilization techniques. Phenol red indicator has been co-immobilized with asparaginase and color visualization approach has been optimized for various asparagines ranges. The detection limit of asparagines achieved with nitrocellulose membrane is 10^{-1} M with silicone gel is 10^{-10}–10^{-1} M, and with calcium alginate beads is 10^{-9}–10^{-1} M. The calcium alginate bead system can be coupled to ISE (ion selective electrode). Furthermore, the calcium alginate bead system of immobilization has been applied for the asparagines range detection in normal and leukemia serum samples. Asparagine biosensor for leukemia based on L-asparaginase obtained from *Erwinia caratovora* has been developed. For this different immobilization strategies were applied to immobilize the enzyme along with phenol red and to improve its stability. Asparagine level studied with nitrocellulose membrane and pH strips is 10^{-1} M and with calcium alginate beads is 10^{-9}–10^{-1} M. In comparison to normal blood samples there was increased pH change in leukemic patient blood samples because of production of more ammonium ions. The above results can be attributed to high levels of asparagine in tumor cells when compared to asparagine level in normal cells. Asparagine range detection in normal and leukemia serum samples is achieved by using both pH strips and calcium alginate bead system of immobilization (Verma et al. 2007). Asparagine has been immobilized in polyacrylamide gel. Detection limit of asparagine achieved was 10^{-9}–10^{-1} M. Response time for concentration level of 10^{-1} M was 15–16 min higher than calcium alginate bead method. Developed biosensor has been applied to monitor asparagines in normal healthy subjects and leukemic patients. Response time for change in color of the gel pieces, till purple color appears was 3 min 35 sec for the normal blood sample corresponding to 10^5 M–10^6 M asparagine. Response time for change in color of the gel pieces till purple color appears was 8–11 min for leukemic blood samples. The asparagine concentration level was 10^{-2} M (Table 11.1, Fig. 11.1). Thus, asparagine levels were found to be higher in leukemic blood than normal blood (Table 11.2, Fig. 11.2). The biocomponent was stable for 5 mon.

Table 11.1. Response time and mV reading of different asparagines concentrations (polyacrylamide gel system).

Concentration of Asparagine (M)	mV reading	Response Time
10^{-1}	–27.8	15 min 30 sec
10^{-2}	–55.6	10 min 25 sec
10^{-3}	–63.0	6 min 12 sec
10^{-4}	–71.2	5 min 35 sec
10^{-5}	–71.6	4 min 42 sec
10^{-6}	–72.5	3 min 08 sec
10^{-7}	–73.8	2 min 45 sec
10^{-8}	–75.2	2 min 28 sec
10^{-9}	–77.5	2 min 10 sec

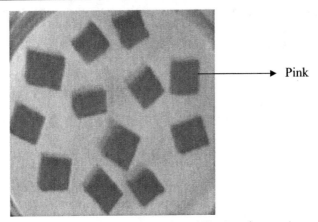

Pink

Figure 11.1. Color of Polyacrylamide gel pieces, co immobilization of asparaginase and phenol red before the Reaction.

Table 11.2. Response time and mV reading of leukemic and healthy blood samples (Polyacrylamide gel).

Samples	mV reading	Response Time
Normal	–73.1	3 min 35 sec
Leukemia-1	–51.8	10 min
Leukemia-2	–50.4	9 min 30 sec
Leukemia-3	–54.8	9 min 51 sec
Leukemia-4	–54.2	8 min 09 sec
Leukemia-5	–49.5	9 min 14 sec

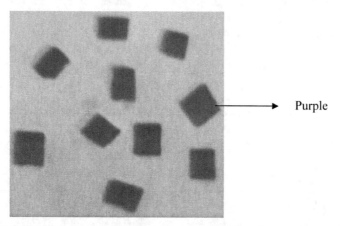

Purple

Figure 11.2. Color of Polyacrylamide gel pieces, co immobilization of asparaginase and phenol red after the Reaction.

DEVELOPMENT OF A MICROBIAL BIOSENSOR FOR MONITORING L-ASPARAGINE IN LEUKEMIC BLOOD

At the start of the stationary phase, the biomass was harvested and centrifuged at 5000 rpm for 20 min at 4°C. The supernatant was discarded and the pellet was retained and suspended in 0.05 M phosphate buffered saline (PBS) pH 7.5 and the O.D.$_{600}$ was set 1.00. The pellet was dissolved in 2 ml of phosphate buffered saline (PBS) pH 7.5. This biomass was used for the development of whole cell biosensor. The whole cells were co-immobilized with phenol red in calcium alginate beads. Detection limit of asparagine achieved was 10^{-9}–10^{-1}M. Response time for concentration level of 10^{-1} M was 3–4 min. Response time for concentration levels of 10^{-9}–10^{-2}M was in the range of 1–3 min (Table 11.3, Fig. 11.3). The response time for whole cell biosensor is slightly higher than the enzyme based biosensor.

Table 11.3. Response time and mV reading of different asparagines concentrations (calcium alginate system).

Concentration of Asparagine (M)	mV reading	Response Time
10^{-1}	−35.6	3 min 58 sec
10^{-2}	−63.7	2 min 40 sec
10^{-3}	−68.8	2 min 15 sec
10^{-4}	−70.3	1 min 45 sec
10^{-5}	−71.2	1 min 28 sec
10^{-6}	−72.5	1 min 25 sec
10^{-7}	−74.4	1 min 20 sec
10^{-8}	−75.2	1 min 10 sec
10^{-9}	−76.1	1 min

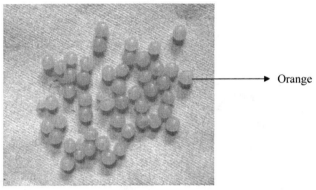

Orange

Figure 11.3. Color of Beads, co-immobilization of whole cells containing asparaginase and phenol red before the Reaction.

Decrease in mV reading with decrease in concentration of asparagine was observed. This is directly related to decrease in NH_4^+ produced after the reaction due to increasingly lesser concentration of the reactant. Developed biosensor has been applied to monitor asparagines levels in leukemic and normal blood samples. Response time for change in color of the beads, till purple color appears was 1 min 14 sec, for the normal blood sample. The asparagine concentration level was in the range of 10^{-5} M. Response time for change in color of the beads, till purple color appears was 2-3 min for the leukemic blood samples. The asparagines concentration level was 10^{-2} M (Table 11.4, Fig. 11.4). Thus, asparagine levels were found to be high in leukemic blood and tumor samples than normal blood. The immobilized whole cells are stable for 9 mon.

Table 11.4. Response time and mV reading of leukemic and healthy blood samples (calcium alginate beads system).

Samples	mV reading	Response Time
Normal	−73.2	1min 14 sec
Leukemia-1	−63.2	2min 47 sec
Leukemia-2	−62.5	2 min 29 sec
Leukemia-3	−60.0	2 min 33 sec
Leukemia-4	−61.2	2min 30 sec
Leukemia-5	−58.8	2 min 41 sec
Leukemia-6	−57.1	2 min 48 sec
Leukemia-7	−60.6	2 min 35 sec
Leukemia-8	−60.7	2 min 34 sec
Leukemia-9	−61.4	2 min 22 sec
Leukemia-10	−60.5	2 min 52 sec

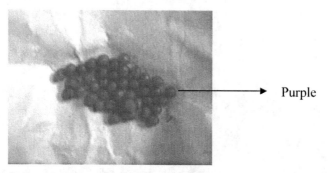

Purple

Figure 11.4. Color of Beads, co-immobilization of whole cells containing asparaginase and phenol red after the Reaction.

RELIABILITY CHECK FOR THE CONSTRUCTED BIOSENSOR

Calculation of response times for change in color of 10^{-2} M and 10^{-5} M was done to check reliability of the developed biosensor, 25 µl of serum sample (leukemic and normal) was mixed with 25 µl of synthetic L-asparagine (10^{-2}M and 10^{-5}M). The mV and time response was studied with the help of calcium alginate beads method (Table 11.5). The results are comparable.

Table 11.5. Reliability check of the constructed biosensor (calcium alginate bead system).

Concentration + Serum Samples	mV reading	Time Response
10^{-2}	−63.2	2 min 42 sec
10^{-5}	−71.4	1 min 27 sec

1/2x +1/2y = X

Where, x= Serum sample

Y= Synthetic sample of L-asparagine

The developed biosensor is quite reliable and comparable. Hence, the visualization approach and ISE transducer coupling can be opted for monitoring L-asparagine concentration in blood samples of leukemia and normal samples.

Future scope for asparagine biosensors

The potential of carbon nanotubes (CNT) as molecular scale biosensor has been investigated for asparagines. This is promising for the prospect of CNT-based single molecule sensors that might depend on devices that respond to changes in either conductance or electroluminescence (Abadir et al. 2008).

APPLICATIONS TO OTHER AREAS OF HEALTH AND DISEASE

L-asparagine is an essential amino acid required for the growth of tumor cells whereas growth of normal cells is independent of its requirement. Normal tissues mainly synthesize L-asparagine in amounts sufficient for their metabolic needs with their own enzyme asparagine synthetase but malignant cells require an external source of L-asparagine for growth and multiplications. In the presence of L-asparaginase, the tumor cells get deprived of an important growth factor and cannot survive. When L-asparaginase destroys asparagines, ammonia is the by product. In patients with compromised liver function, the transient high levels of ammonia in the blood could pose a toxic effect. Liver disease does not omit the use of L-asparaginase but it is recommended to watch symptoms related to liver disease, neurologic abnormalities and hepatic disorders.

KEY FACTS

- People of all ages can be affected by leukemia and approximately 85% of leukemia in children is of the acute type.
- ALL is more common in children, while AML, CLL and CML usually occur in adults.
- Both qualitative and quantitative changes in blood proteins and amino acid nitrogen levels have been observed in patients with leukemia.

- ALL accounts for 75% of all cases of childhood leukemia, and is a malignant proliferation of lymphoid cells blocked at an early stage of differentiation.
- The incidence of this disease mostly occurs between the ages of 2 and 5 yr in children.
- Chemotherapy treatment in ALL includes multi drug, the combination of prednisone, vincristine and L-asparagine.
- L-asparagine is an essential amino acid required for the growth of tumor cells whereas growth of normal cells is independent of its requirement.
- Monitoring of asparagines levels in leukemic patients is desirable.
- Hence biosensor development can be important to detect asparagines levels in nano molar levels in leukemic patients.

DEFINITIONS

- *Leukemia*: is a blood forming cells cancer in the bone marrow.
- *Biosensor*: is an analytical tool or system consisting of an immobilized biological material in intimate contact or in proximity to or coupled with a suitable transducer that converts the biological signal in quantifiable electrical signal.
- *Transducer*: is a device that converts the biochemical signal in to an electrical signal.
- *Immobiliozation*: physical or chemical fixation of cells, organelles, antibodies, nucleic acids, enzymes or other proteins on to a solid matrix or retained/confined by a membrane to increase the stability.

SUMMARY

- ALL is more common in children, while AML, CLL and CML usually occur in adults.
- Biosensors are attracting the attention of many investigators in the field of analytical biotechnology.
- L-asparaginase is an enzyme widely used on the clinical level as an antitumor agent for the treatment of acute lymphoblastic leukemia and lymphosarcoma. It is a relatively wide spread enzyme found in many animal tissues, microbes and plants and in the serum of certain rodents but not in man.
- A wide range of bacteria, fungi, yeast, algae and plants are very efficient producers of L-asparaginase.

- Purification, kinetic characterization and immobilization of L-asparaginase is discussed for the construction of asparagine biosensor.
- Asparagine biosensor based on L-asparaginase obtained from *Erwinia caratovora* and a novel, diagnostic *E. coli* K-12 asparaginase based asparagine biosensor, whole cell biosensor for monitoring asparagines levels in leukemia have been highlighted.

ABBREVIATIONS

ALL	:	Acute Lymphocytic leukemia
AML	:	Acute Myeolocytic Leukemia
CLL	:	Chronic Lymphocytic Leukemia
CML	:	Chronic Myeolocytic Leukemia
CSF	:	Cerebrospinal Fluid

REFERENCES

Abadir GB, K Walus, R Turer and D Pulfrey. 2008. Biomolecular Sensing Using Carbon Nanotubes: A Simulation Study. Int J High Speed Electron Syst 18: 879–887.

Balco VM, C Mateo, LR Fernandez, MF Xavier and JM Guisan. 2001. Co-immobilization of L-asparaginase and glutamate dehydrogenase onto highly activated supports. Enz Microbiol Technol 28: 696–704.

Baskar G, MD Kumar, AA Prabu, S Renganathan and C Yoo. 2009. Optimization of Carbon and Nitrogen Sources for L-asparaginase Production by *Enterobacter aerogenes* using Response Surface Methodology. Chem Biochem Eng Q 23(3): 393–397.

Bessoumy AA, M Sarhan and J Mansour. 2004. Production, isolation, and purification of L-asparaginase from *Psedomonas aeruginosa* 50071 using solid state fermentation. J Biochem Mol Biol 37(4): 387–393.

Borkotaky B and R Bezbaruah. 2002. Production and properties of asparaginase from a new *Erwinia* sp. Folia Microbiol 47: 473–476.

Broome JD 1961. Evidence that the L-asparaginase activity of guinea pig serum is responsible for its antilymphoma effects. Nature 171: 1114–1118.

Cedar H and JH Schwartz. 1967. Localization of the two L-asparaginases in anaerobically grown *Escherichia coli*. J Biol Chem 242: 3753–3754.

Conter V, C Rizzari, A Sala, R Chiesa, M Citterio and A Biondi. 2004. Acute Lymphoblastic Leukemia. Orphanet Encyclopedia. http://www.orpha.net/data/patho/GB/uk-ALL.pdf.

Dhavala P, J Krasotkina, C Dubreuil and AC Papageorgiou. 2008. Expression, purification and crystallization of *Helicobacter pylori* L-asparaginase. Acta Crystallogr. Sect F Struct Biol Cryst Commun 64: 740–742.

Dhevagi P and E Poorani. 2006. Isolation and characterization of L-asparaginase from marine actinomycetes. Indian J Biotechnol 5: 514–520.

Driscoll K, R Korus, T Ohnuma and M Walczack. 1975. Gel entrapped L-asparaginase EC-3.5.1.1 Kinetic behavior and anti tumor activity. J Pharma Exp Therapeu 195: 382–388.

Edman P, U Nylen and I Sjoholm. 1983. Use of immobilized Lasparaginase in acrylic micro particles in an extracorporeal hollow fiber dialyzer. J Pharmacol Exp Ther 225: 164–167.

Fisher SH and VL Wray. 2002. *Bacillus subtilis* 168 Contains Two Differentially Regulated Genes Encoding L-Asparaginase J Bacteriol 184: 2148–2154.

Fraticelli YM and ME Meyerhoff. 1983. Online gas analyser for automated enzymatic analysis with potentiometric ammonia detection. Anal Chem 55: 359–364.

Galaev YV, EG Chuplygina and TA Klement'Eva. 1981. Immobilization of L-asparaginase from *Citrobacter* on Polyacrylamide gel. Voprosy Meditsinskoi Khimii 27: 534–537.

Ghasemi Y, A Ebrahiminezhad, S Rasoul-Amini, G Zarrini, MB Ghoshoon, M Javad Raee, MH Morowvat, F Kafilzadeh and A Kazemi. 2008. An Optimized Medium for Screening of L-Asparaginase Production by *Escherichia coli*. Am J Biochem Biotech 4: 422–424.

Gombotz W and S Hoffman. 1985. The immobilization of L-asparaginase on porous hollow plasma filters. J Controlled Release 2: 375–383.

Heeschen V, J Matlok, S Schrader and H Rudolph. 1996. Asparagine catabolism in bryophytes: Purification and characterization of two L-asparaginase isoforms from *Sphagnum fallax*. Physiol Plantarum 97: 402–410.

Jean F J and G Fortier. 1996. Immobilization of L-asparaginase into a biocompatible polyethylene glycol albumin hydrogel 1: Preparation and *in vivo* characterization. Biotechnol Appl Biochem 23: 221–226.

Kameoka D, T Ueda and T Imoto. 2003. A Method for Detection of Asparagine Deamidation and Aspartate Isomerization of Proteins by MALDI/TOF-Mass Spectroscopy using Endoproteinase Asp-N J Biochem 134: 129–135.

Kelley JJ and HA Waisman. 1957. Quantative plasma amino acid value in leukemic blood. Blood 12: 635–643.

Kim SJ, GM Kim, Y J Bae, EY Lee, MH Hur and MK Ahn. 1995. Determination of L-asparagine using a garlic tissue electrode. Yakhak Hoeji 39: 113–117.

Kumar S, E Poorani, K Sivakumar, T Thangaradjou and L Kannan. 2007. Partial purification and anti-leukemic activity of L-asparaginase enzyme of the actinomycete strain LA-29 isolated from the estuarine fish, *Mugil cephalus*. J Envir Biol 28: 645–650.

Kumar S, VV Dasu and K Pakshirajan. 2010. Localization and production of novel L-asparaginase from Pectobacterium carotovorum MTCC 1428. Process Biochem 45: 223–229.

Ladiwala A and S Gokhale. 2000. Effects of internal and external mass transfer systems on immobilized enzyme systems. www.lib.rpi.edu/dept/chem-eng/biotech-environ/intro.htm.

Lapmak K, S Lumyong, S Thongkuntha, P Wongputtisin and U Sardsud. 2010. L-Asparaginase Production by *Bipolaris* sp BR438 Isolated from Brown Rice in Thailand. Chiang Mai Journal of Science 37: 159–163.

Mardashev SR, AY Nikolaev, NN Sokolov, EA Kozlov and ME Kutsman. 1975. Isolation and properties of a homogeneous L-asparaginase preparation from *Pseudomonas flourescens* AG. Biokhimiya 40: 984–989.

Mashburn L and J Wriston. 1964. Tumor inhibitory effect of L-asparaginase from *Escherichia coli*. Arch Biochem Biophy 104: 450–452.

Minim LA and RM Filo. 1994. Modeling and adaptive control of L-asparaginase reactor. Comp Chem. Eng. 18: 5693–5697.

Moharam M, AM Gamal-Eldeen and ST El-Sayed. 2010. Production, Immobilization and Anti-tumor Activity of L-Asparaginase of *Bacillus* sp. R36. J Am Sci 6: 157–165.

Mohsen MS and M Youssri. 2008. Purification and characterization of L-asparaginase from *Erwinia carotovora*. Bulletin of the National Research Centre (Cairo) 33: 379–390.

Mukherjee J, S Majumdar and T Scheper. 2000. A simple method for the isolation and purification of L-asparaginase from *Enterobacter aerogenes*. Appl Microbiol Biotech 53: 180–184.

Orsonneau JL, EA Brassart, M Lecame, P Thomare, O Delaroche and O Dudouet. 2004. Automated kinetic assay of plasmatic L-asparaginase during therapy of acute lymphoblastic leukemias. Annales-de-Biologie Clinique 62: 568–572.

Pritsa AA and DA Kyriakidis. 2001. L-asparaginase of *Thermus thermophilus*: purification, properties and identification of essential amino acids for its catalytic activity. Mol Cellu Biochem 216: 93–101.

Ramaiah N and D Chandramohan. 1992. Production of L-asparaginase from marine luminous bacteria. Ind J Marine Sci 21: 212–214.

Rizzari C, M Citterio, M Zucchetti, V Conter, R Chiesa, A Colombini, S Malguzzi, D Silvestri and MD' Incalci. 2006. A pharmacological study on pegylated asparaginase used in front line treatment of children with acute lymphoblastic leukemia. Heamatologica 91: 24–31.

Sakamoto T, C Araki, T Beppu and K Arima. 1977. Partial purification and some properties of extracellular Asparaginase from *Candida utilis*. Agri Biol Chem 41: 1359–1364.

Sarkar P, IE Tothhill, SJ Setford and APF Turner. 1999. Screen printed amperometric biosensor for the rapid measurement of L- and D- amino acids 124: 865–870.

Sarquis MI, EM Oliveira, AS Santos and GL Costa. 2004. Production of L-asparaginase by filamentous fungi. Mem Inst Oswaldo Cruz 99: 489–492.

Savitri NA and A Wamik. 2003. Microbial L-asparaginase: A potent antitumour enzyme. Ind J Biotech 2: 184–194.

Sheng SM, JJ Kraft and SM Schuster. 1993. A Specific Quantitative Colorimetric Assay for L-Asparagine. Anal Biochem 211: 242–249.

Stein K, B Shi, G Schwedt. 1996. Determination of -asparagine using flow-injection systems with spectrophotometric and potentiometric detection. Anal Chim Acta 336: 113–122.

Subramanian A, J Kennel, I Oden, K Jacobson, J Woodward and J Mitchel. 1999. Comparison of techniques for enzyme immobilization on silicon supports. Enz Microbiol Tech 24: 26–34.

Sunitha M, P Ellaiah and RB Devi. 2010. Screening and optimization of nutrients for L-asparaginase production by *Bacillus cereus* MNTG-7 in SmF by plackett-burmann design. Afr J Microbiol Res 4: 297–303.

Tagami S and K Mastuda. 1990. An enzymatic method for the kinetic measurement of L-asparaginase an activity and L-asparagine with an ammonia gas sensing electrode. Chem Pharm Bull 38: 153– 155.

Teodor E, G Truica and I Lupescu. 2008. The release of L-asparaginase from hydrogelmagnetic nanoparticles. Roumanian Biotech Letters 13: 3907–3913.

Teodor E, S Litescu, V Lazar and R Somoghi. 2009. Hydrogel-magnetic nanoparticles with immobilized L-asparaginase for biomedical applications. J Mater Sci Mater Med 20: 1307–1314.

Tsurusawa M, M Chin, A Iwai, K Nomura, H Maeba, T Taga, T Higa, T Kuno, T Hori, A Muto and M Yamagata. 2004. L-asparagine depletion levels and L-asparaginase activity in plasma of children with acute lymphoblastic leukemia under asparaginase treatment. Cancer Chemother Pharmacol 53: 204–208.

Venil CK, K Nanthakumar, K Karthikeyan and P Lakshmanaperumalsamy. 2009. Production of L-asparaginase by *Serratia marcescens* SB08: Optimization by response surface methodology. Iranian J Biotech 7: 10–18.

Verma N, K Kumar, G Kaur and S Anand. 2007. L-Asparaginase: A Promising Chemotherapeutic Agent. Critical Reviews in Biotechnology 27: 45–62.

Verma, N, K Kumar, G Kaur and S Anand. 2007. *E. Coli* K-12 based Asparaginase-based Asparagine biosensor for leukemia. Artificial Cells, Blood Substitutes, and Biotechnology 35: 449–456.

Verma N, K Kumar, G Kaur and S Anand. 2007. Asparagine Biosensor for Leukemia Based on L-asparaginase obtained from *Erwinia carotovora*. National J life Sci 4: 1–5.

Vinogradova N, IA Vina and RA Zhagat. 1977. L-asparaginase bound in a Polyacrlamide gel. Chem Nat Comp 12: 331–333.

Wang J, J Li and LG Bachas. 2002. Biosensor for asparagine using a thermostable recombinant asparaginase from *Archeoglobus fulgidus*. Anal Chem 74: 3336–3341.

Wang R, B Xia, B Li, S Peng, L Ding and S Zhang. 2008. Semi-permeable nanocapsules of konjac glucomannan-chitosan for enzyme immobilization . Int J Pharm 364: 102–107.

Woo MH, LJ Hak, MC Storm, AJ Gajjer, JT Sandlund, PL Harrison, B Wang, CH Pui and MV Relling. 1999. Cerebrospinal fluid asparagine concentrations after *Escherichia coli* asparaginase in children with acute lymphoblastic leukemia. J Clin Oncol 17: 1568–1573.

Youssef MM and AM Al-Omair. 2008. Cloning, purification, characterization and immobilization of l-asparaginase ii from *E. coli* W3110. Asian J Biochem 3: 337–350.

Zaho F and J Yu. 2001. L-asparaginase release from *E. coli* cells with K_2HPO_4 and Triton X-100. Biotechnol Program 17: 490–494.

Zhou X, H Chung, MA Arnold, M Rhie and DW Murhammer. 1996. Selective measurement of glutamine and asparagine in aqueous media by near infrared spectroscopy. pp 116–132. *In:* KR Rogers, A Mulchandani and W Zhou (eds.) Biosensor and Chemical Sensor Technology. American Chemical Society.

www.emedicinehealth.com

12

Breast Cancer Detection Using Surface Plasmon Resonance-Based Biosensors

Chii-Wann Lin[1,a,*] and Chia-Chen Chang[1,b]

ABSTRACT

Breast cancer is one of the most common tumors and a major leading cause of cancer-related deaths in women worldwide. Although regular screening with mammography has been routinely applied in clinical diagnosis for many years, the assessment of early breast cancer for prognosis and the prediction of treatment benefit remains a challenge. Therefore, the detection of tumor biomarkers, including genetic and proteomic tumor markers, plays an important role in the determination of prognosis and the individualization of treatment strategies for breast cancer. There are many commercial kits available that utilize enzyme and fluorescent substrates in the clinical diagnosis. However, these conventional approaches always have some drawbacks, leading to the need of other new automated detections. Immunosensors, showing promise as alternatives, are already used for breast cancer screening. Application of immunosensors in cancer testing offers several distinct advantages over other clinical analyses. Surface plasmon resonance (SPR) is one of the popular transducers among the immunosensing approaches. Such optical transducers are

[1]Institute of Biomedical Engineering, National Taiwan University, Taipei, Taiwan.
[a]E-mail: cwlinx@ntu.edu.tw
[b]E-mail: ccchang.ibme@gmail.com
*Corresponding author

List of abbreviations after the text.

extraordinarily useful for giving the targeted information in a simple and fast manner in connection to analyzers. This chapter focuses on the current developments in SPR biosensor technologies for breast cancer-associated biomarkers. It involves the fundamental principle, biomedical applications, and future challenges.

INTRODUCTION

Breast cancer accounts for over 350,000 deaths per year worldwide, and therefore, this disease has a major impact on the health of women (Ferlay et al. 2000). Table 12.1 summarizes some key points related to breast cancer. Early diagnosis and treatment are critically important in affecting the outcome of breast cancer. Until now, many screening methods have been applied to the routine diagnosis of breast tumors, either benign or malignant, which include clinical examination, ultrasound, and mammography for identification. Among these screening modalities, mammography is most effective in screening asymptomatic women of different ages and acceptable to most women. Nevertheless, mammography has a few intrinsic limitations regarding the size of tumor. Unless a tumor becomes at least a few millimeters in size, it is difficult to detect the clonal origin of cancer by using mammographic screening (Ding et al. 2008). Thus, there remains a need for the use of tumor markers in the diagnosis, monitoring, and classification of breast cancer.

Table 12.1. Key facts of breast cancer.

1.	Most early stage breast carcinomas are asymptomatic, and do not cause pain.
2.	Breast cancer often appears outside the top in the breast because the top of the breast tissues are more than in other parts of the breast.
3.	Breast cancer occurs frequently in women and rarely in men.
4.	The rates of breast cancer rise sharply in women over 50 yr of age.
5.	Women with a strong family history of breast cancer, high bone density, or high breast density are at higher than average risk of developing breast tumors.
6.	Smoking, alcohol, and obesity may be associated with an elevated incidence of breast cancer as well as other cancers.
7.	Regular exercise can help lower the risk of developing breast cancer.
8.	Breast cancer can be cured by surgery, radiation therapy, chemotherapy, and hormone therapy.

This table illustrates the features of breast cancer summarizing the characteristics, risk factors, and treatments of cancer.

Various approaches have been routinely applied for the determination of breast cancer markers, including the use of radioimmunoassay (RIA), enzyme immunoassay (EIA), and fluoroimmunoassay (FIA). Before the development of the EIA, the RIA is the first assay to measure tumor makers quantitatively. Nevertheless, this method suffers from drawbacks: radiation hazards, long analysis time, and sophisticated instrumentation. Alternatively, the EIA has replaced the radioisotopic assay toward biomarker determination and is a successful immunoassay especially for the clinical laboratory. Although the conventional assays are sensitive and precise, they also require time-consuming procedures entailing expensive instrumentation, complicated separation and labeling steps methods. Compared to the previously developed immunoassays, biosensors provide a more rapid and efficient procedure. The definition of a biosensor is an analytical device which tightly associates a molecular recognition element with a physical transducer for target detection (Homola et al. 1999). Accordingly, biosensors also combine the advantages of the high sensitivity of sensors and the high specificity of these immunoreactions. Thus, biosensors have been considered as a major development in clinical diagnosis. Since then, numerous biosensors based on various physical transducers have been reported and applied to detect breast cancer markers. Among these biosensor devices, optical devices have attracted considerable attention in biosensor development. Surface plasmon resonance (SPR), for example, is one of the most popular optical biosensors for bioanalysis. Recent advances in SPR technique have made SPR biosensors a promising candidate for development in medical diagnostics (Chiu et al. 2007; Huang et al. 2006). In this chapter, we will focus on the recent SPR development for applications as breast cancer biomarkers and the outlook in clinical diagnosis.

TUMOR MARKERS

Numerous biomarkers have been described for breast cancer (Table 12.2). Clinically approved and experimental biological markers can be classified into two major categories, genetic and proteomic biomarkers. Although DNA markers remain poorly characterized at an early stage due to the low concentrations of cancer biomarkers, they can provide useful information for

Table 12.2. Breast tumor-associated tumor markers.

Types of tumor markers	Tumor marker	Cutoff Value
Genetic	*BRCA1, BRCA1*	-
	p53	-
Proteomic	CEA	2.5 ng/ mL
	HER-2	15 ng/mL
	CA 12-5	35 U/mL
	CA 15-3	30 U/mL
	CA 27.29	38 U/mL

This table lists specific tumor marker of breast cancer that could predict the prognosis and monitor the progress of the cancer. The types of tumor markers, the main tumor markers, and the cutoff values are summarized.

the process of tumor growth (van 't Veer et al. 2002). Also, the spread of breast cancers is generally caused by the overexpression, mutation, or deletion of specific genes. Therefore, lowering the minimum detectable concentration by improving the detection approaches provides good possibilities for assistance in the early detection of cancer. Compared to DNA markers, protein markers are the main auxiliary indicator for breast cancer diagnosis. These tumor markers can be divided into two categories: predictive and prognostic biomarkers. Predictive markers give information about the effect of a particular therapeutic intervention such as human epidermal growth factor receptor 2 (HER-2). Conversely, prognostic markers provide the overall outcome of the patient, regardless of therapy, such as carbohydrate antigen 15-3 (CA 15-3). While predictive factors are the effect of treatment on the tumor, prognostic factors are the effects of tumor characteristics on the patient.

Typically, tumor markers can remain in normal body fluids at trace levels in the absence of a tumor. As a small tumor increasingly grows, the levels of some biomarkers also increase in the body fluids. Thus, the minimum detectable levels of the proposed approaches are important for screening of a small tumor. Most cancers have at least one biomarker associated with their incidence. In other words, most markers do not have sufficient sensitivity or specificity to a particular tumor. Thus, the use of a panel of tumor makers can help to identify the origin of the tumor (Ferlay et al. 2000) and the format of the multi-analyte assay is becoming a promising field of research.

SPR IMMUNOSENSOR

SPR has been attracting much attention because of several important properties. The main advantage of SPR-based assay is that it is an extremely sensitive mass sensor, capable of detecting subnanogram levels in real time without any specific label. Moreover, SPR biosensor can detect trace amounts of specific analytes from complex fluids without sample preparation. Due to these advantages, SPR has emerged as a powerful optical tool that can greatly provide valuable information on biomedical and chemical analysis. In addition, several groups have developed multispot SPR for studying the biomolecular interaction with an array format. This technique provides a possible means of quick and simultaneous detection for observing many interaction events, and is thus considered a promising technique for proteome profiling methods.

The fundamental principle and experimental configurations have been given in several review articles (Homola et al. 1999). Based on the excitation of surface plasmons, there are three commonly used coupling methods including prism, grating and waveguide coupling. For the sake of simplicity, here we only describe a simplified explanation of the prism coupler-based SPR system due to the most widely used configuration for easy preparation and assembly. Briefly, a SPR immunosensor consists of the following components: a light source, an SPR coupler (prism), a transduction layer (gold or silver film), a biomolecule, and a detector. The plane of polarized light first passes through the prism to the metal/dielectric interface on an incident-angle larger than critical angle. Then, the intensity of reflected light is monitored against the incident light angle with a detector. At the specific incident wavelength and resonant angle, the electromagnetic waves interact with the free electrons of thin metallic film resulting in a reduction in the intensity of the reflected light. The angle at the minimum reflectivity (referring to the maximum dip) is denoted as the SPR angle. This critical resonance condition is extraordinarily sensitive to the refractive index of the sample. Consequently, it is both influenced by the density and the thickness, i.e. the amount of biomolecules, of the analytes attached on the transduction layer. Not only biomolecule immobilizations but molecular interactions on the gold substrate will cause a change in the refractive index near the surface, thus leading to a resonance angle shift. This shift is largely proportional to the mass increase and the concentration of the binding biomolecule. Hence, information on the affinity of analyte and the binding kinetics of molecules can be obtained.

Combined with the advances in sensor technology, SPR has been regarded as one of the most used detection systems for optical immunosensors. Therefore, this section will be devoted to the description of the most recent developments in this immunosensors for breast cancer diagnosis.

APPLICATIONS IN BREAST CANCER DETECTION

Tumor-Associated DNA Markers

In the past decade, two major genes, *BRCA1* and *BRCA2*, have been reported to be connected to breast cancer susceptibility. They are tumor suppressor genes involved in repair of DNA double-strand breaks which are responsible for breast cancer. The mutations in these genes result in instability of the human genome and will increase the risk for breast cancer with substantial risk beginning at the age of 30 yr (Narod and Foulkes 2004). Thus, the identification of the *BRCA* mutations is of relevance because prospective interventions can reduce morbidity and mortality for breast cancer patients.

Li and co-workers developed a combination of surface hybridization, surface ligation and nanoparticle amplification for single nucleotide polymorphism (SNP) genotyping in the *BRCA1* gene (Li et al. 2006).

Figure 12.1 shows the operation principle for SNP detection. As shown in Fig. 12.1, two 20-mer oligonucleotides, referred to as P_G and P_A, were immobilized onto the array. The difference of these probes was only in the last nucleotide at their 3′ ends. When the perfect matched target DNA was employed as the ligation template, a 16-mer ligation probe and an immobilized probe (P_G) can be connected by the enzyme of Taq DNA ligase. Thus, a probe of P_G would form stable duplexes with the target DNA. Conversely, a probe (P_A) was mismatched complementary to the target DNA so no ligation was performed. Although duplexes are formed for both of the probes, double-stranded DNA (dsDNA) of P_G was more stable than those of P_A. When the addition of 8 M urea led to denature and remove any target from the surface, the 16-mer ligation probe still linked to the P_G array probe , whereas the ligation probe did not attach to the P_A probe containing the SNP. Then, the introduction of nanoparticles with oligonucleotides complementary to the ligation probe DNA was to enhance the SPR signal. Using this approach, single mismatches of *BRCA1* were readily detected at concentrations as low as 1 pM with nonspecific adsorption of DNA–nanoparticle conjugates.

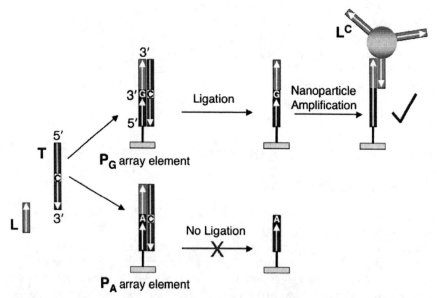

Figure 12.1. Schematic of the SNP genotyping approach with the combination of surface ligation and nanoparticle amplification. The array probes (P_A and P_G) differ only in the last nucleotide at their 3′ ends. Ligation only occurs when the probe is perfectly complementary to the target DNA. After denaturation with 8 M urea, the ligation DNA (L) is still linked to the P_G array probe, while L does not attach to the P_A probe containing the SNP. The presence of L is then detected by the nanoparticles with oligonucleotides complementary to the L. SNP: single nucleotide polymorphism [Figure reproduced with permission from Li et al. (2006)].

The use of the conventional SPR biosensor is difficult in achieving this low detection limit (1 pM) without the amplification of nanoparticles because the direct detection limit of SPR for DNA mutation is about 100 nM (Jiang et al. 2005). Label-free detections provide simpler procedures than label techniques so a minimum detectable concentration for analyzing mutations without labeling is relevant to optimize the SPR methodology. Recently, Carrascosa and co-workers optimized the differentiation between perfect and mismatched duplexes of *BRCA1* (Carrascosa et al. 2009). Different kinds of spacers with either lateral or vertical were employed. They found that a lateral spacer such as mercaptohexanol (MCH) with short target sequences provided a means to prepare surfaces with tunable hybridization response and yield. However, this spacer was not suitable for DNA hybridization with long DNA sequence such as PCR targets due to the decrease in the number of available probes after MCH treatment. To increase the target accessibility with PCR sequences, 15 thymidines as vertical spacers were found to be crucial in improving hybridization. Under the optimal sensor conditions, SPR biosensor without any labeling exhibited a high degree of discrimination with detection levels below 50 nM.

Tumor suppressor *p53* is the most commonly mutated gene in human cancers. The main function of *p53* is to mediate either cell cycle arrest or apoptosis. The loss of its activation is required for new oncogenic activities to promote tumorigenesis and drug resistance. In breast cancer, *p53* mutations can occur in around 30–35% of women with worse overall and disease-free survival (Petitjean et al. 2007). A DNA-based SPR biosensor was developed to analysis *p53* gene binding activity toward various *p53* response elements (REs) (Maillart et al. 2004). A single-stranded oligonucleotide probe was first covalently bound on the surface and then was hybridized with a mix containing the various *p53* target sequences leading to the active chip. On injection, the *p53* REs interacted with active oligonucleotide probes. The affinity properties of REs and *p53* gene are characterized by serial injection of REs above the active oligonucleotide probes. These assays reveal affinity differences between each ligand and REs. Wilson and co-workers described the development of single strand binding protein (SSB)-based biosensor detected mutant *p53* (Wilson et al. 2005). MutS protein specifically recognizes double-stranded DNA (dsDNA) containing mismatched or unpaired nucleobases. Thus, this protein has been deemed as a potential probe to detect mismatched dsDNA. The mismatch detection by MutS has been reported in various forms of detection systems. Interestingly, in this work, MutS could not efficiently react with mismatched dsDNA (Fig. 12.2). Namely, MutS did not increase in discrimination between a matched and a mismatched substrate probably because of the steric hindrance of bulky DNA probe on the sensing surface. In contrast, when SSB was introduced, SPR immunosensor improved mutation detection sensitivity by up to three-fold.

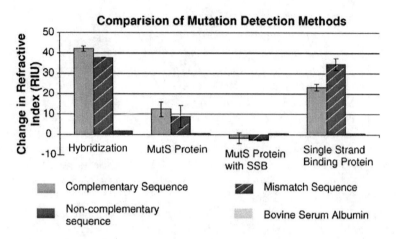

Figure 12.2. Comparison of the mutation detection approaches. There is no obvious discrimination in SPR response between mismatch and complementary DNA sequences after MutS protein is employed to the detection. However, SSB can increase three-fold mismatch discrimination over the hybridization alone. This is because the high probe density creates a steric effect that may influence the interaction of the relatively large (91 kDa) MutS protein to DNA, thus inhibiting the mismatch recognition of MutS protein. SPR: surface plasmon resonance, SSB: single strand binding protein [Figure reproduced with permission from Wilson et al. (2005)].

In the event of the binding condition being optimized for the probe density, it is possible that MutS could be utilized in this application. Nevertheless, if low-molecular-weight molecules such as short DNA sequences resulted in slight resonance angle shifts, SPR is no longer sensitive enough to monitor these binding events accurately. There is a demand for the incorporation of signal amplifications that enable in monitoring all of these interactions. Recently, Yao and co-workers reported a method for detecting *p53* by a combination of a bicell detector and nanoparticles (Yao et al. 2006). In terms of eliminating interference adsorption and providing higher binding capacity, the carboxymethylated dextran was immobilized onto the surface (Fig. 12.3). The aminated DNA can be immobilized to the carboxyl groups of dextran via chemical coupling. The use of DNA-labeled nanoparticles on the SPR sensor resulted in a remarkable DNA detection level as low as 1.38 fM in a 15 μL solution.

Protein Markers in Breast Cancer

In contrast to genetic markers, protein markers provide a rigorous evaluation for clinical applications therefore protein-based assays are being significantly developed.

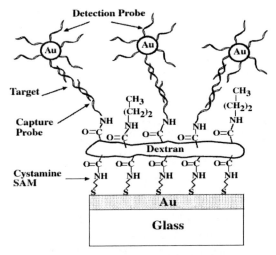

Figure 12.3. Schematic representation of the capture of target (*p53*) by the SPR sandwich gene assay and the following amplified detection of *p53* via the oligonucleotide-modified nanoparticles. An activated cystamine SAM is immobilized onto the gold surface and is then attached via the reaction of the amine groups with the carboxyl groups of the dextran film. The addition of the DNA probe within or on top of the dextran is followed by the detection of DNA hybridization. After hybridization with target DNA, the nanoparticle probes are used to amplify the detection sensitivity. SAM: self-assembled monolayer [Figure reproduced with permission from Yao et al. (2006)].

CEA

Carcinoembryonic antigen (CEA) is the first human cancer-associated antigen and serologic tumor biomarker for clinical diagnosis of breast tumors and others. CEA in serum is related to the negative prognostic factor (Guadagni et al. 2001). Thus, CEA level is mainly used in the postoperative follow-up of breast cancer patients to identify recurrences after surgical resection. The normal CEA level in healthy adults is given in the range 3–5 ng/mL. Accordingly, a sensitive immunosensor for the detection of a subnanogram per milliliter level is required to satisfy this threshold level.

The SPR immunosensor for CEA was reported by Tang and co-workers, which was based on a protein A-conjugated immunosensor (Tang et al. 2006). Monoclonal anti-CEA assembled on the protein A monolayer to obtain an optimal spatial orientation. The detection limit of the sensor for purified CEA was 0.5 ng/mL. Another strategy was proposed by (Su et al. 2008), based on a sandwich assay. The covalent coupling was employed as an antibody immobilization of CEA due to its high resistance to noise of the serum sample. In the presence of the second and third antibodies, the SPR response of immunosensor would significantly enhance upon addition of CEA that bound to the immobilized antibody, leading to the increase in detection sensitivity and specificity. The detection limit for CEA was 25 ng/mL in serum samples. (Hu et al. 2010) prepared an optical immunosensor which was based on the development of a new copolymer brush for immobilization. Antibodies could be covalently attached to the epoxy groups of the poly[oligo(ethylene glycol) methacrylate-*co*-glycidyl methacrylate] (POEGMA-*co*-GMA) brush side chains. The main advantage of this polymer brushes was a high antibody loading and antigen binding activity. Additionally, POEGMA-*co*-GMA brush-based SPR showed remarkable resistance to non-specific adsorption in serum.

HER-2

HER-2 is a member of the ErbB (epidermal growth factor receptor) family which stimulates several downstream signaling cascades. The amplification of the corresponding gene and consequent overexpression of the HER2 protein is associated with poor survival in breast tumors. The cutoff value for HER-2 is determined to be below 15 ng/mL. For the detection of HER-2, Bayer Immuno 1 assay based on a magnetic particle separation has been applied for many years. Although this immunoassay provides the reliable sensitivity, it needs labeled compounds and the assay time is more than 1 hr (Payne et al. 2000). Martin and co-worker proposed a biosensor for direct and label-free detection of HER-2 with only a few preparation steps (Martin et al. 2006). The immunosensor was prepared by capturing anti-HER-2 in a protein G layer to modify the antibody orientation. Compared with an EIA, this SPR biosensor could detect HER-2 more rapid and sensitive.

ESTROGEN RECEPTOR

Estrogen receptor (ER) α is a principal element in human physiology, and its level of expression is a major determinant of response to prognosis and endocrine therapy in ERα-positive breast cancer. Also, it regulates gene expression by directly binding itself to the specific estrogen receptor element (ERE) sequences. The more ERα that appear in the tumor cell, the higher the likelihood of a beneficial response to hormonal therapy (Glass et al. 2007). However, little is known about the ERα-associated regulation of human breast cancer. Yang and co-workers utilized a two-dimensional (2D) and a three-dimensional (3D) streptavidin (SA) chip architecture to study the interactions of ERα and ERE in Fig. 12.4 (Yang et al. 2007). They found that mass transfer effects should be considered in the development of a 3D-based SPR biosensor that achieve a more accurate detection. Although the 3D matrix provided an elevated probe loading resulting in a high biomolecule-

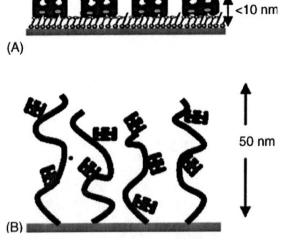

Figure 12.4. Schematic representation of **(A)** the 2D SA monolayer surface and **(B)** the 3D carboxylated hydrogel dextran with SA. The thickness in the 2D manner is less than 10 nm so that several binding sites are blocked by the steric hindrance. However, all the biotin binding sites are available in the dextran since the 3D chip provides more flexibility, resulting in the increase of the amount of biotin-DNA probe. 2D: two-dimensional, 3D: three-dimensional, SA: streptavidin [Figure reproduced with permission from Yang et al. (2007)].

binding capacity, it did not give a sufficiently high binding. Inversely, a 2D platform had more selectivity for sequence dependent protein.

Carbohydrate Antigens

For the development of diagnostic agents, carbohydrate-associated tumor antigens are suitable for tumor screening because they are often observed on the surface of cancer cells.

CA15-3, a mucin-type glycoprotein having a molecular mass of ca. 450 kDa, is found in several other malignant conditions with tumors. It has been approved for use in diagnosis of breast carcinoma. Unfortunately, CA15-3 is not suitable for breast cancer screening in an early stage due to its low sensitivity and specificity. It is useful in combination with clinical examination for making treatment decisions in cancer patients with metastatic disease (Harris et al. 2007). According to the report of De La Lande et al., the level of CA15-3 increased in 80% of patients with metastatic breast cancers (De La Lande et al. 2002). Therefore, it may be adapted as a valuable screening factor to judge recrudescence or metastasis of breast carcinoma.

Fernández-González and co-workers introduced a CA15-3 immunosensor using polyglycerol (PEG) as a covalent linker and protein G as a sublayer for immunoglobulin orientation (Fernández-González et al. 2007). This provided rigid material with good sensitivity and low signal background. When real saliva-sample testing was performed, the sample from a normal individual and cancer patient could be distinguished using this sensor. Our group had used multiple SPR transduction layers to improve sensitivity (Lin et al. 2006a,b). Recently, we described a novel sensor for CA15-3 detection based on a gold/zinc oxide (Au/ZnO) thin film SPR (Chang et al. 2010). For a SPR chip, chromium (Cr) is the most frequently used material to improve the adherence between gold films and glass substrates. Due to a high imaginary part of the refractive index, Cr may cause low optical transmission to the gold surface, thus affecting the optical properties of the plasmon resonance. Consequently, such a conventional structure would reduce the sensitivity of SPR biosensor. In our work, ZnO was applied to replace Cr as an adhesive layer due to its unique optical properties. Our system yielded a two-fold sensitivity and a four-fold detection limit improvement over the convention SPR (Fig. 12.5). Also, our assay developed for the CA15-3 antigen, with a detection limit of 0.025 U/mL, is feasible to detect CA15-3 in clinical diagnostics.

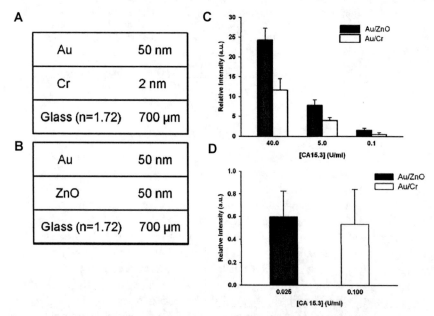

Figure 12.5. Schematic representation of the structure in **(A)** Au/Cr and **(B)** Au/ZnO and SPR intensity changes upon binding of CA15-3 to antibody **(C)** at different concentrations and **(B)** at the detection limit of concentration on Au/ZnO and Au/Cr. Although the intermediate thickness of ZnO is significantly greater than the Cr layer thickness, the intensity changes of CA15-3 binding on the Au/ZnO layers are at least two-fold higher than those on the Au/Cr layers. Additionally, the detection limit of 0.025 U/mL is noticeably better than that obtained using the Au/Cr thin films. Cr: chromium, ZnO: zinc oxide, CA15-3: Carbohydrate antigen 15-3 [Figure reproduced with permission from Chang et al. (2010)].

In addition to the detection of CA15-3, Suwansa-ard and co-workers presented a label-free optical immunosensor for CA12-5 based on monitoring the change in the SPR signal of antibody upon the antigen binding (Suwansa-ard et al. 2009). After each reaction, a CA12-5 assay was regenerated by rinsing HCl solution at pH 2.60 which led to a reusable ability of greater than 96 ± 4 % up to 32 times in succession. The detection range of the CA12-5 assay was 0.1–40 U/mL, and the minimum detectable concentration was 0.1 U/mL, which was sufficient to measure clinically relevant CA12-5 levels (35 U/mL). Thus, their work established an effective platform for developing the simple, rapid, and cost-effective SPR immunosensor.

However, regeneration is not always accomplished as the expected result since the bioactivity of the ligands may be denatured with harsh reagents after several repeats of regeneration. It is one of the main challenges to retain the stability of the immobilized ligands for multiple sample injections. To overcome the surface regeneration problem, the additive assay has attracted an increasing interest for the development of immunosensors (Chung et al. 2006). The additive approach involving successive injection of the equivalent dilutions could calculate the concentration of CA19-9 sample from the SPR signal actually measured. It is based on the calculation of the analyte concentration by using the correlation curve between the accumulated sensor response and the accumulated analyte level. With an additive protocol, the immunosensor reduced the number of regeneration cycles, consequently diminishing the effect of sensor instability. Additionally, using the additive protocol could reduce the total analysis time compared to using the regeneration agents. The sandwich detection formats with secondary antibodies was also employed to enhance the additive assay. As a result, the detection limit for CA19-9 was increased by about a factor of six with the sandwich immunoassay.

Multi-Analyte SPR Immunosensor

Immunosensors for a single biomarker have been well established for breast cancer screening. However, in clinical testing, the diagnostic value of a single tumor marker measurement is not sufficient for the evaluation of cancer screening or therapy due to their limited specificity. The biosensors based on the single-marker diagnosis are facing great challenges. Alternatively, multianalyte biomarker-based tests are rapidly emerging as powerful tools in clinical applications. The major advantage of these assays is to obtain higher accuracy than would be possible from the detection of a single tumor marker. The multi-biomarker analysis also shows promise in improving assay efficiency, lowering sample consumption, and reducing overall cost per assay.

Piliarik and co-workers developed a simultaneous measurement method for tumor markers in human sera by using a high-performance SPR imaging sensor with polarization contrast and internal referencing (Piliarik et al. 2010). Using the polarization contrast measurement, the SPR array offered a superior resolution and extended operating range (Fig. 12.6). To avoid signal interference such as light intensity fluctuations and nonspecific protein interaction, the use of internal referencing diminished the noise of SPR images by an order of magnitude and 1% bovine serum albumin (BSA) reduced the interference binding of serum proteins. The results showed that this proposed method had high sensitivity and specificity.

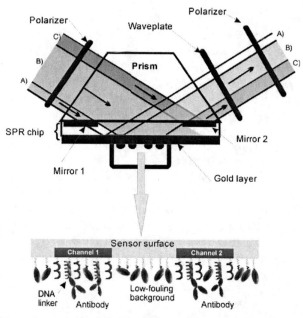

Figure 12.6. Schematic representation of the SPR imaging sensor with advanced polarization contrast and self-referencing. The system consists of two referencing areas (Mirror 1 and Mirror 2). The light is blocked by mirror 1 provides; **(A)** the dark reference signal and is reflected by mirror 2 provides; **(B)** the bright reference signal for real-time compensation [Figure reproduced with permission from Piliarik et al. (2010)].

Campbell and co-workers reported an automated multiplex immunoassay system based on the SPR technology (Campbell et al. 2011). The system provided the quantitative analysis of up to 16 different analytes simultaneously and had a relatively simple fluidic system. Additionally, the sensing surface could be regenerated for the next sample analysis. This proposed array possessed attractive characteristics such as simple, convenient, rapid, high-throughput, and low-cost and could measure biological entities over a wider-angle of sizes.

CONCLUSION AND FUTURE OUTLOOK

The levels of tumor markers show a correlation with the stage of breast tumor development in patients. As described previously, SPR immunosensors hold unique characteristics for the detection of breast tumor markers. Given the nucleic acid and protein applications, such biosensors have great potential to provide the targeted information in a direct, rapid, and simple manner. Research for advanced technologies, including anti-biofouling matrixes, immobilization strategies, and nanomaterials still remain to be developed. Also, multi-analyte SPR biosensors help in detecting many cancer markers simultaneously. The remarkable sensitivity of the SPR-based sensors opens up the possibility for facilitating early breast cancer detection and the treatment of the disease. The use of SPR sensors for breast cancer clinical testing may be fast and flexibile, enabling automatic multi-target analyses, and bringing the cost down. Although SPR immunosensors have the capacity to replace conventional methods in the determination of the breast cancer markers in simple ways, there are still several challenges related to the achievement of reliable screening. The major problem is to bring SPR devices to non-laboratory personnel without compromising accuracy and reliability. Furthermore, interference adsorptions in complex matrix such as undiluted serum have continued to be completely overcome. Other concerns relate to the difficulty with variability of quality control in chips, and portability, or on-site analysis in devices. Up to now, the SPR immunosensors for breast cancer have been limited only to research laboratories. Therefore, besides further technical improvements, the standardization of SPR devices, and training of lay persons should meet the requirement in accepted analysis protocols.

DEFINITIONS

- *Breast cancer*: A group of neoplastic growth appears from cells in the breast.
- *Tumor marker*: A biological molecule produced by tumor cells that is indicative of the existence of cancer in an individual.
- *Dextran*: A large family of glucose polymer composed of chains of varying lengths can be employed as immobilization matrix to fabricate a biosensor.
- *Self-assembled monolayer*: A monolayer is spontaneously formed on the surface and uniformly oriented along the specific direction.
- *Regeneration*: Regeneration is the process that can deactivate a biological binding event and then ideally return the sensor response to the initial baseline.

- *Resonance unit*: The response unit of the SPR measurement. The unit is defined as 1 RU = 1 pg/mm² and is also directly proportional to the amount of biomolecules on the sensor surface.
- *Immobilization*: Immobilization is a permanent or temporary attachment of biomolecules such as enzymes, antibodies or nucleic acids onto a solid matrix by adsorption, entrapment or covalent linkage.
- *Anti-biofouling*: Anti-fouling is the process that resists the undesirable accumulation of adsorbed biomolecules on the surface. Thus, the anti-biofouling matrix for the biosensor can ensure high detection selectivity without the interference of non-specific adsorption.

SUMMARY POINTS

- SPR immunosensors for breast cancer can be used in the following applications:
  - (a) single-base-pair mismatch discrimination
  - (b) characterization of signaling pathways
  - (c) measurement of expression of tumor-associated antigens
  - (d) identification of binding partners to protein markers
- Several kinds of nanomaterials and structures such as nanoparticles, nano thinfilm (ZnO), and brush (POEGMA-*co*-GMA), have been applied in SPR immunosensors for signal amplification, surface transduction, and biomolecular conjugation, etc.
- The combined detection of several specific breast cancer markers is necessary in order to provide high sensitivity for the diagnosis.
- Some challenges that remain in the development and application of SPR biosensor for breast cancer include
  - (a) low accuracy and reproducibility in the clinical use
  - (b) poor performance in undiluted body fluids
  - (c) lack of a clinical standardization and calibration
- Overall, future advances in SPR technology will focus on the design of portable and automated simultaneous multiple analyte whole-blood analyzers for breast tumor marker examinations to achieve the clinical requirements.

ABBREVIATIONS

Au	:	Gold
BSA	:	Bovine serum albumin
CA15-3	:	Carbohydrate antigen 15-3
CEA	:	Carcinoembryonic antigen

Cr	:	Chromium
dsDNA	:	double-stranded DNA
EIA	:	Enzyme immunoassay
Erα	:	Estrogen receptor α
ErbB	:	Epidermal growth factor receptor
ERE	:	Estrogen receptor element
FIA	:	Fluoroimmunoassay
HER-2	:	Human epidermal growth factor receptor 2
MCH	:	Mercaptohexanol
PEG	:	Polyethylene glycol
POEGMA-co-GMA	:	poly[oligo(ethylene glycol) methacrylate-co-glycidyl methacrylate]
RE	:	Response element
RIA	:	Radioimmunoassay
SA	:	Streptavidin
SAM	:	Self-assembled monolayer
SSB	:	Single strand binding protein
SNP	:	Single nucleotide polymorphism
SPR	:	Surface plasmon resonance
ZnO	:	Zinc oxide
2D	:	Two-dimensional
3D	:	Three-dimensional

REFERENCES

Campbell K, T McGrath, S Sjölander, T Hanson, M Tidare, Ö Jansson, A Moberg, M Mooney, C Elliott and J Buijs. 2011. Use of a novel micro-fluidic device to create arrays for multiplex analysis of large and small molecular weight compounds by surface plasmon resonance. Biosens Bioelectron 26: 3029–3036.

Carrascosa LG, A Calle and LM Lechuga. 2009. Label-free detection of DNA mutations by SPR: Application to the early detection of inherited breast cancer. Anal Bioanal Chem 393: 1173–1182.

Chang CC, NF Chiu, DS Lin, Y Chu-Su, YH Liang and CW Lin. 2010. High-Sensitivity Detection of Carbohydrate Antigen 15-3 Using a Gold/Zinc Oxide Thin Film Surface Plasmon Resonance-Based Biosensor. Anal Chem 82: 1207–1212.

Chiu NF, C Yu, SY Nien, JH Lee, CH Kuan, KC Wu, CK Lee and CW Lin. 2007. Enhancement and tunability of active plasmonic by multilayer grating coupled emission. Opt Express 15: 11608–11615.

Chung JW, R Bernhardt and JC Pyun. 2006. Additive assay of cancer marker CA19-9 by SPR biosensor. Sens. Actuator B-Chem 118: 28–32.

De La Lande B, K Hacene, JL Floiras, N Alatrakchi and MF Pichon. 2002. Prognostic value of CA15.3 kinetics for metastatic breast cancer. Int J Biol Markers 17: 231–238.

Ding J, R Warren, I Warsi, N Day, D Thompson, M Brady, C Tromans, R Highnam and D Easton. 2008. Evaluating the Effectiveness of Using Standard Mammogram Form to Predict Breast Cancer Risk: Case-Control Study. Cancer Epidemiol. Biomarkers Prev 17: 1074–1081.

Ferlay J, F Bray, P Pisani and DM Parkin. 2000. GLOBOCAN 2000: Cancer Incidence, Mortality and Prevalence Worldwide. IARC Press, Lyon.

Fernández-González A, J Rychłowska, R Badía and R Salzer. 2007. SPR imaging as a tool for detecting mucin—anti-mucin interaction. Outline of the development of a sensor for near-patient testing for mucin. Microchim Acta 158: 219–225.

Glass AG, JV Lacey, JD Carreon and RN Hoover. 2007. Breast Cancer Incidence, 1980–2006: Combined Roles of Menopausal Hormone Therapy, Screening Mammography, and Estrogen Receptor Status. J Natl Cancer Inst 99: 1152–1161.

Guadagni F, P Ferroni, S Carlini, S Mariotti, A Spila, S Aloe, R D'Alessandro, MD Carone, A Cicchetti, A Ricciotti, I Venturo, P Perri, F Di Filippo, F Cognetti, C Botti and M Roselli. 2001. A Re-Evaluation of Carcinoembryonic Antigen (CEA) as a Serum Marker for Breast Cancer. Clin Cancer Res 7: 2357–2362.

Harris L, H Fritsche, R Mennel, L Norton, P Ravdin, S Taube, MR Somerfield, DF Hayes and RC Bast. 2007. American Society of Clinical Oncology 2007 Update of Recommendations for the Use of Tumor Markers in Breast Cancer. J Clin Oncol 25: 5287–5312.

Homola J, SS Yee and G Gauglitz. 1999. Surface plasmon resonance sensors: review. Sens Actuator B-Chem 54: 3–15.

Hu W, Y Liu, Z Lu and CM Li. 2010. Poly[oligo(ethylene glycol) methacrylate-*co*-glycidyl methacrylate] Brush Substrate for Sensitive Surface Plasmon Resonance Imaging Protein Arrays Adv Funct Mater 20: 3497–3503.

Huang JG, CL Lee, HM Lin, TL Chuang, WS Wang, RH Juang, CH Wang, CK Lee, SM Lin and CW Lin. 2006. A miniaturized germanium-doped silicon dioxide-based surface plasmon resonance waveguide sensor for immunoassay detection. Biosens Bioelectron 22: 519–525.

Jiang T, M Minunni, P, Wilson, J Zhang, APF Turner and M Mascini. 2005. Detection of TP53 mutation using a portable surface plasmon resonance DNA-based biosensor. Biosens Bioelectron 20: 1939–1945.

Li Y, AW Wark, HJ Lee and RM Corn. 2006. Single-Nucleotide Polymorphism Genotyping by Nanoparticle-Enhanced Surface Plasmon Resonance Imaging Measurements of Surface Ligation Reactions. Anal Chem 78: 3158–3164.

Lin CW, KP Chen, CN Hsiao, S Lin and CK Lee. 2006a. Design and fabrication of an alternating dielectric multi-layer device for surface plasmon resonance sensor. Sens Actuator B-Chem 113: 169–176.

Lin CW, KP Chen, MC Su, TC Hsiao, SS Lee, S Lin, XJ Shi and CK Lee. 2006b. Admittance loci design method for multilayer surface plasmon resonance devices. Sens Actuator B-Chem 117: 219–229.

Maillart E, K Brengel-Pesce, D Capela, A Roget, T Livache, M Canva, Y Levy and T Soussi. 2004. Versatile analysis of multiple macromolecular interactions by SPR imaging: application to *p53* and DNA interaction. Oncogene 23: 5543–5550.

Martin VS, BA Sullivan, K Walker, H Hawk, BP Sullivan and LJ Noe. 2006. Surface Plasmon Resonance Investigations of Human Epidermal Growth Factor Receptor 2. Appl Spectrosc 60: 994–1003.

Narod SA and WD Foulkes. 2004. BRCA1 and BRCA2: 1994 and beyond. Nat Rev Cancer 4: 665–676.

Payne RC, JW Allard, L Anderson-Mauser, JD Humphreys, DY Tenney and DL Morris. 2000. Automated Assay for HER-2/neu in Serum Clin Chem 46: 175–182.

Petitjean A, MIW Achatz, AL Borresen-Dale, P Hainaut and M Olivier. 2007. TP53 mutations in human cancers: functional selection and impact on cancer prognosis and outcomes. Oncogene 26: 2157–2165.

Piliarik M, M Bocková and J Homola. 2010. Surface plasmon resonance biosensor for parallelized detection of protein biomarkers in diluted blood plasma. Biosens Bioelectron 26: 1656–1661.

Su F, C Xu, M Taya, K Murayama, Y Shinohara and SI Nishimura. 2008. Detection of Carcinoembryonic Antigens Using a Surface Plasmon Resonance Biosensor Sensors 8: 4282–4295.

Suwansa-ard S, P Kanatharana, P Asawatreratanakul, B Wongkittisuksa, C Limsakul and P Thavarungkul. 2009. Comparison of surface plasmon resonance and capacitive immunosensors for cancer antigen 125 detection in human serum samples. Biosens Bioelectron 24: 3436–3441.

Tang DP, R Yuan and YQ Chai. 2006. Novel immunoassay for carcinoembryonic antigen based on protein A-conjugated immunosensor chip by surface plasmon resonance and cyclic voltammetry. Bioprocess Biosyst Eng 28: 315–321.

van't Veer LJ, H Dai, MJ van de Vijver, YD He, AAM Hart, M Mao, HL Peterse, K van der Kooy, MJ Marton, AT Witteveen, GJ Schreiber, RM Kerkhoven, C Roberts, PS Linsley, R Bernards and SH Friend. 2002. Gene expression profiling predicts clinical outcome of breast cancer. Nature 415: 530–536.

Wilson PK, T Jiang, ME Minunni, APF Turner and M Mascini. 2005. A novel optical biosensor format for the detection of clinically relevant TP53 mutations. Biosens Bioelectron 20: 2310–2313.

Yang N, X Su, V Tjong and W Knoll. 2007. Evaluation of two- and three-dimensional streptavidin binding platforms for surface plasmon resonance spectroscopy studies of DNA hybridization and protein-DNA binding. Biosens Bioelectron 22: 2700–2706.

Yao X, X Li, F Toledo, C Zurita-Lopez, M Gutova, J Momand and F Zhou. 2006. Sub-attomole oligonucleotide and *p53* cDNA determinations via a high-resolution surface plasmon resonance combined with oligonucleotide-capped gold nanoparticle signal amplification. Anal Biochem 354: 220–228.

13

Detection of miRNA with Silicon Nanowire Biosensors

Guo-Jun Zhang

ABSTRACT

MicroRNA, a small non-coding RNA molecule that regulates gene expression, is involved in cancer initiation and progression. It is believed that miRNA gene alterations play a critical role in almost all kinds of human cancers. The small size of miRNA makes not only its detection challenging, but also its selective pairing difficult. Currently, major methods of detecting miRNA are dependent on hybridization, in which a target miRNA molecule is hybridized to a complementary labeled probe molecule. Recently developed detection methods introduce nanomaterials to the hybridized duplex to greatly enhance the sensitivity. However, all of them are indirect, involving labeling or the conjugating process. On the other hand, most of the current assays suffer from low sensitivity. To get sufficient miRNA for detection, enrichment and amplification in the process of isolation of miRNA from the cell are needed prior to detection. However, the additional steps may lead to loss of miRNA, increase the analysis time, and involve large sample volume. In this chapter, we propose a new approach that enables highly sensitive, specific, label-free direct detection of miRNA by using peptide nucleic acid (PNA)-functionalized silicon nanowires (SiNWs)

Institute of Microelectronics, A*STAR (Agency for Science, Technology and Research), 11 Science Park Road, Singapore Science Park II, Singapore 117685;
E-mail: zhanggj@ime.a-star.edu.sg

List of abbreviations after the text.

biosensor. The biosensor is capable of detecting target miRNA as low as 1 fM, as well as identifying fully matched versus mismatched miRNA sequences, especially discriminating between signal base differences, as in single nucleotide polymorphism (SNP). More importantly, the SiNW biosensor enables miRNA direct detection in total RNA extracted from cancer cells, providing a promising tool for early cancer detection in which the species of miRNAs in the cancer cells are different from those of normal cells. The developed PNA-functionalized SiNW biosensor shows potential applications in label-free, early detection of miRNA as a biomarker in cancer diagnostics with very high sensitivity and good specificity.

INTRODUCTION

Over the past decade, small ribonucleic acids (RNAs), including microRNA (miRNA) and small interfering RNA (siRNA), have been demonstrated as specific regulators for gene expression (Kennedy 2002). Due to the big impact of small RNAs, the 2006 Nobel Prize was awarded to two scientists, Andrew Fire and Craig Mello. miRNA is a small noncoding regulatory RNA molecule ranging in size from 17 to 25 nucleotides, which was first discovered in worms in 1993 (Lee et al. 1993), and observed in a number of animals, plants, and viruses several years later (Reinhart et al. 2000). To date, it has been found that a number of miRNAs were implicated and miRNA expression was deregulated in cancer. However, the mechanism of why and how miRNA becomes deregulated remains uncertain. As cancer is a complex genetic disease caused by the accumulation of mutations, leading to deregulation of gene expression and uncontrolled cell proliferation, the cancer-associated miRNAs, as effective cancer biomarkers, are attracting more and more attention for diagnosis and prognosis.

Since tumor origin, stage, and other pathological variables can be reflected by miRNA expression profiles, miRNA is being used as diagnostic or prognostic tools. miRNA is playing a more and more important role in functioning as accurate molecular markers because it is relatively stable and resistant to RNase degradation. Due to its small size, detection of miRNA is challenging and ultrasensitive miRNA quantitation techniques are lacking. Northern blot analysis is a well-established technique for detecting miRNAs in cells or tissues (Valoczi et al. 2004). Although Northern blot allows gene expression quantification and miRNA size determination, the low sensitivity and time-consuming laborious procedures of Northern blot make it difficult for routine miRNA analysis. Subsequently, miRNA microarrays were developed, which allow for detection of multiple miRNAs simultaneously across various samples in a single run (Liu et al. 2004). In addition, quantitative reverse transcriptase polymerase chain reaction (RT-PCR) has also been developed, allowing for the analysis of miRNAs in small tissue samples or even single cells (Miska et al. 2004). Not only can these quantitative RT-PCR assays analyze mature miRNAs, but they can analyze miRNA precursors and primary transcripts. Despite the many advantages, PCR-based assay is neither cost-effective nor feasible for small or rare samples. Likewise, microarrays still suffer from low sensitivity and specificity because of the short nature of mature miRNAs. A novel microarray strategy to improve the specificity was developed by performing hybridization in solution using polystyrene capture beads that are coupled to oligonucleotide probes complementary to the miRNAs of interest, and analyzing the hybridization event using a multicolor flow cytometer measuring bead color (Lu et al. 2005). Besides, surface plasma resonance (SPR) is a surface-sensitive optical technique that has widely been used to the real-time monitoring of various bioaffinity interactions. A combination of surface enzyme chemistry and DNA-coated nanoparticles using SPR imaging has generated a quantitative detection of multiple miRNAs in a microarray format at attomolar level (Fang et al. 2006). Nevertheless, all the methodologies are optical-based detection, requiring additional labeling to visualize the hybridization event.

Compared to optical detection, electrical detection, on the other hand, is more advantageous. The electrical detection directly transduces nucleic acid hybridization events into useful electrical signals. The method is able to provide high sensitivity with multiplexing capability. Because the method is compatible with semiconductor technology, the readout can be miniaturized at low-cost, exempt from the problems encountered in the optical detection systems. Furthermore, the detection system is easy to be integrated, which is suitable for development of point-of-care (POC) device. As an example, an electrochemical method employing electrocatalytic nanoparticle tags for ultrasensitive detection of miRNA was developed (Gao and Yang 2006). The use of nanoparticles enhances the signals, thus improving detection sensitivity. The method was able to ultra-sensitively detect miRNA down to 80 fM levels. Recently, a nanogapped microelectrode-based biosensor array has been fabricated for ultrasensitive electrical detection of miRNAs (Fan et al. 2007). Different from the employment of metal nanoparticles for labeling the target, the *in situ* signal amplification method used in the method simplifies the detection procedure and greatly enhances the sensitivity. Under optimized conditions, the target miRNA could be quantified in a range from 10 fM to 20 pM with a detection limit of 5.0 fM.

It is apparent that the reported methods still require additional labeling and conjugating steps for detection, and are thus time-consuming and indirect. Therefore, there is a demand to develop a sensitive, direct, simple, rapid and label-free assay for miRNA analysis. Direct and label-free electrical readout systems provide an extremely attractive sensing modality, which is widely applicable for miRNA detection. Silicon nanowires (SiNWs) are proven to be ultrasensitive electrical biosensors which are capable of detecting nucleic acids (Bunimovich et al. 2006; Cattani-Scholz et al. 2008; Gao et al. 2007; Hahm and Lieber 2004; Li et al. 2004; Zhang et al. 2008a,b, 2010a,b), proteins (Chua et al. 2009; Cui et al. 2001; Stern et al. 2007; Zhang et al. 2009b; Zheng et al. 2005) and protein-DNA interactions (Zhang et al. 2010c). In this chapter, we describe a new method of directly detecting miRNA by excluding labeling and conjugating processes using peptide nucleic acid (PNA)-functionalized SiNW biosensor with high sensitivity and good specificity. As PNA does not have an anionic phosphate backbone, the hybridization between PNA and miRNA eliminates repulsion, resulting in increased melting temperature and subsequently enhanced hybridization efficiency. The SiNW biosensors functionalized with PNA are capable of discriminating between single base differences, as in single nucleotide polymorphisms (SNPs). Furthermore, miRNA in total RNA extracted from cancer lines are detectable by the developed SiNW biosensors. Due to high surface-to-volume ratio that the nanowire dimensions confer, the sensitivity is greatly enhanced and the detection limit can be lowered to femtomolar concentrations.

APPLICATIONS TO OTHER AREAS OF HEALTH AND DISEASE

This chapter will be particularly focus on utilization of the PNA-functionalized SiNW biosensor for detection of miRNA related to cancer. In parallel, the SiNW biosensor has also been used to diagnose other diseases such as cardiovascular disease, prostate cancer, and infectious diseases. The association of unique properties of the SiNW materials and fabrication of the device using semiconductor technology makes the SiNW biosensor useful as a disease diagnosis tool. Moreover, the development of surface chemistry on SiNW surface allows various receptor molecules to be functionalized on the surface, enabling the SiNW biosensor to detect different species. Important protein biomarkers, indicative of cardiovascular disease, have been detected by the SiNW biosensor, in which real-time detection of troponin T and multiplexed detection of troponin T, creatine kinase MM, and creatine kinase MB in serum were conducted (Chua et al. 2009; Zhang et al. 2009b). In addition, the simultaneous detection of multiple prostate cancer protein biomarkers in a single and versatile detection platform has been studied using the SiNW biosensor (Zheng et al. 2005). Moreover, the SiNW biosensor modified with specific antibodies has yielded selective detection of different viruses like influenza A and adenovirus in parallel, which are significant for infectious disease diagnosis (Patolsky et al. 2004). More recently, the PNA-functionalized SiNW biosensor is capable of detecting dengue virus with rapid speed and high sensitivity, making it possible to be miniaturized into portable device by integrating with other components (Zhang et al. 2010a).

SILICON NANOWIRE BIOSENSOR FOR DETECTION OF microRNA

Working Principle

Field-effect transistor (FET)-based biosensor has emerged as an important platform for biomolecular sensing. The SiNW biosensor is one of the FET-based sensors, which has the structure of a common three-electrode transistor, where the source and drain electrodes bridge the SiNW used as the sensing component of the device and the gate electrode modulates the SiNW conductance. To detect a target, a receptor molecule which is capable of specifically recognizing the target molecule is immobilized on the SiNW surface. Upon binding, the electrical signal is generated based on the conductance change. Different from the conventional FET sensor that has a thin film-type semiconductor structure as gate insulator, the sensing behavior of the SiNW sensor is enhanced because of the extremely small cross-sectional area of the SiNW. As a result, charge accumulation or depletion near the SiNW surface because of surface charge change gives rise to a change in the significant portion of the SiNW cross-sectional area. Therefore, using the SiNW-based sensor will remarkably increase the detection sensitivity compared to the conventional FET sensors.

Figure 13.1 illustrates the working principle of the PNA-functionalized SiNW biosensor for detection of miRNA. PNA is covalently immobilized on the electrically addressable SiNW surface via conventional silane chemistry. Electrical bio-sensing by the SiNW biosensor is based on change in resistance of the SiNWs due to depletion of charge carriers in its "bulk" when negatively charged miRNA originating from the phosphate groups on the miRNA backbone is bound to the PNA-functionalized surface via hybridization. When the targeted species, miRNAs complementary to the immobilized PNA, are present, resistance change occurs whereas, when they are non-complementary, resistance change is minimal. As each wire is provided with independent metal contacts, resistance can be individually measured.

PNA (N-AACCACACAACCTACTACCTCA-C) is immobilized on the SiNW surface as capture probes. Three miRNA sequences are employed as targets in this work. Let-7b (5'-UGAGGUAGUAGGUUGUGUGGUU-3') is a complementary target, let-7c (5'-UGAGGUAGUAGGUUGUAUGGUU-3') is a one-base mismatched target, and control (5'-AUGCAUGCAUGCAUGCAUGCAA-3') is a non-complementary target.

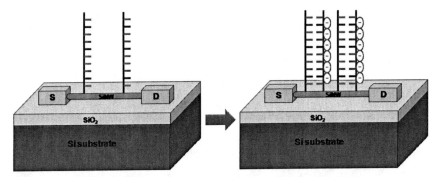

Figure 13.1. Schematic diagram of the SiNW biosensor developed for ultrasensitive, label-free direct detection of miRNA. The SiNW biosensor is a FET-based sensor, which has the structure of a common three-electrode transistor, where the source and drain electrodes bridge the SiNW used as the sensing component of the sensor and the gate electrode modulates the SiNW conductance. PNA immobilized on the SiNW surface is hybridized with miRNA to be detected. Because miRNA is negatively charged, binding of miRNA to PNA on the SiNW surface repels the negative charges in the region of nanowire, resulting in an increase in resistance (Unpublished materials).

Fabrication of Silicon Nanowire Biosensor

Top-down and bottom-up are the two methods for nanofabricating semiconducting SiNW biosensor. Top-down methods start with patterns made on a large scale and reduce its lateral dimensions before forming nanostructures. On the other hand, bottom-up methods begin with atoms or molecules to build up nanostructures, in some cases through smart use of self organization.

Bottom-up techniques like vapor-liquid-solid (VLS) to grow SiNWs have been widely reported along with their applications as biosensors (Lu and Lieber 2006). 20 nm n-type or p-type SiNWs in diameter have been produced by the VLS method using Au nanoclusters as a catalyst and diborane or phosphine as dopant precursors. In principle, the technique allows the growth of NWs on a wide range of substrates, i.e. the most common substrate is a Si wafer. High quality of NWs could be produced, but the NWs grown on the substrate are in random orientation and vary in dimension, leading to poor device uniformity and low fabrication yield. So it is a challenging task by itself to bring such techniques to manufacturing maturity. To reap the potential of SiNW in sensor applications on a large scale, it is important to develop technologies that can reliably produce them.

Top-down technologies use nanofabrication tools like e-beam lithography, or photolithography combined with size-reducing strategies, such as self-limiting oxidation, or superlattice NW pattern transfer (SNAP) method to produce NW structures. The resulting NWs are uniform and well aligned. Moreover, the technologies produce NWs in high yields and in a well-ordered orientation on the Si substrate, simplifying them into various functional devices. Various types of SiNWs have been produced by the top-down methods. The NWs fabricated by e-beam lithography have a width of 50 nm and lengths ranging from 20 μm to 1 mm (Stern et al. 2007a,b; Li et al. 2004). The SNAP method created highly aligned, 20-nm-wide NWs on the n- or p-doped silicon-on-insulator (SOI) wafer (Bunimovich et al. 2006).

Compared to other SiNW sensors, complementary metal-oxide semiconductor (CMOS) compatible SiNW biosensors are definitely promising in terms of their manufacturability and commercialization. We have thus developed a top-down approach to the precise fabrication of individually addressable SiNWs in a perfectly aligned array format using CMOS compatible technology. The SiNWs are formed through conventional optical lithography, etching and oxidation and thus is fully compatible with CMOS technology. Figure 13.2 is a schematic diagram of process

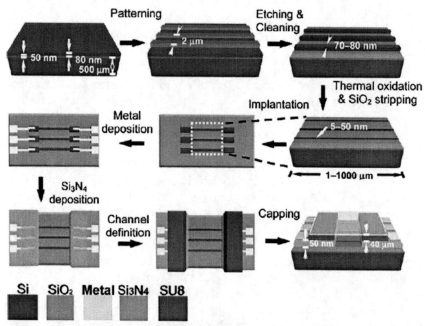

Figure 13.2. Schematic illustration of process flow for fabrication of the SiNW biosensor array. 8-inch SOI wafers with a 50–100 nm buried oxide layer and a 50–80 nm silicon layer are patterned and etched, and the resulting fin structures are further oxidized to realize nanowire arrays, followed by contact metal deposition and passivation. Microfluidic channels are realized on the SiNW array wafer using SU-8 photoresist by thermal compression at low temperatures. Isolation of all electrical contacts from the aqueous solution is achieved by encapsulating only the SiNW arrays in a fluidic channel. (Reprinted with permission [Gao et al. 2007]. Copyright 2009 American Chemical Society).

flow for the fabrication of SiNW biosensor array. 8-inch SOI wafers were doped with n-type phosphorous impurities using an ion implanter where implant dose varied from 1×10^{13} to 1×10^{15} and energy from 30 to 50 keV. The dopants were then activated in rapid thermal annealing furnace and NW-fins were patterned using standard deep ultra-violet (DUV) lithography in the array format. Silicon was etched in reactive ion etcher and resulting fins (60–80 nm wide) were oxidized in O_2 at 900°C (for 2–6 hr) to realize NW array. The two ends of the NWs were further doped to obtain n+ regions, followed by connecting to contact metal and alloying to realize Ohmic contacts. The biosensor was then passivated by silicon nitride film except for the active nanowire sensor area and metal pads. Micro-fluidic channels were realized on the passivated SiNW array wafers using SU-8 photo resist. The channel depth up to 40 μm were obtained, which were capped by polydimethyl-siloxane (PDMS) using thermal compression at low temperatures (<60°C).

A SiNW sensor chip has two portions of SiNW arrays for sensing, and each portion has 100 SiNWs in parallel. Typical scanning electron microscopy (SEM) images of the SiNW arrays are illustrated in Fig. 13.3, in which highly uniform and regular SiNWs are fabricated in parallel. The SiNWs used in this experiment are ~50 nm in diameter and 100 μm in length. As Fig. 13.3B shows, the fine lines on the left side correspond to the NWs, and the broad lines on the right side correspond to the metal pads for electrical contacts.

Surface Functionalization of Silicon Nanowire

In addition to the SiNW dimensions, surface chemistry of the SiNW biosensor also plays a significant role. Because the SiNW is tiny at the nanoscale level, high surface density of the probe molecules is desirable, which is anticipated to capture more target molecules. By doing so, the detection sensitivity can be improved. To date, two methods, electrostatic adsorption and covalent binding, have mainly been developed for the SiNW biosensor based on the nature of silicon surface.

Electrostatic adsorption is an attractive force responsible for adsorbing ionic solute on an oppositely charged adsorbent. Heath group demonstrated DNA detection in electrolyte solution using a SiNW sensor, in which a primary DNA strand was electrostatically adsorbed onto an amine-terminated organic monolayer on top of the NW surface (Bunimovich et al. 2006). Although electrostatic adsorption for immobilization of biomolecules is effective in many applications, the binding efficiency is low if the surfaces are neutrally charged since biomolecules passively adsorb to surfaces through ionic interactions. Furthermore, the biomolecules immobilized via

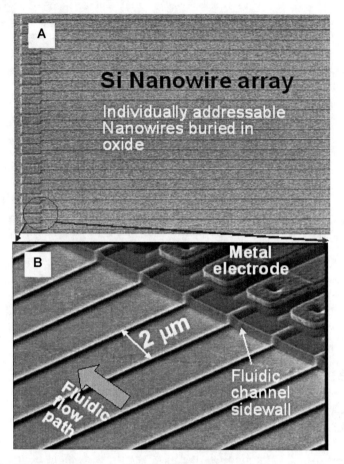

Figure 13.3. SEM micrographs of the SiNW biosensor arrays with metal contacts. **(A)** 200 SiNW arrays are fabricated in two portions (100 NWs each) on one chip by the top-down method, which are individually addressable buried in oxide. The SiNWs are ~50 nm in diameter and 100 μm in length. The distance in between the two NWs is 2 μm; **(B)** A zoom image of the SiNW arrays and electrical contacts. (Reprinted with permission from [Zhang et al. 2008a]. Copyright 2008 Elsevier Science).

electrostatic adsorption are random in orientation and conformation, which further lowers the binding efficiency for the target molecules.

To immobilize the affinity receptor on the SiNW surface, covalent attachment is preferable compared to electrostatic adsorption method. Covalent immobilization is able to bind biomolecules through chemical bonds, which are specific, strong and stable. In addition, proper orientation and conformation can be controlled by selecting the self-assembled monolayers (SAMs) as functional surfaces. Covalent immobilization thus leads to better biomolecule activity, more ordered molecule conformation, less nonspecific adsorption, and greater stability. Due to the fact that the oxide grows on the SiNW surface naturally, a number of methods have been developed by functionalizing the oxide-coated SiNW surface with biomolecules. In general, the most well-known linker molecules are alkoxysilane, of which 3-aminopropyltriethoxysilane (APTES) is the popular one. Amine groups are yielded on the surface by the reagent, which can be used to immobilize PNA, DNA and antibodies for various types of sensing (Chua et al. 2009; Zhang et al. 2010a,b). Likewise, reaction of the SiNW surface with 3-mercaptopropyltrimethoxysilane (MPTMS) gives rise to a thiol-termination. This –SH terminated SiNW biosensor can be used to detect DNA by immobilizing DNA probes modified with acrylic phosphoramidite at the 5' end (Li et al. 2004). In addition, another common reagent terminated with aldehyde groups, 3-(trimethoxysilyl) propyl aldehyde (APTMS), can be functionalized with the SiNW surface. The aldehyde-terminated SiNW surface can directly be immobilized with PNA, DNA and antibodies (Cui et al. 2001; Hahm and Lieber 2004; Zheng et al. 2005). Besides the alkoxysilane, phosphonate derivatives are the alternative molecules to functionalize the SiNW surface with hydroxyl groups, enabling PNA to be attached (Cattani-Scholz et al. 2008). Apart from the native oxide-based method, oxide-free chemistry has also been investigated by etching away the thin oxide on the SiNW surface using dilute hydrofluoric acid (HF). The stable Si-C bonds can subsequently be formed on the generated hydrogen-terminated SiNW via photochemical hydrosilylation, resulting in SiNW coated with amine groups. Subsequently, the probe molecules can be immobilized on the SiNW surface to detect protein and DNA (Stern et al. 2007a; Zhang et al. 2008a,b).

In order to immobilize PNA on the SiNW surface in the study, APTES was used to convert the silanol groups of the SiNW surface to amines. Since APTES is amine-terminated, a bifunctional linker is required to bind the amine-terminated PNA probe onto the surface. The bifunctional linker employed in this study is glutaraldehyde, which constitutes of two aldehyde terminals. One end would bind to the anime-terminated APTES and the other end free to immobilize the amine-terminated PNA. PNA can serve as a favorable sensing element because it has a neutral backbone, which reduces electrostatic repulsion between the PNA and miRNA duplex, hence resulting in superior PNA–miRNA recognition with higher stability and affinity, and greater specificity. In brief, the array was thoroughly cleaned by ethanol and acetone to remove contaminants. The silanation was performed by immersing the chips into 2% APTES in a mixture of ethanol/water (95%/5%, v/v) for 2 hr. The chips were washed with absolute ethanol three times and blow dried. Then they were treated with 2.5% glutaraldehyde solution in water for 1 hr, and thoroughly washed with water. 10 µM PNA in 1× SSC was incubated with the arrays in a humid atmosphere at room temperature overnight. Unreacted PNA probes were removed by washing the chips with 1× SSC three times after immobilization of the PNA.

Electrical Detection

The Debye length is an important parameter in the SiNW biosensor, which affects the sensing performance. The Debye length is the distance over which significant charge separation can take place. In other words, longer Debye length is expected to be long enough to ensure less charge screened by using dilute buffer solution with low electrolyte concentrations. Hence the detection sensitivity can be maximized by choosing the appropriate buffer for measurement. As the SiNW biosensor is used to detect miRNA from the total RNA extracted from cancer cells, a steady-state measurement rather than a real-time detection is employed in this study. To enable direct detection of miRNA in the impurity, the sample does not need to be desalted for replacing the high ionic strength buffer in the sample with low ionic strength buffer, and can directly be incubated with the PNA-functionalized SiNW biosensor. After PNA-miRNA hybridization, the measurement could be conducted in 0.01 × SSC, which has low ionic strength and in reverse long Debye length. The sensor response is referred to as resistance change before and after miRNA hybridized to the PNA immobilized on the SiNW surface.

The sensing experiments for miRNA were performed by measuring the resistance change of SiNWs before and after PNA-miRNA hybridization. The SiNW resistances were measured between the two terminals, source (S) and drain (D) electrodes with Alessi REL-6100 probe station (Cascade Microtech, Beaverton, OR). The resistance change before and after the hybridization is caused by the introduction of negatively charged miRNA since PNA is neutral. Hybridization and electrical measurements were carried out in 0.01× SSC (0.15 mM sodium citrate, 1.5 mM NaCl, PH 7.4) buffer. Hybridization was conducted by incubating the sensor chips with varying concentrations of miRNA in 0.01 × SSC at room temperature for 1 hr. Unhybridized miRNAs were removed by washing the chips with the same buffer for three cycles of 5 min. The attachment methods used in the experiment are covalently binding, which provides better stability and less non-specific hybridization for DNA sensing. In this experiment, a different SiNW chip was used for each individual measurement. Each chip consists of 100 NWs in an array format. Data were analyzed as an average of the responses from 25 parallel measurements.

Specificity of Silicon Nanowire Biosensor

As with other types of biosensors, high specificity is crucial for the success of miRNA biosensors. Specifically, the detection of miRNA sequence variations plays an important role in the diagnosis of genetic-related diseases like cancer, especially for early stage treatment and monitoring. Among the different types of cancers caused by sequence alterations, sequence-specific mismatch has the most importance, yet is extremely difficult to detect, especially for SNP.

First of all, some control experiments were carried out to assess the nature of the SiNW biosensor. The basal signal of the devices in which only the hybridization buffer ($0.01 \times$ SSC) was added was conducted. Addition of the buffer solution exhibited negligible change in resistance. No substantial change in resistance was observed when a target miRNA was applied to the devices that did not have a PNA probe covalently attached, which means that barely any non-specific adsorption of miRNA on the SiNW surface is found. These control experiments suggest that addition of abundant buffer solution and non-specific interaction of negatively charged miRNA is negligible, which make it easy for ultrasensitive detection of miRNA.

The hybridization specificity of the SiNW biosensor for detection of miRNA was demonstrated using let-7b, let-7c and non-complementary miRNA sequence. When the targeted species, miRNAs complementary to the immobilized PNA, are present, resistance change occurs whereas, when they are non-complementary, resistance change is minimal. As each wire is provided with independent metal contacts, resistance can be individually measured. The miRNAs for hybridization were complementary let-7b, one-base mismatched let-7c, and noncomplementary control. As expected, the specific resistance change was obtained from hybridization of let-7b to the SiNW biosensor immobilized with PNA. As can be seen in Fig. 13.4, a significant change (~47.2%) was observed when 1 nM let-7b was used, whereas only a negligible change was obtained when the same concentration of control was applied to the SiNW biosensor. To evaluate the capability of the SiNW biosensor for discrimination of single base mismatch in miRNAs, let-7c was tested at the same concentration. The increase in resistance for let-7c was ~7.9% which is much lower than that of let-7b. The high specificity suggests that the SiNW biosensor allows for label-free discrimination between the fully matched and mismatched miRNAs, especially discrimination between signal base differences, as in SNP, offering a unique advantage over other technologies which require labeling and additional tags.

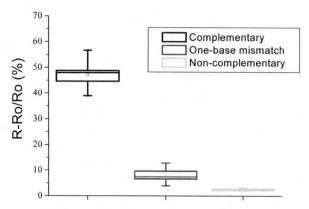

Figure 13.4. Sequence specificity of the PNA-functionalized SiNW biosensor for detection of miRNA. Hybridization specificity demonstrated by distinguishable response of the PNA-functionalized SiNW biosensors to fully complementary, one-base mismatched, and non-complementary miRNA sequences. (Reprinted with permission from [Zhang et al. 2009a]. Copyright 2009 Elsevier Science).

Detection Sensitivity of Silicon Nanowire Biosensor

Because of the significance of miRNA in carcinogenesis, miRNAs in blood may be unique biomarkers for early diagnosis of human cancers. To assist early detection of miRNA, the development of techniques allowing highly sensitive and specific direct detection will ultimately be desirable.

The sensitivity for detection of miRNA is investigated by applying various concentrations of miRNA to the PNA-functionalized SiNW biosensor. The sensor response is referred to as the resistance change before and after hybridization of miRNA with PNA. In the study, different known concentrations of let-7b were applied to the SiNW biosensor immobilized with PNA. The SiNW resistance was then recorded before and after hybridization, and the change between the two values was monitored. Concentration-dependent detection of let-7b by the PNA-functionalized SiNW biosensor is shown in Fig. 13.5. In theory, the resistance change before and after PNA-miRNA hybridization primarily depends on the amount of charge layer contributed by miRNA. The more the target miRNA molecules hybridized, the more negative charges accumulated on the SiNW surface, thus the higher the resistance increase. As described above, an obvious resistance increase was obtained when 1 nM let-7b was hybridized to the PNA-functionalized SiNW biosensor. It was observed that resistance change drops as a function of varying concentrations of let-7b. A 7.3% response was still observed while 1 fM let-7b was employed, which is distinguishable from the control signals (S/N>3). This indicates that ultralow concentrations of miRNA can effectively be detectable down to 1 fM with the biosensor

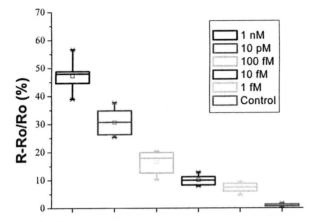

Figure 13.5. Sensitivity of the PNA-functionalized SiNW biosensor for detection of miRNA. Response of the PNA-functionalized SiNW biosensors to the complementary miRNA (let-7b) of varying concentrations. The response drops as a function of decreasing concentrations of let-7b. Ultralow concentrations of miRNA down to 1 fM can effectively be detected with the SiNW biosensor. (Reprinted with permission from [Zhang et al. 2009a]. Copyright 2009 Elsevier Science).

used in the work without labeling/tagging. Remarkably, the detection limit demonstrated in the study is one order of magnitude lower than that demonstrated by other indirect approaches such as nanoparticle-based (Gao and Yang 2006) detection of miRNA. Moreover, the sensitivity is one order of magnitude higher than that reported for detection of DNA (Zhang et al. 2008a). This phenomena can probably be explained by higher thermal stability and melting temperature (Tm) of the PNA-RNA duplex than that of a PNA-DNA duplex. Practically, the ultrahigh sensitivity of the assay allows for direct miRNA expression profiling application.

PNA, an artificially-synthesized polymer similar to DNA, is commonly used in biological research, especially in DNA or RNA hybridizations. Because PNA has no phosphate groups in its backbone, the binding of PNA/DNA or PNA/RNA strands is stronger than that of DNA/DNA or DNA/RNA duplexes due to the lacking of electrostatic repulsion. To compare the sensing performance between the PNA-functionalized SiNW biosensor and the DNA-functionalized SiNW biosensor, a DNA molecule, whose sequence is same as that of PNA, modified with amine groups at its 5′ end (sequence of DNA used: 5′-NH$_2$-AACCACACAACCTACTACCTCA-3′), was utilized to be attached to the SiNW surface and the DNA-functionalized SiNW biosensor was used to detect 1 nM let-7b using the same experimental conditions as mentioned above. As shown in Fig. 13.6, a smaller resistance change (~14.3%) was observed compared to that generated by PNA-miRNA hybridization. Because DNA, as a probe molecule, is negatively charged, thereby decreasing the signal-to-noise ratio, The DNA-functionalized SiNW

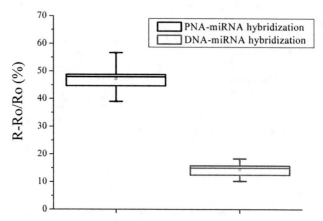

Figure 13.6. Different sensing performance of the PNA-functionalized and the DNA-functionalized SiNW biosensors for detection of miRNA. Comparison of response of the PNA-functionalized and the DNA-functionalized SiNW biosensors to the complementary miRNA. The PNA-functionalized SiNW biosensor generates higher change than the DNA-functionalized SiNW biosensor does, pointing to a higher sensitivity (Reprinted with permission from [Zhang et al. 2009a]. Copyright 2009 Elsevier Science).

biosensor generates lower change than the PNA-functionalized SiNW biosensor does, pointing to a lower sensitivity. This experiment implies that PNA is more preferable to be functionalized with the SiNW biosensor for detection of miRNA than DNA, in case one expects a higher sensitivity of a biosensor. Also, this PNA-functionalized SiNW biosensor could be applied in medical diagnosis of various miRNAs in cancer cells by simply varying the sequences of the PNA capture probes.

Detection of miRNA in Total RNA from Cancer Cell

In view of miRNA importance in cancer diagnostics, miRNA detection methods should be rapid, sensitive, selective, and direct, require minimal amounts of sample, and be capable of in situ application. Current assays usually require enrichment and amplification to isolate miRNA from the cell. However, the overall analysis time is increased by this step, and the sensitivity is also affected by the efficiency of the isolation procedure. Furthermore, large samples are required to enable the isolation process. Consequently, development of the label-free, direct, ultrasensitive method for miRNA detection in real samples is of great significance.

To demonstrate the direct detection using the PNA-functionalized SiNW biosensor, the assay was further identified for detection of miRNA in real sample by analyzing let-7b in total RNA extracted from Hela cells. Aliquots of the total RNA were diluted with 0.01×SSC and subsequently applied to the PNA-functionalized SiNW biosensor for 1 hr. A resistance increase was achieved and the results were normalized with respect to the total RNA. The concentration of let-7b detectable in the total RNA extracted from Hela cells is found to be $2.15 \pm 0.25 \times 10^7$ copies/µg RNA, which is in agreement with previously published data of miRNA expression profiling (Nelson et al. 2004), and also consistent with recently reported data of miRNA detection using target-guided formation of conducting polymer nanowires in nanogaps (Fan et al. 2007). The results suggest that the PNA-functionalized SiNW biosensor enables direct detection of miRNA in total RNA from cancer cell without introducing tagging steps, and is suitable for the demand for early detection of miRNA in cancer diagnostics due to its high sensitivity. The relative standard deviation of the SiNW biosensors was found to be <15%, which indicates a satisfactory reproducibility for label-free and direct detection of miRNA by using the assay.

KEY FACTS OF microRNA

- miRNA was discovered in 1993 by Victor Ambros, Rosalind Lee and Rhonda Feinbaum during a study of the gene lin-14 in C. elegans development.
- miRNA is a class of small endogenous noncoding RNA molecule, on average only 22 nucleotides long and is found in all eukaryotic cells.
- miRNA fine tunes the gene expression at the posttranscriptional level through binding to complementary sequences on target messenger RNA transcripts (mRNAs).
- miRNAs play important roles in diverse aspects of cancer such as proliferation, apoptosis, invasion/metastasis, and angiogenesis.
- miRNAs exhibit an expression pattern characteristic of tumor type, stage, or other clinical variables. Thus miRNAs can be used for cancer diagnosis and prognosis.

DEFINITIONS

- Silicon nanowire. One of semiconducting NWs, can be prepared as single-crystal structures with several nanometers. Compared to planar silicon devices produced by microelectronic technology, they can be prepared as p- or n-type materials and configured as field effect transistors that exhibit higher sensitivity due to very small dimension of NWs10s of nanometers or less, and thus resulting in large surface-to-volume ratio.
- Biosensor. An analytical device that uses specific biochemical reactions mediated by isolated enzymes, DNA, immunosystems,

tissues, organelles or whole cells to detect chemical compounds usually by electrical, thermal or optical signals.

- Cancer. A class of disease in which a group of cells display uncontrolled growth through division beyond normal limits, invasion that intrudes upon and destroys adjacent tissues, and sometimes metastasis, in which cancer cells spread to other locations in the body via the lymph or blood.

- miRNA in cancer. It is considered as a clinically-relevant good biomarker for important tumor behavior. It now appears that at least some of the more than 200 miRNA sequences discovered in the human genome contribute to the development of cancer. It is demonstrated that miRNAs are not only part of the process that leads to cancer but in some cases may act as oncogenes or tumor suppressors in their own right. Furthermore, miRNA levels in tumors may possibly be used to classify cancers, even those of ambiguous origin.

- Early disease detection. The use of screening tests to find health problems before symptoms appear and diagnostic tests, medical exams, and self-exams to find a disease or other health problem early in its course.

SUMMARY POINTS

- An ultrasensitive, label-free and direct hybridization assay for detection of miRNA based on the SiNW biosensor is described.

- The assay shows a label-free hybridization method for direct detection of miRNA by eliminating sophisticated processes for labeling/conjugating and simplifying the detection steps.

- The PNA-functionalized SiNW biosensor is capable of detecting 1 fM miRNA, which is one order of magnitude higher than that demonstrated by other indirect approaches like nanoparticle-based detection of miRNA.

- The biosensor is capable of identifying fully matched versus mismatched miRNA sequences, especially discriminating between signal base differences, as in SNP.

- The developed SiNW biosensor enables high sensitive and direct detection of miRNA in total RNA from the cancer cell, which is suitable for the demand of early detection of miRNA in cancer diagnostics.

ACKNOWLEDGMENT

The author would like to thank Dr. Ajay Agarwal and Ms. She Mein Wong for SiNW biosensor chip fabrication; Mr. Huiyi Chua Jay and Ms. Ru-Ern Chee for biotesting.

ABBREVIATIONS

APTES	:	3-Aminopropyltriethoxysilane
APTMS	:	3-(Trimethoxysilyl)propyl aldehyde
CMOS	:	Complementary metal-oxide semiconductor
DNA	:	Deoxyribonucleic acid
DUV	:	Deep Ultra-Violet
FET	:	Field-effect transistor
HF	:	Hydrofluoric acid
LOD	:	Limit of detection
MPTMS	:	3-Mercaptopropyltrimethoxysilane
mRNA	:	Messenger RNA
miRNA	:	microRNA
NW	:	Nanowire
PBS	:	Phosphate buffered saline
PDMS	:	Polydimethylsiloxane
PNA	:	Peptide nucleic acid
POC	:	Point-of-care
RNA	:	Ribonucleic acid
RT-PCR	:	Reverse transcriptase polymerase chain reaction
SAM	:	Self-assembled monolayer
SEM	:	Scanning electron microscopy
Si	:	Silicon
SiNW	:	Silicon nanowire
siRNA	:	Small interfering RNA
SNAP	:	Superlattice NW pattern transfer
SNP	:	Single nucleotide polymorphism
SOI	:	Silicon-on-insulator
SPR	:	Surface plasmon resonance
Tm	:	Melting temperature
VLS	:	Vapor-liquid-solid

REFERENCES

Bunimovich YL, YS Shin, W-S Yeo, M Amori, G Kwong and JR Heath. 2006. Quantitative real-time measurements of DNA hybridization with alkylated nonoxidized silicon nanowires in electrolyte solution, J Am Chem Soc 128: 16323–16331.

Cattani-Scholz A, D Pedone, M Dubey, S Neppl, B Nickel, P Feulner, J Schwartz, G Abstreiter and M Tornow. 2008. Organophosphonate-based PNA-functionalization of silicon nanowires for label-free DNA detection. ACS Nano 2: 1653–1660.

Chua J, RE Chee, A Agarwal, SM Wong and G-J Zhang. 2009. Label-free electrical detection of cardiac biomarker with CMOS-compatible silicon nanowire sensor arrays. Anal Chem 81: 6266–6271.

Cui Y, QQ Wei, HK Park and CM Lieber. 2001. Nanowire nanosensors for highly sensitive and selective detection of biological and chemical species. Science 293: 1289–1292.

Fan Y, XT Chen, AD Trigg, C-H Tung, JM Kong and ZQ Gao. 2007. Detection of microRNAs using target-guided formation of conducting polymer nanowires in nanogaps. J Am Chem Soc 129: 5437–5443.

Fang S, HJ Lee, AW Wark and RM Corn. 2006. Attomole microarray detection of microRNAs by nanoparticle-amplified SPR imaging measurements of surface polyadenylation reactions. J Am Chem Soc 128: 14044–14046.

Gao ZQ and ZC Yang. 2006. Ultrasensitive detection of microRNA using electrocatalytic nanoparticle tags. Anal Chem 78: 1470–1477.

Gao Z-Q, A Agarwal, AD Trigg, N Singh, C Fang, C-H Tung, Y Fan, KD Buddharaju and J-M Kong. 2007. Silicon nanowire arrays for ultrasensitive label-free detection of DNA. Anal Chem 79: 3291–3297.

Hahm J-I and CM Lieber. 2004. Direct ultrasensitive electrical detection of DNA and DNA sequence variations using nanowire nanosensors. Nano Lett 4: 51–54.

Kennedy D. 2002. Breakthrough of the year. Science 298: 2283.

Lee RC, RL Feinbaum and V Ambros. 1993. The *C. elegans* heterochronic gene *lin-4* encodes small RNAs with antisense complementarity to *lin-14*. Cell 75: 843–854.

Li Z, Y Chen, X Li, TI Kamins, K Nauka and RS Williams. 2004. Sequence-specific label-free DNA sensors based on silicon nanowires, Nano Lett 4: 245–247.

Liu CG, GA Calin, B Meloon, N Gamliel, C Sevignani, M Ferracin, DC Dumitru, M Shimizu, S Zupo, M Dono, H Alder, F Bullrich, M Negrini and CM Croce. 2004. An oligonucleotide microchip for genome-wide microRNA profiling in human and mouse tissues. Proc Natl Acad Sci USA 101: 9740–9744.

Lu J, G Getz, EA Miska, E Alvarez-Saavedra, J Lamb, D Peck, A Sweet-Cordero, BL Ebert, RH Mak, AA Ferrando, JR Downing, T Jacks, HR Horvitz and TR Golub. 2005. MicroRNA expression profiles classify human cancers. Nature 435: 834–838.

Lu W and CM Lieber. 2006. Semiconductor nanowires, J Phys D: Appl Phys 39: R387–R406.

Miska EA, E Alvarez-Saavedra, M Townsend, A Yoshii, N Sestan, P Rakic, M Constantine-Paton and HR Horvitz. 2004. Microarray analysis of microRNA expression in the developing mammalian brain. Genome Biol 5: R68.

Nelson PT, DA Baldwin, LM Scearce, JC Oberholtzer, JW Tobias and Z Mourelatos. 2004. Microarray-based, high-throughput gene expression profiling of microRNAs. Nat Methods 1: 155–161.

Patolsky F, G Zheng, O Hayden, M Lakadamyali, X Zhuang and CM Lieber. 2004. Electrical detection of single viruses. Proc Natl Acad Sci USA 101: 14017–14022.

Reinhart BJ, FJ Slack, M Basson, AE Pasquinelli, JC Bettinger, AE Rougvie, HR Horvitz and G Ruvkun. 2000. The 21-nucleotide let-7 RNA regulates developmental timing in Caenorhabditis elegans. Nature 403: 901–906.

Stern E, JF Klemic, DA Routenberg, PN Wyremebak, DB Turner-Evans, AD Hamilton, DA LaVan, TM Fahmy and MA Reed. 2007a. Label-free immunodetection with CMOS-compatible semiconducting nanowires. Nature 445: 519–522.

Stern E, R Wagner, FJ Sigworth, R Breaker, TM Fahmy and MA Reed. 2007b. Importance of the Debye screening length on nanowire field effect transistor sensors. Nano Lett 7: 3405–3409.

Valoczi A, C Hornyik, N Varga, J Burgyan, S Kauppinen and Z Havelda. 2004. Sensitive and specific detection of microRNAs by northern blot analysis using LNA-modified oligonucleotide probes. Nucleic Acids Res 32: e175.

Zhang G-J, J Chua, RE Chee, A Agarwal, SM Wong, KD Buddharaju and N Balasubramanian . 2008a. Highly sensitive measurements of PNA-DNA hybridization using oxide-etched silicon nanowire biosensors. Biosens Bioelectron 23: 1701–1707.

Zhang G-J, G Zhang, J Chua, RE Chee, EH Wong, A Agarwal, KD Buddharaju, N Singh, ZQ Gao and N Balasubramanian. 2008b. DNA sensing by silicon nanowire: charge layer distance dependence. Nano Lett 8: 1066–1070.

Zhang G-J, J Chua, RE Chee, A Agarwal and SM Wong. 2009a. Label-free direct detection of miRNAs with silicon nanowire biosensors. Biosens Bioelectron 24: 2504–2508.

Zhang G-J, ZH Luo, M Huang, GK Tay, E-J Lim and Y Chen. 2009b. Highly sensitive and selective label-free detection of cardiac biomarkers in blood serum with silicon nanowire biosensors. IEDM Tech Dig P 607–609.

Zhang G-J, L Zhang, MJ Huang, ZHH Luo, GKI Tay, E-J A Lim, TG Kang and Y Chen. 2010a. Silicon nanowire biosensor for highly sensitive and rapid detection of dengue virus. Sens Actuators B: Chem 146: 138–144.

Zhang G-J, ZHH Luo, MJ Huang, GKI Tay and E-J A Lim. 2010b. Morpholino-functionalized silicon nanowire biosensor for sequence-specific label-free detection of DNA, Biosens Bioelectron 25: 2447–2453.

Zhang G-J, MJ Huang, ZHH Luo, GK Tay, E-J A Lim, ET Liu and JS Thomsen. 2010c. Highly sensitive and reversible silicon nanowire biosensor to study nuclear hormone receptor protein and response element DNA interactions. Biosens Bioelectron 26: 365–370.

Zheng G, F Patolsky, Y Cui, WU Wang and CM Lieber. 2005. Multiplexed electrical detection of cancer markers with nanowire sensor arrays. Nat Biotechnol 23: 1294–1301.

14

Biosensors for BCR-ABL Activity and Their Application to Cancer

Yusuke Ohba,[1,a,*] Stephanie Darmanin,[1,2] Tatsuaki
Mizutani,[1,3] Masumi Tsuda[1,b] and Takeshi Kondo[4]

ABSTRACT

The emergence of imatinib mesylate; designed to inhibit the causative
protein of chronic myeloid leukemia—BCR-ABL, has radically
innovated the treatment of this disease, making it now controllable by
oral drugs. However resistance and intolerance are still of concern in a
substantial number of patients. A recently developed biosensor, which
utilizes the major BCR-ABL substrate CrkL, green fluorescent protein
technology, and the principle of Förster resonance energy transfer,

[1]Laboratory of Pathophysiology and Signal Transduction; Hokkaido University Graduate
School of Medicine, N15W7, Kita-ku, Sapporo 060-8638, Japan.
[a]E-mail: yohba@med.hokudai.ac.jp
[b]E-mail: tsudam@med.hokudai.ac.jp
[2]*Current Affiliation:* Centre for Infectious Medicine F59, Department of Medicine, Karolinska
Institutet, Karolinska University Hospital Huddinge, Stockholm 14186, Sweden;
E-mail: stephanie.darmanin@ki.se
[3]*Current Affiliation:* Ludwig Boltzmann Institute for Cancer Research, Waehringerstrasse
13A, A-1090, Vienna, Austria; E-mail: Mizutani.Tatsuaki@lbicr.lbg.ac.at
[4]Department of Hematology & Oncology, Hokkaido University Graduate School of
Medicine, N15W7, Kita-ku, Sapporo 060-8638, Japan.
E-mail: t-kondoh@med.hokudai.ac.jp
*Corresponding author

List of abbreviations after the text.

to overcome these issues in chronic myeloid leukemia treatment is introduced here. This novel diagnostic method for the measurement of BCR-ABL activity has a higher sensitivity than that of established techniques. It can be used as an accurate gauge of BCR-ABL kinase activity in small numbers of living cells, and is a useful tool for the detection of minor drug-resistant populations, as well as the prediction of the clinical course after drug treatment and future onset of drug resistance using patient cells. In consideration of its quick and practical nature, this method is potentially a promising tool for the prediction of both current and future therapeutic responses in individual patients with chronic myeloid leukemia, which will surely be beneficial for both patients and clinicians. Moreover, the biosensor now provides a new window for the application of fluorescent proteins in the practical scene of clinical medicine, whereas to date, their contributions have only been limited to basic research fields.

INTRODUCTION

Cancer is a disease characterized by the autonomous, aimless and excessive proliferation of cells, in which genetic abnormality is accumulated. The cells invade their surrounding tissues and metastasize to distant organs (expansion of cancer), leading to disturbance of normal homeostasis and, in turn, death of host human beings. Due to these DNA abnormalities the proteins are synthesized based on a flawed blueprint, and either leave the mitogenic signal switched on or suppress cell death, resulting in cancer cell transformation. Therefore, cell signaling, especially that regulating proliferation, is intimately associated with oncogenesis—cancer cells possess a chaotic signal transduction system compared to the organized one in normal cells.

Molecular targeted drugs are developed based on accumulating evidence from cell signaling research, and are aimed at a specific protein identified as the one causing cell signaling irregularity in a certain disease or condition. They were therefore perceived as quixotic medicines, with greater benefits and fewer side effects thanks to their direct action. While this strategy sounds simple, previously available cancer therapy has been far from ideal. As for conventional cancer treatments, both anti-cancer drugs that globally obstruct cell proliferation and radiation therapy are utilized based on the premise that the proliferation of cancer cells is faster than that of healthy cells, which is a phenotype consequently obtained by cancer cells. Thus, these conventional drugs, apart from suppressing cell proliferation, have more or less negative effects on normal cell homeostasis, causing different side effects. On the other hand, the mechanism-based nature of molecular targeted drugs may help balance the competing goals of efficacy and safety. Therefore, the development of such medicine is urgently needed to supplement, and someday possibly replace, currently available agents, which is already a reality for the treatment of chronic myeloid leukemia (CML), as described below.

CML is a hematological malignancy involving the transformation of hematopoietic stem cells in the bone marrow and is characterized by the formation of an abnormal chromosome (Philadelphia chromosome, Ph1) and the expression of its transcript BCR-ABL (Kurzrock et al. 1998). About 8,000 people in Japan and 63,000 worldwide, who represent about 1/5 to 1/4 of all leukemia patients, suffer from this disease. Emergence of the molecular targeted drug, imatinib mesylate (IM), the therapeutic outcomes of which are better than other options, radically innovated therapy for CML, and provides a way to control the disease other than bone marrow transplantation. On the other hand, it is also true that there are a considerable number of patients for whom IM does not work (this can either occur from the beginning or also during IM treatment). The mechanisms of IM resistance can be in a manner dependent on or independent of mutations in the Abl kinase domain, and these are reported to happen at approximately a 1:1 ratio. In the former case, because the second-generation drugs nilotinib (NL) and dasatinib (DS) are now available for treatment of IM-resistant patients, the effectiveness of these medicines might be predicted according to the kind of mutation present. When however, there is no mutation, the only way in which to evaluate drug efficacy is to actually prescribe the drug and follow the course of treatment by blood and bone marrow tests for several months, a year, or more. Given that treatment with an ineffective medicine cannot be expected to hamper progression of the disease, ideally the suitable medication should be used from the start. To solve this problem and to optimally select the effective drug for each individual patient, it is required to develop a technique/s that deciphers the effect of every medicine separately on patients' leukemic cells and detects the presence of any resistant cells before starting therapy. To overcome this issue we hereby introduce a novel diagnostic method based on the use of bio-imaging technology and fluorescent proteins.

BASIC TECHNOLOGIES FOR THE DEVELOPMENT OF THE DIAGNOSTIC METHOD

First, we want to briefly review the basic technologies that support the diagnostic method presented here.

Green Fluorescent Protein (GFP)

Green fluorescent protein (GFP) is a fluorescent protein, isolated from the luminous organ of the jellyfish *Aequorea victoria* by Dr. Osamu Shimomura (Morise et al. 1974). It is probably no exaggeration that GFP has been shedding light on cell biology since its cDNA was isolated in 1992 (Prasher et al. 1992). By now, many mutants of the original GFP as well as a range of fluorescent proteins originating from cnidarians other than jellyfish are commercially available, which together build a palette of abundant color variations. The main reason why GFP is so revolutionary is the fact that it can be easily introduced into cells by means of DNA transfection. It has therefore been widely used to visualize protein dynamics and environmental changes in living cells, though uptil now its use was restricted to the basic research field.

Förster Resonance Energy Transfer (FRET)

FRET in its abbreviated form might be more familiar than fully spelling it out: Förster resonance energy transfer. FRET is a phenomenon of non-irradiation excitation energy transfer from a donor chromophore to an acceptor chromophore (Miyawaki 2003). A niche in molecular biological research was established for it by the TaqMan probe for real-time PCR, which utilizes this principle. In most cases of GFP-based FRET, a pair of cyan- and yellow-emitting mutants of GFP (CFP and YFP) is used as the donor and the acceptor, respectively. FRET can be observed only when CFP and YFP are very close to each other, ca. 10 nm (Fig. 14.1A).

PICKLES (PHOSPHORYLATION INDICATOR OF CrkL *EN* SUBSTRATE)

Design

The causative protein of CML, BCR-ABL, is a protein tyrosine kinase which activates a range of signaling pathways related to malignant transformation through the phosphorylation of tyrosine residues on various substrates in CML cells. CrkL is an all-star representative of the substrates of BCR-ABL, and participates in various processes of the malignant transformation, including cell proliferation, invasion, and cell death, through its phosphorylation.

CrkL harbors one Src homology 2 (SH2) domain and two SH3 domains in addition to the tyrosine residue that is phosphorylated by BCR-ABL (Fig. 14.1B). Of these, the SH2 domain possesses the ability

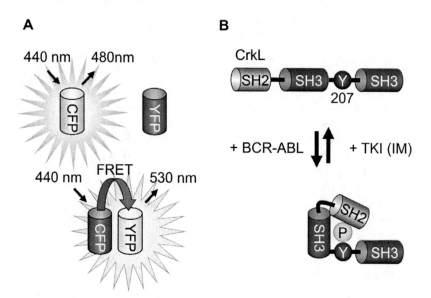

Figure 14.1. Schematic representation of the principle of Förster resonance energy transfer (FRET) and the conformational change in CrkL. **(A)** The principle of FRET. When cyan-emitting mutant of fluorescent protein (CFP) exists alone, and is excited by light having a wavelength of 440 nm, it will emit light at a wavelength of 480 nm. In contrast, when yellow fluorescent protein (YFP) exists close to CFP, radiation-less energy transfer between CFP and YFP acts as a converter from 440 nm light to 530 nm light. As a result, this phenomenon can be used as a molecular ruler to measure the distance between CFP and YFP in living cells; **(B)** Structure of CrkL. CrkL consists of a Src homology 2 (SH2) domain, an SH3 domain, a tyrosine residue phosphorylated by BCR-ABL, and another SH3 domain. Due to SH2 domain binding to phosphorylated tyrosine, CrkL phosphorylation by BCR-ABL results in its conformational change into a compact form. CrkL reverts to an open form upon BCR-ABL inactivation by tyrosine kinase inhibitors (TKIs) such as imatinib (IM). *Unpublished.*

to bind to phosphorylated tyrosine, leading to structural changes upon phosphorylation by BCR-ABL or the inhibition of BCR-ABL activity in response to drug treatment (Fig. 14.1B). The biosensor for BCR-ABL activity, Pickles, was designed based on this characteristic of CrkL; CrkL is sandwiched between CFP and YFP. CrkL phosphorylation by BCR-ABL triggers a structural change in CrkL, leading to an increase in FRET efficiency due to the close proximity of CFP and YFP, and vice versa, inhibition of the kinase activity by inhibitors results in a decrease in FRET (Fig. 14.2).

Specifications

The final construct of this biosensor molecule could not be made just by adding CFP and YFP to both ends of CrkL. Some fine-tuning, including

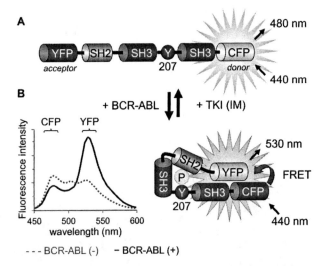

Figure 14.2. A prototype of phosphorylation indicator of CrkL *en* substrate (Pickles). **(A)** An acceptor, YFP, and a donor, CFP, are added to N- and C-termini of CrkL, respectively. A conformational change induced by tyrosine phosphorylation of CrkL results in the close proximity of CFP and YFP, leading to an increase in FRET efficiency. Dephosphorylation of CrkL in contrast results in low FRET efficiency. **(B)** Typical spectra of Pickles in the presence (solid line) or absence (dashed) of BCR-ABL are shown. *Modified from Clin. Cancer Res. 16: 3964–3975, 2010. Note: Authors of articles published in AACR Journals are permitted to reproduce parts of their article, including figures and tables, in books, reviews, or subsequent research articles they write without requesting permission from the AACR.*

a truncation in CrkL, circular permutations in CFP, and a monomeric mutation in YFP, was required for its development for clinical application, and detailed procedures are described in our research paper (Mizutani et al. 2010). As for the final product, version 2.31 (Pickles_2.31), its FRET efficiency increased along with phosphorylation by BCR-ABL by about 80~100%, in a manner specific for BCR-ABL (and its cellular counterpart c-Abl) as opposed to other non-receptor type tyrosine kinases tested. In addition, when we tested its dose-dependent response to IM, Pickles could detect the drug effect at lower concentrations than those of other existing techniques e.g. the western blotting method, resulting in a wider measureable range (Fig. 14.3A). Moreover, a faithful time-dependent decrease in FRET efficiency could be observed in the drug-treated cells compared to the control cells with time-lapse microscopy for the evaluation of drug efficacy in tumor cells (Fig. 14.3B). Figure 14.3B represents data of five cells, which means that just five cells are enough to obtain accurate evaluation of the drug efficacy. Furthermore, the time required for evaluation can be assumed to be about 12 hr; BCR-ABL activity reached a nadir 3–6 hr after drug treatment. The diagnosis project that we are currently setting up aims to obtain results

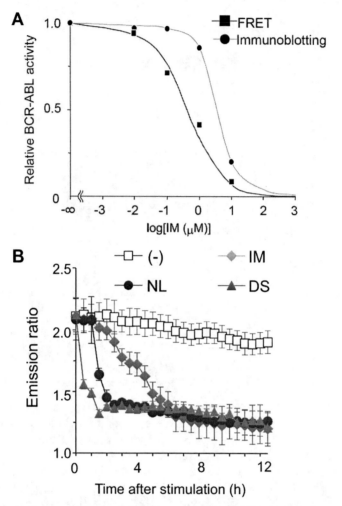

Figure 14.3. Properties of Pickles. **(A)** Higher sensitivity of Pickles than immunoblotting. 293F cells expressing Pickles along with BCR-ABL were treated with various doses of imatinib (IM) for 24 h. The cells were then lysed in buffer and subjected to fluorescence spectrometry and immunoblotting using anti-phosphorylated CrkL (pCrkL) antibody, where BCR-ABL activities were calculated by the emission ratio of Pickles and the intensities of the bands representing pCrkL, respectively. BCR-ABL activity relative to control, untreated samples is plotted at each concentration of IM. **(B)** K562 chronic myeloid leukemia cells were transfected with the expression vector for Pickles and, after 24 hr, subjected to time-lapse fluorescence microscopy. During the observation period, indicated drugs were added into culture media, and emission ratio, which represents FRET efficiency and thus BCR-ABL activity, were plotted against time. Values represent mean ± SD of five cells analyzed. *(A) is unpublished and (B) is modified from Clin. Cancer Res. 16: 3964–3975, 2010. Note: Authors of articles published in AACR Journals are permitted to reproduce parts of their article, including figures and tables, in books, reviews, or subsequent research articles they write without requesting permission from the AACR.*

within 48 hr, including the time required for protein expression, after the patients' tumor cells are collected.

Pickles—Special Features

Originally, GFP-based FRET technology has been used to observe spatiotemporal protein activation in living cells. Therefore, the most prominent feature of our Pickles system is that we can perform evaluation of drug responsiveness at a single cell level by using FRET technology. In fact, a drug-resistant cell population of 1% or less could be distinguished from other drug-sensitive cells. In our system, in which a researcher manually observes a few hundreds of cells with a microscope, 1% is the highest sensitivity. In this regard, we also tried using similar analyses by combining immunofluorescence with an antibody specific for phosphorylated CrkL and a flow cytometer, which can simultaneously analyze significantly higher cell numbers; however, unexpectedly, the detectability of resistant cells was the same as that in our system. A possible reason why better sensitivity was not achieved using the flow cytometer might be the noise of the detector per se (unpublished data). Therefore, this fact consequentially highlights the low noise and high potential of our system, indicating that a less resistant cell can be identified if, in the future, the number of analyzed cells is increased by the automation of image acquisition with computer-controlled architecture. Moreover, it is also possible to examine whether any other medicines are effective for drug-resistant cells, if these tumor cells, which are alive after analysis, are inspected again with another medicine. From a diagnostics viewpoint it is good that fewer cells are required for analysis, but more importantly, it is advantageous that a next therapeutic option can be offered to a patient who has resistant cells.

Gaining Insight into Disease Mechanics

The mutations of BCR-ABL and their relationship to drug susceptibility have been extensively examined, and if the mutation is typical, one can specify the effective drug in a relatively straightforward manner. However, the effectiveness of the second-generation drug NL on the G250E mutation of BCR-ABL (in which glycine 250 is substituted by glutamate) remains controversial among reports (O'Hare et al. 2005; Redaelli et al. 2009). We therefore attempted to investigate this issue by using Pickles. Each individual cell expressing the G250E mutant of BCR-ABL showed diverse NL sensitivities, resulting in a large standard deviation. When we examined the dose-dependent responses of BCR-ABL, we found that drug responsiveness decreased in a way dependent on the expression level

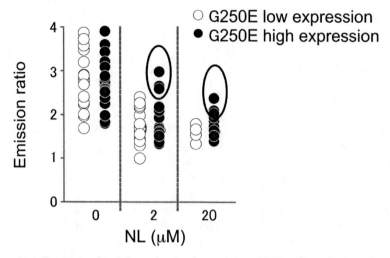

Figure 14.4. Expression level-dependence of sensitivity of BCR-ABL G250E to nilotinib (NL). 293F cells expressing Pickles were transfected with 50 ng (open circle, G250E low) or 2 μg (closed circle, G250E high) of an expression vector for BCR-ABL G250E, treated with 2 or 20 μM NL for 24 h, and analyzed by fluorescence microscopy. *Modified from Clin. Cancer Res. 16: 3964–3975, 2010. Note: Authors of articles published in AACR Journals are permitted to reproduce parts of their article, including figures and tables, in books, reviews, or subsequent research articles they write without requesting permission from the AACR.*

of BCR-ABL only for the G250E mutant and NL combination (Fig. 14.4). Therefore, the expression level of BCR-ABL with the G250E mutation in the patients' tumor cells might have been low in the study that described this mutation as being sensitive to NL, whereas it might have been high in the report that concluded that G250E is a mutation resistant to NL. Although it has already been reported that drug susceptibility decreases in a manner dependent on BCR-ABL expression level (Gorre et al. 2001), this tendency is especially emphasized for the G250E mutant. In either case, it is necessary to take into consideration the expression level of BCR-ABL specifically when this mutation is detected, and drug options may vary according to expression levels.

Evaluation of Drug Efficacy in Patients' Cells

Approval from the Internal Review Board in our research institute has already been obtained for this system, and drug efficacy is being evaluated using patient tumor cells. More than 40 analyses for about 17 cases in all have been executed within the past 2 yr. This project is still ongoing and there are many cases that require careful follow-up hereafter; however from the patients who were incorporated into the study at its earlier stage, we have learnt that our system is able to forecast patients' drug susceptibilities and detects the existence of drug resistant cells by examination prior to starting treatment (except for patients whose drug intolerance was not due to tumor cell drug sensitivity per se e.g. withdrawal due to side effects). Because the examination uses peripheral blood or bone marrow samples obtained by blood specimen collection or bone marrow aspiration, which, although is invasive, is included in conventional tests for CML, no specific burdens are added to patients for analyses to be performed. For each sample, after the separation of mononuclear cells (including the tumor cells) by density gradient centrifugation, cDNA encoding Pickles is introduced into the

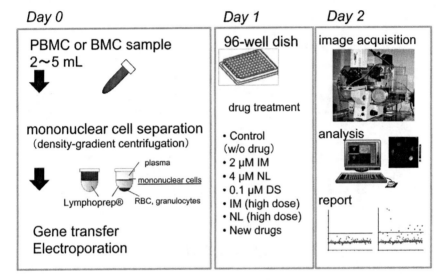

Figure 14.5. Flow chart for the analysis of clinical samples by Pickles. Samples are subjected to density-gradient centrifugation to separate mononuclear cells. The separated cells are then transfected with the expression vector for Pickles using electroporation. On day 1, drug treatment is started, followed by image acquisition and analysis on day 2. *Unpublished.*

cells by electroporation. After confirming fluorescence emission through the expression of Pickles at 24 hr, drug treatment is started and the FRET efficiency in individual cells is calculated from the image data obtained with fluorescence microscopy (Fig. 14.5).

Given that tumor cells in the chronic phase of CML contain cells at each step of differentiation, it is not necessarily the case that BCR-ABL activity is high in all leukemia cells. This phenomenon is reflected in the range of distribution of FRET efficiency. For this reason, a threshold value D-FRET was utilized to identify cells in which BCR-ABL activity is high. This value was mathematically decided from the mean and standard deviation of the FRET efficiency in cells that did not express BCR-ABL. Given that the probability for cells with low BCR-ABL activity to exceed D-FRET is less than 0.003, the BCR-ABL activity of cells that exhibit higher FRET efficiencies than this value is significantly high.

We are currently engaged in drug efficacy evaluation according to the aforementioned processes and criteria. If the cells from both peripheral blood and bone marrow that are above D-FRET disappear by drug treatment, the patient is considered to be sensitive, whereas if they remain above this value we can say that the patient is resistant (Fig. 14.6). In addition, when the distribution pattern of FRET efficiency was carefully compared with the clinical course, we saw that we were able to anticipate the patients' reactivity to drugs, albeit in part, by the analysis performed at the initial stage of the disease. For instance, we experienced a case where drug-resistant cells existed only in the bone marrow sample, while the peripheral blood showed drug susceptibility. At the beginning of treatment, a decrease in the number of tumor cells was observed; however, the patient could achieve neither a complete cytogenetic response nor a major molecular

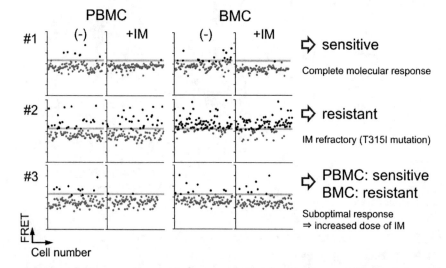

Figure 14.6. Evaluation of drug efficacy in primary CML patient cells using Pickles. Peripheral blood mononuclear cells (PBMC) and bone marrow cells (BMC) were obtained from three CML patients (cases #1–3), transfected with Pickles, and incubated in the presence or absence of 2 µM IM. After 24 hr, the cells were subjected to dual-emission fluorescence microscopy to determine the FRET efficiency. The scatter diagrams show data for 150 randomly chosen cells, which are representative of the total cell population analyzed. Orange lines represent D-FRET. *Modified from Clin. Cancer Res. 16: 3964–3975, 2010. Note: Authors of articles published in AACR Journals are permitted to reproduce parts of their article, including figures and tables, in books, reviews, or subsequent research articles they write without requesting permission from the AACR.*

response after 12 months of therapy (a sub-optimal response) and had to be put on different dosage and ultimately different drugs. One can speculate that the resistant cells that had been detected during the initial examination remained and relapsed.

APPLICATIONS TO AREAS OF HEALTH AND DISEASES

Because of the specific nature of the current technology that is targeted to the chimeric tyrosine kinase BCR-ABL, its application is so far limited to hematological malignancies expressing BCR-ABL: chronic myeloid leukemia and Philadelphia chromosome-positive acute lymphocytic leukemia. However, a similar concept can theoretically be applicable to every cancer for which molecular targeted drugs (preferably small compounds inhibiting tyrosine kinases) are available. Given the inoperability and sample availability of hematological malignancies, these are preferred by us to develop techniques that provide more therapeutic benefits to patients and clinicians.

Future Tasks

In our system, the biosensor is introduced into tumor cells via DNA transfection, and its expression totally depends on the ability of the tumor cell to synthesize the protein. An issue to be solved, therefore, is the fact that the success or failure of this diagnosis can be influenced by the gene introduction efficiency. From our knowledge, different transfection efficiencies can be observed in different patients, even those whose leukemia stage or leukemic cell population is similar to each other. The development of a suitable congenic method is unquestionably needed and this issue is also being looked into.

Another problem is the distribution of this technology to a broad range of clinical sites. As for the analysis, the processes have already been automated by the image processing software MetaMorph (Universal Imaging); most of the image acquisition processes depend on handiwork with a microscope, therefore requiring skilled researchers. The establishment of a system, through which anyone can easily analyze samples e.g. automated image acquisition by a computer-controlled microscope, is also being developed. Alternatively, there is a plan to build up a center to collect samples and analyze them. In this case, because fresh samples are better for gene transfer, it would also be necessary to overcome the problem of preservation and transportation of the samples. After overcoming these issues, we aim to establish this technology for use in leukemia diagnostics as soon as possible.

CONCLUDING REMARKS

Up to now, the fluorescent protein has literally brought a lot of light to biology research. GFP-based FRET is an epoch-making imaging technology; events occurring in living cells can be captured as a color change! However, it has been purely limited to the basic research field until now. The research introduced here is the first step to help GFP widen its appeal on a clinical stage, and is a "pioneer study" for tailor-made medicine (Lu and Wang 2010). However, we believe that for our work to be indeed useful, its use should be made widespread, and we will therefore make a zealous effort to achieve this. The advantage of this technology does not only include the improvement of therapy, but also less time is required to obtain the maximum treatment effect. Moreover, given the high cost of molecular-targeted drugs, the spread of this technology to clinical sites will definitely lead to the practice of both efficient and economical medicine. In addition to the clinical benefits, the specific feature of this system, enabling analysis in living cells may contribute to basic research that gains insight into the mechanism of drug resistance in CML cells.

KEY FACTS

- CML can occur in all age groups, but most commonly in the middle-aged and the elderly with an annual incidence of 1–2 per 100,000 people. The only well-described risk factor for CML is exposure to ionizing radiation e.g. increased rates of CML were seen in people from Hiroshima and Nagasaki who experienced the atomic bombs (Moloney 1987).
- CML is diagnosed by detecting the Philadelphia chromosome (Ph1), formed through the reciprocal translocation t(9;22). It is so named because it was first discovered in 1960 by scientists in Philadelphia (Nowell 2007). Patients are often asymptomatic and are diagnosed with CML due to the presence of elevated numbers of blood cells in a routine laboratory test. Other major symptoms of CML include low-grade fever, malaise and susceptibility to infection.
- More than 80% of the patients are in the chronic phase of the disease at diagnosis, and usually have no or mild symptoms as described above; however, the disease inevitably regresses and acquires lethality, in the absence of curative treatment.

  Before IM, CML therapy was limited to conventional chemotherapy, interferon, and allo-stem cell transplantation, the efficacies of which were far from satisfactory. IM has radically innovated therapy with an overall survival rate of 89% after 5 yr. However, this amazing value is only obtained for the chronic phase. Once disease progression supervenes this therapeutic efficacy is lost, so it is important to keep the disease status in the chronic phase by selecting the most effective drug for each individual patient.

DEFINITIONS

- *CML*: Chronic myeloid leukemia (CML) is a malignancy of a pluripotent hematopoietic stem cell. The disease is characterized by a stable phase in which there is a massive expansion of myeloid lineage cells with full differentiative capabilities. This disease is associated with a specific chromosomal translocation between the long arms of chromosomes 9 and 22 t(9;22) (q34;q11), resulting in the formation of an abnormal chromosome, the Philadelphia chromosome (Ph1), and the expression of its transcript BCR-ABL,which is identifiable throughout the course of the disease.
- *BCR-ABL*: The *BCR-ABL* oncogene is the product of the Philadelphia chromosome (Ph1), which encodes a chimeric BCR-ABL protein that has constitutively activated ABL tyrosine kinase activity; it is the underlying cause of chronic myeloid leukemia (CML).
- *CrkL*: CrkL, a member of the Crk adaptor molecules, mediates a variety of pathophysiologic signaling involved in cell proliferation, differentiation, migration, and transformation. Like the other family member CrkII, it consists of one src homology (SH) 2 domain, two SH3 domains, and a tyrosine residue that is phosphorylated by cellular tyrosine kinases. In human chronic myeloid leukemia (CML) cells, CrkL is identified as a major substrate of BCR-ABL and is constitutively phosphorylated, playing important roles in oncogenic signal transduction.
- *Imatinib (IM)*: Imatinib (IM) is a small molecule-tyrosine kinase inhibitor that functions by blocking the ATP binding site of BCR-ABL, keeping it in an inactive state. It also inhibits KIT and platelet-derived growth factor receptor (PDGFR) at physiologically relevant concentrations. This targeted therapy has not only changed how newly diagnosed patients with CML are treated and greatly improved their prognosis; it has altered the natural history of the disease.

SUMMARY POINTS

- By utilizing bioimaging techniques, including fluorescent proteins and the principle of Förster resonance energy transfer, a biosensor for the accurate measurement of BCR-ABL activity in small numbers of living chronic myeloid leukemia cells has been successfully developed.
- This biosensor displays higher sensitivity and a wider dynamic range in the evaluation of dose responses to imatinib than previously established techniques.
- Due to this high sensitivity, the biosensor can detect minor drug-resistant populations within heterogeneous ones.
- Drug susceptibility can be assessed regardless of existing drug-resistant mechanisms, such as increased protein expression.
- Pickles enables prediction of the clinical course after drug treatment and future onset of drug resistance using patient cells *ex vivo*.
- Through optimization for more practical and widespread use, this method might be a promising tool for the prediction of both current and future therapeutic responses in individual patients with chronic myeloid leukemia, which will be surely beneficial for both patients and clinicians.

ABBREVIATIONS

CFP	:	cyan-emitting mutant of GFP
CML	:	chronic myeloid leukemia
DS	:	dasatinib
FRET	:	Förster resonance energy transfer
GFP	:	green fluorescent protein
IM	:	imatinib mesylate
NL	:	nilotinib
Ph1	:	Philadelphia chromosome
Pickles	:	phosphorylation indicator of CrkL *en* substrate
SH	:	Src homology
YFP	:	yellow-emitting mutant of GFP

REFERENCES

Gorre ME, M Mohammed, K Ellwood, N Hsu, R Paquette, PN Rao and CL Sawyers. 2001. Clinical resistance to STI-571 cancer therapy caused by BCR-ABL gene mutation or amplification. Science 293: 876–880.

Kurzrock R, JU Gutterman and M Talpaz. 1998. The molecular genetics of Philadelphia chromosome-positive leukemias. N Engl J Med 319: 990–998.

Lu S and Y Wang. 2010. Fluorescence resonance energy transfer biosensors for cancer detection and evaluation of drug efficacy. Clin Cancer Res 16: 3822–3824.

Miyawaki A. 2003. Visualization of the Spatial and Temporal Dynamics of Intracellular Signaling. Dev Cell 4: 295–305.

Mizutani T, T Kondo, S Darmanin, M Tsuda, S Tanaka, M Tobiume, M Asaka and Y Ohba. 2010. A novel FRET-based biosensor for the measurement of BCR-ABL activity and its response to drugs in living cells. Clin Cancer Res16: 3964–3975.

Moloney WC. 1987. Radiogenic leukemia revisited. Blood 70: 905–908.

Morise H, O Shimomura, FH Johnson and J Winant. 1974. Intermolecular energy transfer in the bioluminescent system of Aequorea. Biochemistry 13: 2656–2662.

Nowell PC. 2007. Discovery of the Philadelphia chromosome: a personal perspective. J Clin Invest 117: 2033–2035.

O'Hare T, DK Walters, EP Stoffregen, T Jia, PW Manley, J Mestan, SW Cowan-Jacob, FY Lee, MC Heinrich, MWN Deininger and BJ Druker. 2005. *In vitro* activity of Bcr-Abl inhibitors AMN107 and BMS-354825 against clinically relevant imatinib-resistant Abl kinase domain mutants. Cancer Res 65: 4500–4505.

Prasher DC, VK Eckenrode, WW Ward, FG Prendergast and MJ Cormier. 1992. Primary structure of the *Aequoria victoria* green fluorescent protein. Gene 111: 229–233.

Redaelli S, R Piazza, R Rostagno, V Magistroni, P Perini, M Marega and C Gambacorti-Passerini. 2009. Activity of bosutinib, dasatinib, and nilotinib against 18 imatinib-resistant BCR/ABLmutants. J Clin Oncol 27: 469–471.

15

Optical Fiber Nanobiosensor for Single Living Cell Detections of Cancers

Xin Ting Zheng[1] and Chang Ming Li[1,2,*]

ABSTRACT

Analysis of cancers at a single cell level is essential to understand the heterogeneous nature of cancer cells. Optical fiber based nanobiosensors emerge as a useful nanotool to detect fast biochemical processes in a single cell with high spatio-temporal resolution in a minimally invasive way. A class of nanobiosensors specifically designed for cancer analysis is discussed in detail in this chapter. The optical fiber based nanobiosensor functionalized with specific biomolecules has been demonstrated to successfully detect the over-expression of a general cancer biomarker, telomerase and the release profile of a metabolite maker, lactate. The effect of a monocarboxylate transporter inhibitor on the lactate efflux from cancer cells have also been investigated by the nanobiosensor. Such an optical nanoprobe is further integrated with a nanoring electrode to become a bifunctional electro-optical nanoprobe for localized concurrent measurements of the oxidant generation and the intracellular antioxidant levels in single cells. The optical fiber based

[1]Institute for Clean Energy and Advanced Materials, Southwest University, Chongqing 400715, P.R. China.
E-mail: zhen0012@hotmail.com
[2]School of Chemical and Biomedical Engineering, Center for Advanced Bionanosystems Nanyang Technological University, 70 Nanyang Drive, Singapore 637457.
E-mail: ecmli@ntu.edu.sg
*Corresponding author

List of abbreviations after the text.

nanobiosensor renders a universal approach for detecting a broad range of low expression proteins in a single living cell. It also has potential for evaluating the effect of metabolic agents on cancer metabolism and survival. Finally, the bifunctional electro-optical nanoprobe provides a unique opportunity to probe chemical dynamics in a nanoscopic environment for elucidating key biological processes.

INTRODUCTION

Cancer usually originates from genetic mutations or aberrant epigenetic regulation, subsequently the alteration of transcript and protein expression levels leads to uncontrolled tumor growth (Irish et al. 2006). The resulted tumors are often composed of heterogeneous mixtures of both clonally transformed cancer cells and other cell types. In addition, cancer cells are unstable and the heterogeneous characteristics of many tumors may be enhanced in the course of carcinogenesis or metastasis, leading to multiple subpopulations of cancer cells with marked differences in protein expression, metabolism and signaling characteristics (Cohen et al. 2008). In contrast to conventional population based studies that only report average values, single cell analysis determines the actual distribution of cancer cell characteristics, enables the classification of cancer cells with high resolution, and allows rare cells or rare events to be detected for discriminating deterministic events from stochastic ones in cancer cells (Anselmetti 2009) (Key features of single cell analysis is presented in Table 15.1). Therefore, single cancer cell analysis is critical for understanding the fundamentals of cancer biology, discovering novel cancer biomarkers and improving clinical cancer diagnosis and prognosis.

Table 15.1. Key Facts of Single Cell Analysis.

1.	The cell is the fundamental unit of life and an individual cell differs significantly from one another in the same population.
2.	Classical analytical techniques require large amount of cells (> 1,000 cells) for analysis and only report the population averaged values thus masking the cell-to-cell variations (Cohen et al. 2008).
3.	A typical human somatic cell is around 10 µm in diameter, weights around 0.5 ng and contains approximately 100 pg proteins, 40 pg nucleic acids, 15 pg carbohydrates, 10 pg lipids, and other components even less (Cohen et al. 2008).
4.	Individual cells may show variations in their morphology, biochemical properties, composition, function and behavior (Arriaga 2009).
5.	A plethora of technologies now exist for analyzing single cells, however, further methodological development to achieve high-throughput simultaneous quantifications of multiple cellular analytes in a single living cell is still critical.

This table lists the key facts of single cell analysis including the advantages of single cell analysis when compared with bulk analysis, the approximate content of a single cell, the types of single cell heterogeneity, and future directions for single cell analysis techniques.

Due to the ultra-small size of cells, the trace amount of chemicals and fast chemical reactions in each living cell, single cell analysis is proven to be a challenging task that demands ultra-low sampling volume, high sensitivity, specificity and temporal resolutions (Lu et al. 2004). Through the years, a plethora of technologies has been developed for analyzing single cells including flow cytometry, capillary electrophoresis, electrochemistry, and fluorescence microscopy. Although these single cell technologies have exerted great impact on biomedical research, they have various limitations. For example, flow cytometry cannot be applied for real-time monitoring; capillary electrophoresis is rather destructive; while electrochemical methods employing microelectrodes are usually limited to monitor released electroactive species in the extracellular environment. Therefore, developing a versatile biosensor to readily detect critical changes associated with cancers is important in fundamental studies of cancer biology and in the discovery of drugs for cancer treatment.

The optical fiber nanosensor that has been developed attracts much interest due to its nanoscale size and sub-diffraction limited resolution. The nanoprobe is much smaller than a typical cell (~10 μm), thus it can easily penetrate the cell membrane for intracellular detection. Another advantage of this nanoscale size is the improvement of the spatial resolution to break the diffraction limit. A sub-wavelength nano-aperture at the end surface of a nanosized tapered optical fiber allows only the penetration of an evanescent field. The low penetration depth of this evanescent field allows only the molecule in close vicinity to be excited, thus effectively reduces the detection volume and suppresses the background to achieve high signal-to-noise ratio (Vo-Dinh 2008). Its unique features render it to be suitable for dynamic single cell analysis with minimal invasiveness, good sensitivity and high spatio-temporal resolution. Taking advantage of these unique properties, two classes of optical fiber based nanosensors including chemical nanosensors and nanobiosensors have been developed to reliably detect several important biochemicals or cellular events including intracellular pH (Tan et al. 1992), cytotoxic compounds (Cullum et al. 2000; Vo-Dinh et al. 2000), and apoptosis (Kasili et al. 2004; Song et al. 2004) in single living cells. Recently, this optical fiber nanosensor is further developed by our group to achieve single living cell detection of important cancer biomarkers such as telomerase, lactate and real-time detection of local biochemical processes such as oxidative stress. The layout of this chapter is as follows: The first section focuses on development and characterization of optical fiber based nanobiosensor; subsequently we discuss in detail the applications of this nanobiosensor in cancer investigation. We close with the future outlook of this nanobiosensor in healthcare.

DEVELOPMENT OF OPTICAL FIBER BASED NANOBIOSENSOR

The fabrication of optical fiber nanoprobes is a crucial prerequisite to the successful development of optical fiber nanosensor. Optical fiber nanoprobes with a tip diameter of 50 nm were tapered from multimode fibers by the heating and pulling method using a laser-based micropipette pulling device as reported (Zheng and Li 2010). Two methods can be used to coat the tapered sidewalls of nanoprobes with opaque metals for preventing the leakage of excitation light. One method is to coat the sidewalls with 100–200 nm of silver via silver mirror reaction (Wang et al. 2008; Zheng and Li 2010). After coating, the size of the nanoprobe tip is about 500 nm. Another method is to sputter metals such as 100 nm of aluminum to obtain a coated nanoprobe with diameter around 250 nm. Careful adjustment of the fiber placement angle in the sputter chamber is required to leave the distal end of the nanotip free for light transmission and subsequent chemical modifications (Zheng et al. 2010). Comparing these two methods, sputtering gives a smoother film with better control in film thickness, whereas the silver mirror reaction is more facile and relatively inexpensive.

This optical fiber based nanoprobe is currently being developed into a bifunctional electro-optical nanoprobe, in which the lateral wall of pulled nanotip is sputter-coated with gold and then insulated via electrodeposition of a copolymer (Zheng et al. 2011). The gold nanoring is finally exposed by focused ion beam (FIB) machining. The silica core of the nanoprobe allows optical detection and the gold nanoring enables simultaneous electrochemical detection to obtain more information concurrently. These nanoprobes are further modified with specific biomolecules such as antibodies and enzymes or selected electrocatalysts for target specificity.

The single cell detection system utilized is illustrated in Fig. 15.1. The cell sample is placed on the stage of an inverted microscope. The monochromic light coupled into the optical fiber creates a nanoscale light source at the nanotip to excite the target molecules. The fluorescence emission is then collected by the microscope objective to be detected by the photomultiplier tube (PMT). The optical fiber nanoprobe is attached to a micromanipulator for precise positioning with respect to a target cell. For simultaneous electrochemical detection, the gold nanoring electrode is connected to an electrochemical station. Both the optical signal from the PMT and the electrical signal from the electrochemical station are displayed online on a computer.

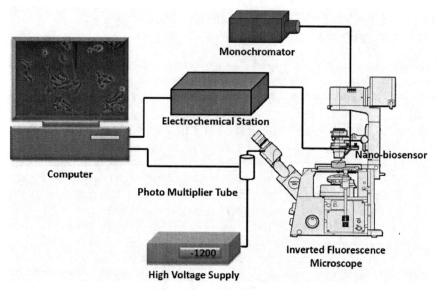

Figure 15.1. Schematics of the single cell analysis platform. This figure depicts the detailed setup of the single cell analysis platform that is capable of simultaneously detecting both optical and electrical signals (Unpublished).

APPLICATIONS TO CANCER DETECTION

Single Living Cell Detection of Telomerase Over-expression

The first demonstration of the optical fiber based nanobiosensor in cancer analysis is the detection of a general cancer biomarker, telomerase, in single living cancer cells. Telomerase is a ribonucleoprotein enzyme that catalyzes telomere maintenance for cellular immortalization (Hiyama and Hiyama 2003). Telomerase expression is up-regulated in 85–90% of human tumors but generally repressed in normal somatic cells (Hiyama and Hiyama 2003). Therefore, telomerase detection is potentially applicable in cancer diagnosis and evaluating anti-cancer therapeutics (Harley 2008). Conventional methods such as telomeric repeat amplification protocol (TRAP) assay and Western Blot require large amount of samples, usually the homogenate from thousands or millions of cells. Moreover, the protein expression distribution, the protein localization and the cell type information are generally not available from population based analysis. In addition, the intensive preparation steps such as lysis, fixation and permeabilization may distort the protein conformation to reduce detection accuracy. Single cell telomerase detection is more advantageous since it can overcome the above difficulties (Zheng and Li 2010).

To detect the endogenous telomerase in the nucleus of single living cells, an optical fiber nanobiosensor is constructed by immobilizing the anti-telomerase antibodies on the silver-free silica end surface of the nanotip end. This anti-telomerase functionalized nanoprobe is first inserted into the nucleus of a single cell to capture the endogenous telomerases via the specific antibody-antigen interaction. It is then manipulated out of the cell and an enzyme-linked immunosorbent assay (ELISA) is performed *in vitro*. For nanoprobes that captured the telomerases, the enzymes on the nanotip can convert the non-fluorescent substrates to fluorescent products for detection. It is worth noting that blocking usually practiced in conventional ELISA is especially critical in this method to eliminate the non-specific adsorptions (Zheng and Li 2010). Figure 15.2 illustrates the detailed procedure for telomerase detection in a single cell.

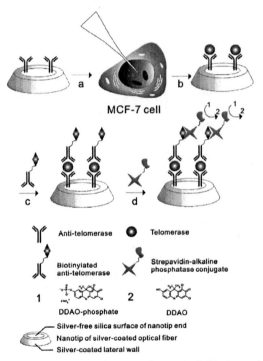

Figure 15.2. Single cell telomerase detection by optical fiber nanobiosensor. After immobilization of polyclonal rabbit anti-telomerases on the nanotip, the optical fiber was inserted into the nucleus of a single living cell to capture endogenous telomerases via antigen-antibody interactions. Then the nanosensor with captured telomerases was incubated to attach biotinylated anti-telomerases. After washing, the biotinylated anti-telomerases were further labeled with strepavidin-alkaline phosphatase conjugates through biotin-strepavidin interactions. Finally, the alkaline phosphatases on the nanotip could catalyze the conversion of DDAO phosphate to DDAO for sensitive fluorescent detection (Reprinted with permission from Zheng and Li 2010 © Copyright Elsevier).

Single cell detection of telomerase is definitely a challenging task since the single cell telomerase expression is extremely low, estimated to be 20 to 50 molecules in single HEK cell (Cohen et al. 2007). The success of this work is mainly attributed to the unique properties of the nanobiosensor (Zheng and Li 2010). The nanoscale size enables easy nuclear penetration and the capture of telomerase via antigen-antibody interaction allows each nanotip to harvest ~50 telomerase molecules. More importantly, the nanoprobe acts as a highly localized nanoscale light source that significantly eliminates possible interferences to achieve high signal to noise ratio. Another key to success is the signal amplification offered by the *in vitro* ELISA step.

The fluorescence intensity upon the addition of the enzyme substrate is monitored in real-time. To eliminate the interference caused by probe-to-probe differences, $(F-F_0)/F_0$ ratio was calculated for comparison, where F_0 and F are detected fluorescence intensities upon addition of substrate at 0 s and 1800 s, respectively. For nanoprobes incubated in MCF7 cells, the fluorescence increases quickly in the first 250 sec and continues to rise gradually until reaching a plateau. The enzyme reaction kinetics is similar to that of conventional ELISA performed in microplates since the concentration of enzymes are in the same order for both cases (Zheng and Li 2010).

Large variations in $(F-F_0)/F_0$ ratios between individual cells of the same cell type is observed (Fig. 15.3A). This variation most probably comes from the large cell-to-cell variability in protein expression which arises from the difference in cell size, cell cycle state and the stochasticity in protein production (Newman et al. 2006). The Student's t-test confirms that the average ratio for MCF7 cancer cell nucleus is significantly larger than that of the negative control, human mesenchymal stem cell (hMSC) nucleus; and the average ratio detected in the MCF7 cytoplasm is significantly smaller as compared to the nucleus (Fig. 15.3B). The high expression level

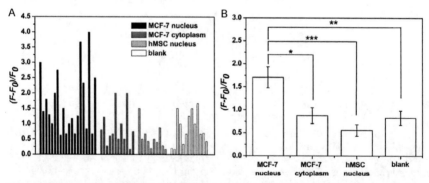

Figure 15.3. Optical detection of telomerase. **(A)** Single cells results; **(B)** Population-averaged results (n = 20 for MCF7 nucleus, n = 12 for MCF7 cytoplasm, n = 10 for hMSC nucleus and n = 13 for blank). Error bars represent standard errors of mean (s.e.m). t-test: *p<0.05, **p<0.01, ***p<0.001 (Reprinted with permission from Zheng and Li 2010 © Copyright Elsevier).

of telomerase in the nucleus of MCF7 cancer cell (Masutomi et al. 2003) can be clearly determined, but the extremely low expression of telomerases in normal stem cells or cytoplasm is not distinguishable by the nanoprobe; thus the as-fabricated nanobiosensor is very useful in distinguishing over-expression of telomerases from normal expression levels in individual cells for cancer detection (Zheng and Li 2010).

Optical Detection of Lactate Release of Single Cells for Cancer Metabolic Analysis

Besides the distinct alterations in the protein expressions, metabolism of the cancer cells also evolves markedly during carcinogenesis (Spratlin et al. 2009). Investigating metabolism at the single cell level has the potential to reveal cellular heterogeneity and deconvolute complicated metabolic interactions, leading to the deciphering of various metabolic pathways. A universal metabolism change in invasive cancers is the increase in glucose uptake and lactate production, known as aerobic glycolysis or "Warburg effect" (Table 15.2). Particularly, lactate, the end product of glycolysis, is considered as an important metabolite marker for malignant cancer (Gatenby and Gillies 2004). Although several techniques have been reported to achieve single cell lactate detection, the invasive and labor-intensive sampling steps limit their practical applications. An enzyme-based optical fiber nanobiosensor is developed to directly measure extracellular lactate concentration profile of a single living cancer cell (Zheng et al. 2010).

As illustrated in Fig. 15.4, lactate secreted from a single cell is catalyzed by the lactate dehydrogenase (LDH) immobilized on the nanotip and the fluorescence of the byproduct, reduced nicotinamide adenine dinucleotide

Table 15.2. Key Facts of Warburg effect.

1.	Warburg effect, also known as aerobic glycolysis, refers to the conversion of glucose to lactic acid in the presence of oxygen.
2.	This phenomenon was first reported by Warburg in the 1920s and has been repeatedly verified since then (Gatenby and Gillies 2004).
3.	While for normal mammalian cells, glycolysis is inhibited in the presence of oxygen, the cancer cells show high level of aerobic glycolysis, where high glucose uptake and high lactate production are usually observed (Gatenby and Gillies 2004).
4.	In order to maintain intracellular homeostasis, lactate needs to be exported from tumor cells to the microenvironment, which results in a lowered extracellular pH and consequently creates a hostile environment for neighboring healthy cells.
5.	A correlation between increased intra-tumoral lactate concentration and the increased incidence of metastasis has been established in many cancer types, thus lactate is considered as an important metabolite marker for malignant cancer (Gatenby and Gillies 2004).

This table lists the key facts of Warburg effect including its definition, the first report, basic concepts, and its implication in cancer diagnosis.

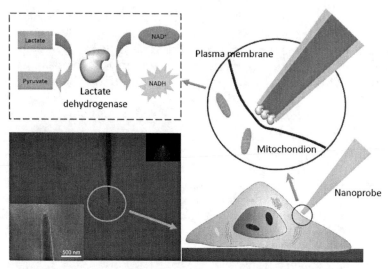

Figure 15.4. Detection of extracellular lactate by an optical fiber based nanobiosensor. The nanobiosensor is parked on the plasma membrane of a single cell. The evanescent field from the nanotip illuminates a spatially confined region. The immobilized lactate dehydrogenases catalyze the conversion of lactate into pyruvate and the fluorescence of the byproduct NADH is monitored by the fluorescence measurement system to determine the lactate concentration. The inset at the top right corner of the figure shows the nanoscale excitation light spot and the inset at the bottom left corner shows the field emission-scanning electron microscope (FESEM) image of the aluminium-coated nanotip (Reprinted with permission from Zheng et al. 2010 © Copyright American Chemical Society).

(NADH), is monitored in real-time. The as-fabricated lactate nanobiosensor has a dynamic range from 0.06–1 mM, a low detection limit of *ca.* 20 µM and a fast response time of 1 sec. These parameters confirm that this nanobiosensor is suitable for measuring single cell release. Furthermore, the lactate release profiles of individual cells can also be spatially mapped by precise positioning of the nanoprobe. The unique properties of the nanobiosensor is critical to achieve high spatial resolution, high signal-to-noise (S/N) ratio and minimize ultraviolet (UV) light damage to the cell. Most remarkably, the detection volume for a nanoprobe with evanescent field excitation is at least three orders smaller than that of a microprobe with free-beam propagation. This significant reduction in detection volume explains the high spatial resolution and high S/N ratio achieved which is critical for mapping the lactate release profile (Zheng et al. 2010).

Lactate secreted from the individual isolated cell creates a lactate concentration gradient around a single cell. The lactate sensitive nanobiosensor is precisely positioned at different distances to the single cell to determine the local lactate concentrations. The single cell lactate release profile (Fig. 15.5) indicates that the highest lactate concentration exists on the cell membrane and it drops exponentially as the distance increases.

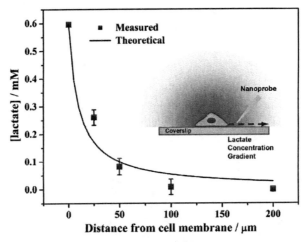

Figure 15.5. Concentration profile of the released lactate around a single cancer cell. Measured (data points with standard deviation bars) and simulated (solid line) diffusion profiles of the released lactate. The inset illustrates the hemispherical lactate diffusion zone around a single cell adhered on a glass coverslip (Reprinted with permission from Zheng et al. 2010 © Copyright American Chemical Society).

At 100 μm or further distances away from a single HeLa cell, the lactate concentration detected is negligible. The experimental diffusion profile of the released lactate also fits well with the theoretical diffusion model (Land et al. 1999; Shiku et al. 2001):

$$C_x = C_b + \frac{(C_s - C_b)R}{R + x} \tag{1}$$

Where R is the cell radius, x represents the distance from the cell and C_b and C_s are the lactate concentrations in the bulk solution and at the single cell surface, respectively.

It is observed that the two human cancer cell lines, HeLa and MCF7 cells, exhibit significantly higher lactate concentrations than that of the normal human fetal osteoblast (hFOB) cells (Fig. 15.6B). This result follows the trend predicted by the Warburg effect (Gatenby and Gillies 2004). In addition, the cell-to-cell variability in metabolism is evident from the spread in the measured extracellular lactate concentrations adjacent to individual cells (Fig. 15.6A). Comparing the two cancer cell lines, HeLa cells of the cervical cancer origin release 70% more lactate than MCF7 cells, a non-metastatic breast cancer cell line (p<0.01). Besides the difference in tissue origins and cancer development stages, the exclusive expression of monocarboxylate transporter 4 (MCT4) (Ullah et al. 2006; Gallagher et al. 2007), a membrane protein for lactate efflux (Ganapathy et al. 2009), in HeLa cell may also account for the higher level of extracellular lactate detected as compared to MCF7 cells.

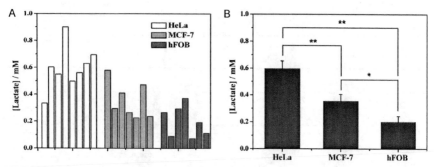

Figure 15.6. Cancerous cells exhibit higher extracellular lactate concentrations in comparison to normal cells. **(A)** Single cell results and; **(B)** statistical analysis of single cell results for HeLa cells ($n = 8$), MCF7 cells ($n = 7$) and hFOB cells ($n = 7$). Error bars represent standard errors; ** and * indicate $p < 0.01$ and $p < 0.05$ respectively (Reprinted with permission from Zheng et al. 2010 © Copyright American Chemical Society).

The alteration in lactate flux after the MCTs are inhibited by α-cyano-4-hydroxycinnamic acid (α-CHC) is also measured at a single cell level. α-CHC application leads to a much faster drop in lactate concentration in MCF7 cells, indicating that α-CHC is three times more effective in inhibiting lactate efflux from MCF7 cells in comparison to HeLa cells (Zheng et al. 2010). This phenomenon is very likely due to the exclusive MCT4 expression in HeLa cell and the five times lower affinity of α-CHC for MCT4 (Fox et al. 2000). The lactate efflux inhibition can cause cytosolic lactate accumulation and subsequent lowering of intracellular pH, which will eventually disturb the cell homeostasis leading to cell death. Thus, monitoring the lactate flux inhibition at a single cell level provides an approach to evaluate the anti-cancer effect of various metabolic agents.

Real-time Detection of Local Biochemical Processes in Single Cells by a Bifunctional Electro-optical Nanoprobe

Cellular processes are usually controlled by multiple signaling pathways (Scott and Pawson 2009). For example, the redox homeostasis reflects the delicate balance of reactive oxygen species (ROS) generation and elimination. The deregulation of such systems leads to oxidative stress that inflicts biological damages and is implicated in cancer initiation and progression (Trachootham et al. 2009). It is critical to monitor the production and the scavenging of ROS simultaneously in real-time to assess the cellular redox status and to understand the fundamental mechanisms for ROS associated cancer development. This requires a bifunctional or multifunctional probe that is capable of simultaneously monitoring at least two targets. In previous works, we have demonstrated that the optical fiber based nanoprobe is a powerful tool for single cell analysis; however, it can only detect one target at a time.

To achieve real-time simultaneous detections, the original nanoprobe is further developed into a unique bifunctional electro-optical nanoprobe as illustrated in the previous section. The optical fiber core efficiently delivers the excitation light to achieve high resolution optical detection of intracellular activities, while the gold nanoring surrounding the silica core as a nanoelectrode can simultaneously monitor the extracellular chemical events by electrochemical detections. Due to the nanoscale sizes of the optical fiber core and the electrode, both the optical and electrochemical detection can achieve high spatial resolution and high S/N ratio (Zheng et al. 2011).

The oxidative stress in three breast cell lines including a normal mammary epithelial cell line (MCF10A), a mammary adenocarcinoma cell line (MCF7) and a drug-resistant HER2-overexpressing MCF7 cell line (MCF7/HER2) upon phorbol 12-myristate 13-acetate (PMA) stimulation (Griner and Kazanietz 2007) were investigated. The target cells were stained with 2', 7' - Dichlorofluorescin diacetate (DCFDA) or CellTracker^{TM} Green diacetate (CMFDA) to indicate the redox status or the reduced thiol level, respectively (Zheng et al. 2011).

By precise positioning of the electro-optical nanoprobe on the cell membrane, concurrent measurements of H_2O_2 release and the intracellular redox status reveals distinct oxidative responses and antioxidant levels in the three breast cell lines (Zheng et al. 2011). While redox homeostasis is maintained in normal cells, the intracellular environments of malignant cells are oxidizing. Furthermore, the drug resistance may be associated with the high antioxidant level that protects the malignant cells from excessive oxidative stress. Simultaneous real-time analysis of oxidant generation and changes in antioxidant level helps to understand the redox changes associated with the cancer progression, which is potentially useful in cancer diagnosis and prognosis.

Analysis of single cancer cell is important but also presents a significant challenge. We have developed the optical fiber based nanosensor to determine the cancer biomarker over-expression, concentration profiles of metabolites and the real-time fluctuations of biochemicals in single cells. This platform still requires further optimization to improve its throughput and multi-functionality; more sensing schemes are to be designed to expand the range of targets detectable. Nevertheless, the preliminary results obtained so far indicate that this technique is promising to unveil cancer cell heterogeneity which may lead to better understanding of cancer progression and consequently the development of novel treatments.

PERSPECTIVES OF POTENTIAL APPLICATIONS IN HEALTHCARE AND DISEASE DIAGNOSIS

Fundamental understanding of the differences between individual cells could result in new diagnostic tools or improvement of existing medical test methods, thus leading to better treatments for cancer patients. Optical fiber based nanobiosensor is an exciting new tool that will allow for a more thorough examination of the variations that influence the predisposition of cancers, and the cellular responses to therapeutic and prevention agents. However, this emerging technique is only at the research stage and has not yet been adopted by the medical community. Several factors need to be addressed. Up to date, this technique has only been applied to investigate cancer cell lines; clinical samples should be tested to establish a correlation between the detection result and the clinical outcome for possible clinical diagnostic applications. Moreover, the throughput of this technique needs to be improved, possibly by integrating with microfluidic platforms and automation with redundant design for high reliability. In addition, the measurement system used is home-built; the commercial availability of a standard robust system is required for broad clinical applications. We expect these addressed points can be accomplished in the near future and wide applications of this technique is envisioned, not only to provide more insights to the fundamentals of oncology, but also to present a way to improve healthcare in terms of better cancer diagnosis and treatment.

DEFINITIONS

- *Evanescent field*: Evanescent field is formed at the nanotip of the optical fiber nanosensor by total internal reflection, to excite only molecules in the vicinity of the nanotip by the means of an exponentially decaying surface energy (Kasili et al. 2004).
- *Capillary electrophoresis*: Capillary electrophoresis utilizes high electric fields for analyst separation based on its charge, size, or hydrophobicity (Borland et al. 2008).
- *Telomeric repeat amplification protocol (TRAP) assay*: TRAP assay is an assay that determines the telomerase activity from cell lysates. It consists of three steps: the extension of the telomerase substrate, followed by polymerase chain reaction (PCR) to amplify the extended product and finally detection of the products (Saldanha et al. 2003).
- *Monocarboxylate transporter (MCT)*: MCTs belong to a family of membrane transporters that catalyzes the proton-coupled transport of monocarboxylates such as lactate and pyruvate across membranes (Ullah et al. 2006).

- *Reactive oxygen species (ROS)*: ROS are broadly defined as oxygen-containing, reactive chemical species including free radicals such as superoxide, nitric oxide and hydroxyl radicals, and non-radicals like hydrogen peroxide and peroxynitrate (Trachootham et al. 2009).

SUMMARY POINTS

- Cancer exhibits significant cellular heterogeneity. Analyzing cancer cells at single cell level is critical to define the role of this heterogeneity underlying cancer initiation and progression.
- Optical fiber based nanobiosensor is a promising tool for single cell detection because of its nanoscale size and the sub-diffraction limited resolution.
- Further development of the nanobiosensor into an electro-optical nanoprobe allows real-time, simultaneous measurements of both optical and electrical signals in single cells.
- Over-expressions of telomerases are successfully detected in single cancer cells due to the unique design of the nanoprobe, *in situ* sampling in a living single cell nucleus and followed *in vitro* sandwich ELISA.
- The optical fiber based nanobiosensors may provide a potential method for cancer detection, and also demonstrate a universal approach that can be used to detect other low expression proteins in a single living cell.
- The optical fiber based nanobiosensors with lactate dehydrogenases immobilized detect higher extracellular lactate levels in cancer cell lines as compared to the normal cell line. Furthermore, different lactate efflux inhibition profiles are obtained for the two cancer cell lines.
- This nanobiosensor provides a powerful tool to noninvasively study the fundamental metabolic processes at a single cell level and could further be used in early cancer diagnosis.
- A bifunctional electro-optical nanoprobe is developed to study the local dynamic cellular oxidative activity at a single cell level by simultaneously detecting the electrical and optical signals.
- This uniquely structured bifunctional electro-optical nanoprobe with ultra-low detection volume is potentially applicable for universal monitoring of intracellular biochemical reactions with enhanced S/N ratio, providing a unique opportunity to probe chemical dynamics in a nanoscopic environment for elucidating key biological processes.

ABBREVIATIONS

α-CHC	:	α-cyano-4-hydroxycinnamic acid
CMFDA	:	CellTracker™ Green diacetate
DCFDA	:	2', 7'-dichlorofluorescin diacetate
DDAO	:	dimethylacridinone
DDAO phosphate	:	9H-(1,3-dichloro-9,9-dimethylacridin-2-one-7-yl) phosphate
ELISA	:	Enzyme linked immunosorbent assay
FESEM	:	field emission- scanning electron microscope
FIB	:	Focused ion beam
HER2	:	Human Epidermal growth factor Receptor 2
hFOB	:	human fetal osteoblast
hMSC	:	human mesenchymal stem cell
LDH	:	lactate dehydrogenase
MCT	:	monocarboxylate transporter
NADH	:	reduced nicotinamide adenine dinucleotide
PMA	:	phorbol 12-myristate 13-acetate
PMT	:	Photomultiplier tube
ROS	:	reactive oxygen species
S/N	:	signal-to-noise
TRAP	:	telomeric repeat amplification protocol
UV	:	ultraviolet

REFERENCES

Anselmetti D. 2009. Single Cell Analysis: Technologies and Applications. Wiley. Weinheim. Germany.

Arriaga A. Single cell heterogeneity. pp. 223–234. *In:* D Anselmetti (ed.) Single Cell Analysis: Technologies and Applications. 2009. Wiley. Weinheim, Germany.

Borland LM, S Kottegoda, KS Phillips and NL Allbritton. 2008. Chemical Analysis of Single Cells. Annual Review of Analytical Chemistry 1: 191–227.

Cohen D, JA Dickerson, CD Whitmore, EH Turner, MM Palcic, O Hindsgaul and NJ Dovichi. 2008. Chemical Cytometry: Fluorescence-Based Single-Cell Analysis. Annual Review of Analytical Chemistry 1: 165–190.

Cohen SB, ME Graham, GO Lovrecz, N Bache, PJ Robinson and RR Reddel. 2007. Protein composition of catalytically active human telomerase from immortal cells. Science 315: 1850–1853.

Cullum BM, GD Griffin, GH Miller and T Vo-Dinh. 2000. Intracellular measurements in mammary carcinoma cells using fiber-optic nanosensors. Anal Biochem 277: 25–32.

Fox JEM, D Meredith and AP Halestrap. 2000. Characterisation of human monocarboxylate transporter 4 substantiates its role in lactic acid efflux from skeletal muscle. J Physiol (London) 529: 285–293.

Gallagher SM, JJ Castorino, D Wang and NJ Philp. 2007. Monocarboxylate transporter 4 regulates maturation and trafficking of CD147 to the plasma membrane in the metastatic breast cancer cell line MDA-MB-231. Cancer Res 67: 4182–4189.

Ganapathy V, M Thangaraju and PD Prasad. 2009. Nutrient transporters in cancer: Relevance to Warburg hypothesis and beyond. Pharmacol Ther 121: 29–40.

Gatenby RA and RJ Gillies. 2004. Why do cancers have high aerobic glycolysis? Nat Rev Cancer 4: 891–899.

Griner EM and MG Kazanietz. 2007. Protein kinase C and other diacylglycerol effectors in cancer. Nat Rev Cancer 7: 281–294.

Harley CB. 2008. Telomerase and cancer therapeutics. Nat Rev Cancer 8: 167–179.

Hiyama E and K Hiyama. 2003. Telomerase as tumor marker. Cancer Lett 194: 221–233.

Irish JM, N Kotecha and GP Nolan. 2006. Innovation—Mapping normal and cancer cell signalling networks: towards single-cell proteomics. Nat Rev Cancer 6: 146–155.

Kasili PM, JM Song and T Vo-Dinh. 2004. Optical sensor for the detection of caspase-9 activity in a single cell. J Am Chem Soc 126: 2799–2806.

Land SC, DM Porterfield, RH Sanger and PJS Smith. 1999. The self-referencing oxygen-selective microelectrode: Detection of transmembrane oxygen flux from single cells. J Exp Biol 202: 211–218.

Lu X, WH Huang, ZL Wang and HK Cheng. 2004. Recent developments in single-cell analysis. Anal Chim Acta 510: 127–138.

Masutomi K, EY Yu, S Khurts, I Ben-Porath, JL Currier, GB Metz, MW Brooks, S Kaneko, S Murakami, J DeCaprio, RA Weinberg, SA Stewart and WC Hahn. 2003. Telomerase Maintains Telomere Structure in Normal Human Cells Cell 114: 241–253.

Newman JRS, S Ghaemmaghami, J Ihmels, DK Breslow, M Noble, JL DeRisi and JS Weissman. 2006. Single-cell proteomic analysis of S-cerevisiae reveals the architecture of biological noise. Nature 441: 840–846.

Saldanha SN, LG Andrews and TO Tollefsbol. 2003. Analysis of telomerase activity and detection of its catalytic subunit, hTERT. Anal Biochem 315: 1–21.

Scott JD and T Pawson. 2009. Cell Signaling in Space and Time: Where Proteins Come Together and When They're Apart. Science 326: 1220–1224.

Shiku H, T Shiraishi, H Ohya, T Matsue, H Abe, H Hoshi and M Kobayashi. 2001. Oxygen consumption of single bovine embryos probed by scanning electrochemical microscopy. Anal Chem 73: 3751–3758.

Song JM, PM Kasili, GD Griffin and T Vo-Dinh. 2004. Detection of cytochrome c in a single cell using an optical nanobiosensor. Anal Chem 76: 2591–2594.

Spratlin JL, NJ Serkova and SG Eckhardt. 2009. Clinical Applications of Metabolomics in Oncology: A Review. Clin Cancer Res 15: 431–440.

Tan WH, ZY Shi, S Smith, D Birnbaum and R Kopelman. 1992. Submicrometer Intracellular Chemical Optical Fiber Sensors. Science 258: 778–781.

Trachootham D, J Alexandre and P Huang. 2009. Targeting cancer cells by ROS-mediated mechanisms: a radical therapeutic approach? Nat Rev Drug Discov 8: 579–591.

Ullah MS, AJ Davies and AP Halestrap. 2006. The plasma membrane lactate transporter MCT4, but not MCT1, is up-regulated by hypoxia through a HIF-1 alpha-dependent mechanism. J Biol Chem 281: 9030–9037.

Vo-Dinh T. 2008. Nanosensing at the single cell level. Spectrochimica Acta Part B-Atomic Spectroscopy 63: 95–103.

Vo-Dinh T, JP Alarie, BM Cullum and GD Griffin. 2000. Antibody-based nanoprobe for measurement of a fluorescent analyte in a single cell. Nat Biotechnol 18: 764–767.

Wang SQ, H Zhao, Y Wang, CM Li, ZH Chen and V Paulose. 2008. Silver-coated near field optical scanning microscope probes fabricated by silver mirror reaction. Applied Physics B-Lasers and Optics 92: 49–52.

Zheng XT and CM Li. 2010. Single living cell detection of telomerase over-expression for cancer detection by an optical fiber nanobiosensor. Biosens Bioelectron 25: 1548–1552.

Zheng XT, HB Yang and CM Li. 2010. Optical Detection of Single Cell Lactate Release for Cancer Metabolic Analysis Anal Chem 82: 5082–5087.

Zheng XT, WH Hu, HX Wang, HB Yang, W Zhou and CM Li. 2011. Bifunctional Electro-optical Nanoprobe to Real-time Detect Local Biochemical Processes in Single Cells. Biosens Bioelectron 26: 4484–4490.

16

Microfluidic Biosensors for Thyroglobulin Detection and Application to Thyroid Cancer

Seokheun Choi[1,a,*] and Junseok Chae[1,b]

ABSTRACT

Thyroglobulin Tg is a unique protein which can only be produced by the thyroid gland. Tg is used as a cancer biomarker in the post-operative management of patients with differentiated thyroid cancer DTC. As high as 20% of patients initially treated for thyroidectomy and radioablation therapy show subsequent persistence or recurrence of the disease; 8% eventually die. It is crucial for clinicians managing patients of DTC to monitor their concentration of Tg in serum. Unfortunately, conventional immunoassay techniques for Tg detection are not satisfactory for clinical use due to variability in between-method and interference by other serum proteins. Effective, accurate and rapid biosensing techniques are urgently needed to measure Tg in serum. This chapter reviews state-of-the-art microfluidic-based biosensors for general disease diagnostics and proposes potential biosensing techniques for detecting Tg. It is critical for clinicians and engineers to understand the technical limitations inherent in Tg measurement so that appropriate biosensors can be developed for accurate Tg monitoring,

[1]School of Electrical, Computer, and Energy Engineering, Arizona State University, Tempe, Arizona, USA.
[a]E-mail: shchoi2@asu.edu
[b]E-mail: Junseok.Chae@asu.edu
*Corresponding author

List of abbreviations after the text.

then used effectively in post-operative DTC patient management. This chapter provides a comprehensive overview of thyroid cancer, Tg as a biomarker, conventional Tg measurement methods, and novel biosensor techniques. It also introduces a potential method for the early diagnosis of thyroid cancer.

INTRODUCTION

Thyroid cancers are the most common malignant tumor associated with the endocrine system. During the past several decades, thyroid cancer has been diagnosed with increasing frequency in clinical practice (Haugen 2005). Up to 90% of all these cases are classified as differentiated thyroid cancer DTC (Rodrigo et al. 2006). DTC includes papillary and follicular cancers, both of which are derived from the follicular epithelium. Papillary thyroid cancers PTCs are more common, and constitute up to 85% of all cases. PTCs are often multifocal and usually metastasize to cervical lymph nodes. Follicular thyroid cancers FTCs are typically solitary and are largely encapsulated. FTCs are single, and more likely to metastasize to distant sites such as the lungs and skeleton. Both PTCs and FTCs are more common in women than men; the ratio is roughly 3:1. Early DTCs often do not generate vivid symptoms. As tumor cells grow, some symptoms are developed, yet they still do not directly signal thyroid cancer. Such difficulties led to combining several diagnostic methodologies, such as ultrasonography, scintigraphy, and fine-needle aspiration biopsy FNA for accurate diagnosis. These diagnostic methods are, however, bulky and costly. They require expertize and time-consuming processes, and include a number of procedures patients find painful. In the past several years, significant progress has been accomplished uncovering thyroid-specific biomarkers in human blood, such as thyroglobulin Tg. These biomarkers can be used as supplementary data to assist disease diagnosis. Recent advancements in biomarker identification support possibilities for clinical diagnosis at the point of care POC; the developments suggest potentially fast, simple and inexpensive tests for many diseases are now commercially available (Wu et al. 2007). The advent of microfluidic systems has revolutionized the methodology for the POC test. Microfluidic systems allow miniaturization of fluidic domains to create unprecedented access to monitor/detect biomolecules of interest. Such features have led integrated advanced biosensors into lab-on-a-chip systems. The combined application using biosensors and microfluidic technology could create a new generation of portable, fully automated POC test kits (Choi et al. 2011). The stringent requirements of POC testing, however, offer new challenges for biosensor technologies. Detecting target analytes with high sensitivity and selectivity, for instance, is a key challenge in microfluidics-based POC devices because of their significantly reduced sample volume.

In this chapter, we first review potential biosensor techniques that could be integrated with microfluidics in POC applications to detect general cancer biomarkers. Then, we describe Tg as a DTC biomarker, and introduce conventional methods for determining Tg. We provide a literature review that addresses potential biosensor techniques for POC applications. Future direction for DTC diagnosis will be discussed at the end of the chapter.

BIOSENSORS AND CANCER DETECTION

This section describes the fundamental structure of biosensors and introduces several sensing techniques with potential for merging with microfluidics in POC testing applications.

A biosensor is a device designed to detect or quantify a biological analyte. The basic structure and function of a biosensor is shown in Fig. 16.1. Biosensors have a specific biomolecular recognition element that selectively recognizes target entities, and a transducer to monitor the recognition event. Recognition elements, such as antibodies, enzymes, aptamers, or DNAs, are immobilized on a solid surface and maintain permanent bonding through linker molecules. Target cancer biomarkers are captured by the recognition elements, which induces an optical, mechanical or electrical signal and is then converted by a transducer into an output-readable signal.

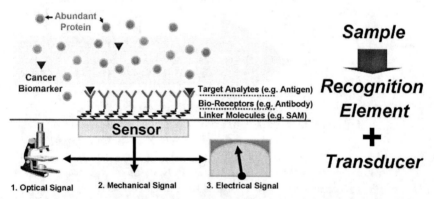

Figure 16.1. General scheme of a protein biosensor. A sample containing many different proteins contacts the sensor surface. Target analytes including cancer biomarkers selectively interact with bio-receptors, such as antibodies, on the sensor surface via linker molecules (SAM: Self-assembled monolayer). Upon binding of the analytes and bio-receptors the sensor transduces the binding to different forms such as optical, mechanical and electrical signals.

Biosensors can be either labeled or label-free systems. Labeling techniques have been broadly employed for biological/chemical analysis, but labeling may modify a target protein's characteristics, altering its behavior (Haab 2003). The labeling procedure is time-consuming and labor-intensive, and variations in labeling efficiency for different proteins make it difficult to achieve accurate quantification. Label-free techniques, by contrast, are a rather attractive alternative for biological/chemical analysis because they can eliminate labeling processes (Yu et al. 2006).

In cancer diagnostics, the analyte to be detected is a cancer biomarker. By measuring levels of certain proteins expressed and/or secreted by cancer cells, biosensors provide information on the presence of a cancer or the effectiveness of a treatment. Significant challenge for biosensors as diagnostic and therapeutic tools in cancer detection, however, exists; the biosensors should be able to detect and characterize relevant biomarkers, comparable to or even better than conventional analytical systems. Biosensor technologies are currently deployed for clinical applications like blood glucose or blood gas measurement, but relatively few biosensors have been developed for cancer-related diagnosis/prognosis. This is mainly because their combined performance of sensitivity and selectivity does not meet the clinical requirements. Recently, however, a number of novel biosensor technologies have been proposed, and their practicability has been demonstrated by detecting actual cancer biomarkers in a complex media such as serum.

Biomolecular Recognition Element

A recognition element is a critical component of any biosensor. These elements have a specific affinity site that captures the target analyte, and this determines the selectivity of the biosensor. Many different biomolecules have been used as recognition elements, including antibodies, enzymes, aptamers, and DNAs. Initially, biosensors used naturally-occurring recognition elements, purified from living systems. With advances in technology and synthetic chemistry, many biosensor recognition elements are now synthesized in the laboratory to support improved stability, and reproducibility for biosensing functions.

Antigen- or antibody-based elements have been extensively studied in biosensor research. A distinct advantage of these elements is the inherent specificity of antibody-antigen interactions. This specificity precludes the need for purification prior to detection. This method became very popular significantly after monoclonal antibody technology was established.

Enzymes are very attractive as recognition elements because a variety of measurable reaction products arise from the catalytic process: protons, electrons, light, and heat. One of the most advanced sensors currently based on enzymes is the glucose sensor, which uses glucose oxidase as the recognition element. In the presence of oxygen glucose oxidase catalyzes glucose oxidation, producing gluconolactone and hydrogen peroxide. An amperometric transducer measures oxygen elimination or hydrogen peroxide formation, and converts that rate into a glucose reading.

Aptamers are nucleic acid ligands isolated from libraries of oligonucleotides by an *in-vitro* combinatorial chemistry-based technology. Aptamers can be synthesized from commercial sources with high reproducibility and purity, and they tend to be highly chemically stable compared to antibodies or enzymes.

Transducer Technologies

Transducers convert recognition events into measurable signals. Many different transducing techniques exist, including mechanical, electrical, and optical. Mechanical sensors monitor stress or mass changes caused by molecular adsorption and interactions on a sensing surface. In stress sensing modes, molecular recognition events induce stress on the surface, resulting in mechanical bending of the surface (Fig. 16.2A). In mass sensing modes, transducing materials are brought into resonance (Fig. 16.2B). Mass variation induced by the recognition events on the materials is then correlated to the concentration of the target analyte. Film bulk acoustic resonators FBARs (Xu et al. 2010), quarts crystal microbalances QCMs (Aizawa et al. 2001) and microcantilever techniques (Wu et al. 2001) are well established as mechanical transducers, and have proven useful in identifying cancer biomarkers, including as prostate-specific antigen PSA and C-reactive

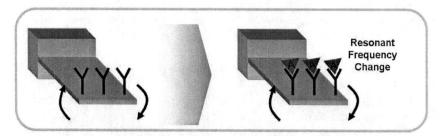

Figure 16.2. Illustration of a microcantilever with or without target molecules. **(A)** Stress sensing mode and **(B)** mass sensing mode. **(A)** Recognition events induce stress on the surface and result in mechanical bending of the cantilever. **(B)** The cantilever is excited mechanically so that it vibrates at its resonant frequency. The change in mass can be detected by monitoring the resonant frequency shift.

protein CRP. Wu et al. demonstrated that a microcantilever-based biosensor achieved a 0.2 ng/mL PSA detection rate from samples containing human serum and plasminogen (Wu et al. 2001). Kurosawa et al. reported a QCM immunosensor that provided pg/mL CRP detection directly from serum samples (Kurosawa et al. 2004).

Optical biosensors are light-based sensors that measure changes in optical characteristics. The transducer can be divided into two categories based on optical characteristics: optical intensity-based (Fig. 16.3A), and surface plasmon resonance SPR-based (Fig. 16.3B). Optical intensity-based measurements characterize some of the simplest and most widely used biosensors today. The optical signal can be either fluorescent or luminescent. Fluorescence detection is used mainly to identify the availability of labels with a large spectral range and different functional groups. Gervasis and Delmarche (2009) demonstrated an impressive fluorescence-based microfluidic device that yielded a ng/mL detection limit for serum sample analysis, and contained various concentrations of the cardiac biomarker, CRP. Luminescence detection relies on the enzymatic reaction of a luminogenic substrate solution, or activation following a highly energetic electron transfer process (during the application of a potential at an electrode surface). More recently, luminescent techniques have been utilized for detecting cardiac-specific biomarkers such as cTnI, myoglobin and CRP, at clinically significant concentrations. Surface plasmon resonance SPR is a very attractive optical transducer that allows real-time monitoring of biochemical

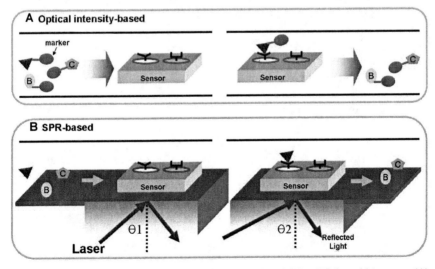

Figure 16.3. Illustration of **(A)** a optical intensity-based and **(B)** a SPR-based biosensor. (A) Optical intensity-based techniques identify the availability of labels with a large spectral range and different functional groups. **(B)** SPR biosensors allow real-time monitoring of biochemical interactions without the need for reagent labeling.

interactions without the need for reagent labeling. SPR provides high analyte sensitivity up to few ppt (pg/mL) (Li et al. 2007). Recently, several research groups have been investigating the use of modified gold surfaces and gold nanoparticle-based sensors to improve detection sensitivities. SPR-based technology has been used to detect several cancer biomarkers: cTnI cardiac troponin I, PSA, CRP, BNP brain natriuretic peptide, and fibrinogen (Mohammed and Desmulliez 2011; Choi et al. 2010).

Portability, miniaturization and cost effectiveness have led the development of electrical or electrochemical detection techniques over the past decades. Electrical biosensors have been downscaled to nanometer dimensions using silicon nanowires or carbon nanotubes, demonstrating integration into CMOS technology up to 512 array positions (Simon 2010). Electrical biosensors fall into four categories: potentiometric, amperometric, conductometric and impedimetric sensors. Potentiometric biosensors are based on measuring changes in the potential induced by recognition events between bioelements and target analytes. The most common form of potentiometric sensors is ion-sensitive field effect transistors ISFETs. Kamahori et al. demonstrated ISFET-based potentiometric immunosensors, which allowed detection of Interleukin 1β, an inflammatory biomarker, at a range of 1 ~250 pg/mL (Kamahori et al. 2007). Amperometric biosensors measure the current generated when electro-active species are either oxidized or reduced at the electrode at a fixed potential. The most widely used examples are glucose biosensors monitoring hydrogen peroxide formation when the hydrogen peroxide is reduced at –600 mV at Ag/AgCl reference electrode. Conductometric biosensors measure the conductance changes associated with changes in the overall ionic medium between two electrodes (Fig. 16.4). Conductometric techniques are attractive due to their simplicity and ease of use since no specialized reference electrode is required. Zheng et al. reported detection of a cancer marker, PSA, using a silicon-nanowire conductometeric biosensor (Zheng et al. 2005). They identified a detection limit of 0.9 pg/mL in undiluted serum samples. Last but not least, impedimetric sensors monitor any change in resistance or capacitance at the sensor surface on which biomolecular reaction occurs. Billah et al. presented a microfluidic impedimetric biosensor capable of

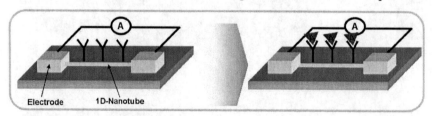

Figure 16.4. Illustration of a conductometric biosensor. A target analyte that binds specifically to its biorecognition element produce a conductance change.

Table 16.1. Summary of various transducer techniques.

		Target Analyte	Recognition element	Labeling	Limit of detection	Real-time detection	Ref.
Mechanical	QCM	CRP	Anti-CRP	No	10 pg/ml	Yes	Kurosawa et al. 2004
	Cantilever	PSA	Anti-PSA	No	0.2 ng/ml	Yes	Wu et a. 2001
Optical	Fluorescence-based	CRP	Anti-CRP	Yes	1 ng/ml	No	Gervasis and Delmarche 2009
	Luminescence-based	cTnI	Anti-cTnI	Yes	0.1 ng/ml	No	Cho et al. 2009
	SPR	cTnT	Anti-cTnT	No	10 pg/ml	Yes	Dutra and Kubota 2007
Electrical	Potentiometric sensor	IL-1β	Anti-IL-1β	Yes	1 pg/ml	No	Kamahori et al. 2007
	Amperometric sensor	H-FABP	Anti-H-FABP	Yes	4 ng/ml	No	O'Regan et al. 2002
	Conductometric sensor	PSA	Anti-PSA	No	0.9 pg/ml	Yes	Zheng et al. 2005
	Impedimetric sensor	Myoglobin	Anti-Myoglobin	No	15 ng/ml	Yes	Billah et al. 2008

detecting the cardiac biomarker, myoglobin, of 15 ng/mL (Billah et al. 2006). The transducer techniques and specifications reviewed here are summarized in Table 16.1.

Microfluidics

Microfluidic technologies have the potential to enable POC testing because they allow the functional integration of biosensors with sample preparation techniques (e.g. valves, mixers, and pumps). Most biological assays require labor-intensive and time-consuming processes, including a series of washing, mixing, and incubation steps, which can add several hours to even several days for testing. Moreover, the reagents for the assay are relatively expensive and sometime bio-hazardous. The usage of the microfluidic systems reduces assay time and sample/reagent consumption, enhancing the reaction efficiency. Microfluidics have been active research since early 1990s, and many review articles on microfluidics have been reported (Choi et al. 2011; Lin et al. 2010)

THYROGLOBULIN (TG)

Tg is a large glycoprotein (660 kDa) produced exclusively by normal follicular cells as the precursor protein for synthesizing the thyroid hormone, thyroxine (T4) and triiodothyronine (T3). The thyroid hormones are formed within the backbone of Tg molecules and liberated into circulation according to the degree of thyro-stimulating hormone TSH receptor stimulation (Lin 2008). With the thyroid hormone secretion, some intact Tg molecules and Tg mRNA are liberated and put into circulation. Most DTC cells also synthesize and secrete Tg. Currently there is no method of determining whether Tg in serum originates from normal follicular or DTC cells. Further, a number of variable factors cause false Tg detections. This does, however, prevent the Tg concentration method from being a sole diagnostic tool for cancer (See the Section 4). Tg is very useful in all phases of DTC patient management. Tg in serum prior to surgery (thyroidectomy) provides information about the ability of the targeted tumor to secrete Tg. As a post-operative cancer biomarker test, serial Tg measurements confirm the efficacy of treatment. After surgery for thyroid tumor tissue, detectable Tg may originate from a small amount of normal thyroid tissue that has not been removed, and the measurement may help determine the need for radioiodine therapy to destroy the remaining thyroid tissue. After radioiodine therapy, the serum Tg level should be reduced. Every 6 to 12 mon after thyroidectomy, regular Tg detection is recommended, augmented with radioiodine therapy to detect metastatic thyroid tissue and tumor recurrence. Changes in the Tg level during the post-operative time period are more important than those in the pre-operative stage. After surgical treatment of patients with DTC, the lack of thyroid hormones and their inhibitory effect elevate TSH levels in serum and cause an increase of Tg concentration. For this reason, TSH suppression therapy is required for acute serum Tg measurements (Haugen 2005).

Conventional Measurement Methods of Tg

The typical mean value of Tg concentration is about 1~2 ng/ml per gram of normal thyroid tissue under normal TSH levels (0.5~2.5 mIU/L) (Haugen 2005). Although there is no baseline "normal" Tg reference level for every DTC patient after surgery, the relationship between thyroid mass and Tg concentrations at a TSH status provides an important reference for monitoring DTC recurrence: 1ng/ml or less for Tg concentration in human serum. Measuring serum Tg can, however, diminish its clinical importance when the methods are too sensitive to other parameters.

There are many commercial diagnostic sets, and these can be divided into two groups, according to detection principle; radioimmunoassay RIA or immunometric IMA assay (Spencer and LoPresti 2008). In the competitive RIA assay, Tg in the patient's serum competes with a trace amount of ^{125}I-labeled human Tg for a limited amount of high-affinity, polyclonal, rabbit antibody raised against human Tg. The amount of radioactivity caused by the labeled Tg-antibody complex is inversely proportional to the Tg concentration in the patient (Fig. 16.5 A). In the non-competitive IMA assay (immunoradiometric IRMA or immunochemiluminometric ICMA), Tg in the patient's serum is captured by an excess of monoclonal TgAbs affixed to the solid surface of the sensor. After uncaptured Tg is washed away, labeled monoclonal TgAbs are added to bind different Tg epitopes, and

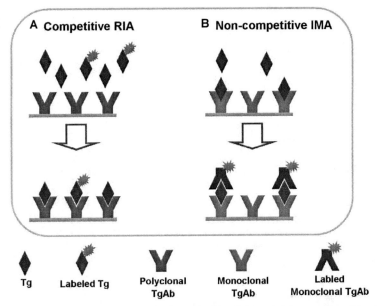

Figure 16.5. Scheme of immunoassay **(A)** competitive RAI and **(B)** non-competitive IMA. **(A)** Tg competes with an amount of labeled Tg for a limited amount of polyclonal TgAbs. **(B)** Tg is captured by monoclonal TgAbs and then, labeled monoclonal TgAbs bind different Tg epitopes.

these form a sandwich of Tg between the unlabeled and labeled monoclonal antibodies. After a short incubation, unbound labeled antibodies are washed away; the number of labeled marks remaining is directly proportional to the concentration of Tg in the examined specimen (Fig. 16.5 B). Recently, most laboratories have abandoned labor-intensive, competitive RIA procedures in favor of the more easily automated, non-competitive IMA methods. IMA methods offer several practical advantages: shorter incubation times, extended dynamic measurement range, and a more stable labeled antibody reagent that is less prone to labeling damage, at least when compared with RIA, which uses antigen labeling. ICMA methods can be automated more easily and flexibly than IRMA, making ICMA more preferable as a method.

Challenges in Determining Tg

Serum Tg measurement techniques remain technically challenging even after three decades of assay research. This is because a number of technical limitations still impact the clinical utility and reliability of Tg measurements. First of all, existing Tg detection methods still have unacceptable variability between methods. A recent study of Tg measurement showed an approximate two-fold difference in mean Tg levels in different detection methods (Spencer and LoPresti 2008). The discrepancies between methods do not allow results comparisons, and practically prevent interpretation of changes in Tg levels. Therefore, serial monitoring of patients' Tg must be performed using the same method and in the same laboratory (Savin et al. 2010). Secondly, the methods have insufficient sensitivity for detecting small DTC (Spencer and LoPresti 2008), and inadequate sensitivity impairs early detection in the event of recurrence. IMA methods are preferable to the RIA method for sensitivity. RIAs use polyclonal antibodies with broader epitope specificities than IMAs, which use monoclonal antibodies with limited epitope specificities. Thirdly, interference from TgAbs or heterophilic human anti-murine-protein antibodies HAMAs can cause false-negative errors (Haugen 2005). Interference occurs in about 3% of specimens sent for Tg testing. HAMA interference arises when antibodies that recognize murine proteins are present in the patients' serum. They interact with the capture and labeled monoclonal antibody reagents. These reactions simulate Tg in the specimen, which can create false negative errors even when Tg is missing from the sample. Interference caused by TgAbs remains the most serious problem, limiting the clinical utility of Tg testing. TgAbs are detected in about 20% of patients with DTC, compared with the 10% incidence reported for the general population. TgAbs tend to bind with Tg, causing an underestimate of Tg levels that may mask markers for a clinically significant disease. As a note, IMA methods are more prone to interference problems caused by HAMA or TgAb than RIA techniques.

Development of Microfluidic Biosensors for Tg Detection

It is common and routine to perform immunoassay (either IMA or RAI) for Tg detection on a microtiter plate with sample wells. However, this diagnostic technology has limitations: sample handling vulnerabilities, long analysis time, and consumption of expensive samples or reagents. The microfluidic biosensor utilizes a nascent bioanalytical technology capable of alleviating the above-mentioned issues, and of greatly advancing the clinical utility of Tg testing. Unfortunately, there has been minimal research on microfluidic biosensor techniques for Tg detection, though immunoassay for Tg testing is compatible with the microfluidic format (Lin et al. 2010). Although thyroid diseases are actually rather rare, thyroid cancer comprises more than 90% of all endocrine cancers, and accounts for the most endocrine cancer deaths each year. In that sense, development of microfluidic biosensor for Tg detection will be meaningful, providing clinicians with essential information for proper patient treatments.

Why do biosensor techniques have great potential for Tg detection? In terms of biorecognition, antibody-based affinity techniques are more appropriate for capturing large glycoprotein (Tg, 660 kDa). Since DTC cells can change the structure of Tg, monoclonal antibodies with several different epitopes mapping on the Tg molecule can provide better selectivity than polyclonal antibodies. As an alternative technique, the indicator displacement assay can also be used to detect Tg without using antibodies. While immunoassay techniques are based on specific recognition of an antibody and/or antigen, displacement assays use the competitive adsorption between indicators and Tg molecules. (Choi and Chae 2009). detected Tg in a cocktailed protein mixture using the competitive protein adsorption. Implemented in a microfluidic system, the Tg molecules displace a pre-adsorbed, weak-affinity protein on one surface; a pre-adsorbed, strong-affinity protein was not displaced by Tg on the other surface (Fig. 16.6). Differential measurement in two channels allows detecting Tg using SPR. This technique avoids relying on bioreceptors as capture probes with attachments to transducers. This contrasts with immunosensing technologies, which require a time-consuming and labor-intensive immobilization process.

Applications in other areas of healthcare and disease diagnosis show huge potential. This technique could be associated with detecting disease-related proteins of having high molecular weight. This is because larger-sized proteins have strong-affinity strength on a hydrophobic surface, displacing a smaller-sized protein which can provide better selectivity in monitoring the larger protein. Choi et al. successfully monitored fibrinogen, one of potential biomarkers for cardiovascular disease, in undiluted human serum using the competitive nature of protein adsorption on a gold hydrophobic surface (Choi et al. 2010).

Electrical-based biosensors normally utilize enzymes as a bioreceptors and need labeling to increase selectivity and sensitivity. When it comes to transducer techniques, however (as mentioned in Section 2), label-free technologies are much more attractive than labeling methods like IMA or RAI. Besides the time and expenses saved by omitting labeling, label-free operations enable detection of target-probe binding in real-time. This is not possible with labeling methods. Real-time sensing improves measurement accuracy by averaging binding time and affinity constants, and curve-fitting the sensor output relative to time. In that sense, mechanical sensors like QCM, FBAR, micro-cantilevers and the SPR optical technique, are excellent candidates for achieving highly sensitive, label-free and real-time Tg testing.

A Pre-adsorbing Proteins   **B Tg Injection**

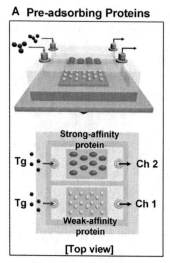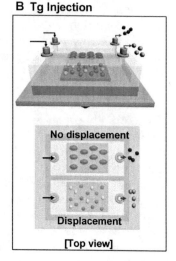

C SPR angle profiles

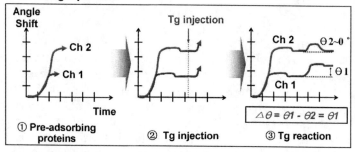

Figure 16.6. Operating principle of the sensor based on the competitive protein adsorption and a schematic of the SPR profiles. **(A)** The sensing surfaces are covered by weak-affinity and strong-affinity proteins, respectively. **(B)** Tg is injected into both channels. Tg displaces weak-affinity protein in channel 1 while no displacement occurs in channel 2. **(C)** The differential measurement of the SPR angle change from Ch 1 and 2 allows the detection of the target analyte, Tg.

FUTURE DIRECTION IN DIAGNOSING THYROID CANCER

Tg in blood is a very specific protein biomarker that can be used for prognosis after a total thyroidectomy and radioiodine ablation of residual thyroid tissue. The questions then remain: Why not use Tg measurement as a sole clinical diagnostic tool for thyroid cancer, and what would be the most potential biosensing technique for cancer diagnosis?

As mentioned in Section 3, several challenges exist to make Tg monitoring very difficult. (1) Tg concentration levels in the blood are very low, at nano grams per mL, and changes can be monitored only by highly sensitive biosensing techniques. Most current biosensors provide ultra-sensitivity, and this has largely eliminated the issue. Significant lingering problems do, however, include false negative/positive errors caused by (2) TgAbs, (3) HAMA, (4) cross-reactivity and (5) non-specific adsorption, which induces over/under-estimation of the Tg level. Another issue is (6) inability to distinguish normal Tg (already in the body) from abnormal Tg (from the DTC). These issues are hard to tackle as long as we remain focused simply on detecting the presence of Tg. First, there is no perfect bioreceptor to capture only Tg molecules. Second, Tg concentration changes vary according to surroundings, and may cause unexpected interactions with other proteins, making accurate detection extremely difficult. These two challenges may be addressed by adopting rapid and efficient identification of total protein imbalances in serum, a method called "Pattern-recognition". This technique is inspired by the sense of taste and smell, where an array of differentially responsive receptors creates patterns to identify and quantify individual analytes when they are present at elevated levels in media (Albert et al. 2000). Figure 16.7 shows the "Pattern-recognition" concept. Each sample produces unique interaction patterns with the array. The distinct advantage of this method is that receptors do not need to be highly specific or selective to an analyte. De et al. detected five proteins in

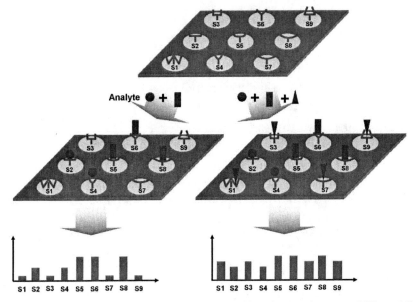

Figure 16.7. General scheme for a "Pattern-recognition"-based sensor. An array of differentially responsive receptors creates patterns to identify and quantify individual analyte when they are newly generated or present at elevated levels in media.

undiluted human serum using the competitive adsorption between green fluorescent proteins on gold nanoparticles and the target proteins (De et al. 2009). The Pattern recognition technique for Tg detection, however, will prove more appropriate in the future because the pattern-based composite signals can arise from an imbalance of blood proteins from thyroid cancer. This signal has more predictive value than the presence of a biomarker Tg concentration.

KEY FACTS

1. Key facts of Thyroid Cancer

- Contributes 1% of the total tumors.
- Makes up more than 90% of all endocrine cancers.
- Estimated new cases (44,670) and death (1,690) in the United States in 2010 (National Cancer Institute).
- Higher frequencies in women and the elderly.
- 20~40% of disease recurrence and metastasis.

2. Key facts of Biosensors

- The history of biosensors started in 1962 with the development of enzyme electrodes by Leland C. Clark.
- Many applications in the area of medicine, biotechnology, environmental monitoring, food industry, and military technology.
- After the September 11, 2001 event, the detection of biohazards in the environment has become an important issue in U.S.A. and other countries.
- Glucose and lactate biosensors and a few other commercial hand-held immunosensors for clinical diagnostic are currently available.

3. Key facts of Thyroglobulin Tg

- Tg was discovered by Roitt and others in 1956.
- Tg is produced by the thyroid epithelial cells.
- Tg is secreted and stored in the follicular lumen.
- Tg functions both as a pro-hormone and a storage site for thyroid hormones.
- Tg has approximately 2,768 amino acid residues including a 19-amino acid signal peptide.

4. Key facts of competitive protein adsorption

- Called Vroman effect in other words.
- Discovered by Vroman and Adams in 1969.

- The exchange process is led by thermodynamics.
- Strong-affinity proteins tend to displace weak-affinity proteins.

5. Key facts of "Pattern recognition"

- Uses Cross-reactivity on differentially responsive arrays.
- Provides a fingerprint that allows classification and identification of an analyte.
- Pattern-recognition-based device: Electronic nose or tongue.
- The opposite conceptual sensing technique: Lock-and-key.

DEFINITIONS

Definition 1. Thyroid Cancer

Thyroid cancer is a cancerous growth of the thyroid gland. There are several types of thyroid cancer:

- Anaplastic thyroid cancer (< 5 % of cases): Most dangerous form of thyroid cancer.
- Papillary thyroid cancer (up to 85 % of cases): Most common type
- Follicular thyroid cancer (up to 30 % of cases): More likely to come back and spread.
- Medullary thyroid cancer (up to 8% of cases): A cancer of non-thyroid cells that are normally present in the thyroid gland.

Definition 2. Quarts crystal microbalances QCMs and film bulk acoustic resonators FBARs

- QCMs and FBARs are mass sensors, capable of measuring mass changes in the nanogram per cm^2 range. Both sensors consist of a piezoelectric material sandwiched between two electrodes and acoustically isolated from the surrounding medium. FRABs improve the sensitivity more than that of QCM by the physical miniaturization provided by the micromachining techniques.

Definition 3. Surface plasmon resonance SPR

- SPR is a surface-based optical technique which utilizes the coupling of excitation light to a thin metallic surface, under exacting experimental conditions, which include the thickness of the metal layer, the wavelength and angle of incidence of the excitation light.

Definition 4. Complementary metal–oxide–semiconductor CMOS

- CMOS is a widely used semiconductor technology for constructing integrated circuits. Both P-type or N-type transistors are used in a complementary way to form a gate. CMOS technology is used in microprocessors, microcontrollers, image sensors, and random access memory.

Definition 5. Microfluidics

- Microfluidics is a new multidisciplinary field intersecting bioengineering, microtechnology, physics, and chemistry aimed at manipulating liquids and particles at ultra-low volumes. It has one or more channels and chambers with at least one dimension-less than 1mm.

SUMMARY

- Tg measurement in serum has been an important tool in post-operative monitoring for patients with DTC.
- Following surgery for DTC, the presence of Tg in serum implies recurring or residual disease; its absence signals a disease-free individual.
- RIA and IMA are routinely used to measure Tg in serum, but have disadvantages of long incubation time, high cost, and limited measurement ranges.
- IMAs became popular with the advent of monoclonal antibody techniques; there are still, however, major problems with the accuracy of Tg estimates.
- Merging microfluidics and advanced biosensor technologies offers new promise for Tg detection. Mechanical biosensors (QCM, FBAR, and microcantilever) and SPR provide real-time, label-free, and sensitive measurements that are more appropriate for Tg detection.
- The microfluidic biosensor for determining whether Tg is present poses challenges in thyroid cancer diagnosis because technical limitations are inherent in Tg measurement.
- Thyroid cancer may be more effectively diagnosed using the "pattern-recognition" technique to monitor protein imbalances. The technique uses an array of differentially responsive receptors to create patterns that reveal how protein concentrations are changed in serum.

ABBREVIATIONS

BNP	:	Brain natriuretic peptide
CMOS	:	Complementary metal–oxide–semiconductor
CRP	:	C-reactive protein
cTnI	:	Cardiac troponin I
cTnT	:	Cardiac troponin T

DTC	:	Differentiated thyroid cancer
FBAR	:	Film bulk acoustic resonator
FNA	:	Fine-needle aspiration biopsy
FTC	:	Follicular thyroid cancer
HAMA	:	Heterophilic anti-mouse antibodies (HAMA)
H-FABP	:	Heart-Fatty Acid Binding Protein
IgG	:	Immunoglobulin G
ICMA	:	Immunochemiluminometric assay
IMA	:	Immunometric assay
IL-1β	:	Interleukin 1β
IRMA	:	Immunoradiometric assay
ISFET	:	Ion-sensitive field effect transistor
PBS	:	Phosphate buffered saline
PDMS	:	Polydimethylsiloxane
POC	:	Point-of-care
PSA	:	Prostate-specific antigen
PTC	:	Papillary thyroid cancer
QCM	:	Quarts crystal microbalance
RIA	:	Radioimmunoassay
SAM	:	Self-Assembled Monolayer
SPR	:	Surface plasmon resonance
Tg	:	Thyroglobulin
TgAb	:	Anti-thyroglobulin antibody
TSH	:	thyrostimulating hormone
T3	:	thiiodothyronin
T4	:	Thyroxine

REFERENCES

Aizawa H, S Kurosawa, K Ogawa, M Yoshimoto, J Miyake and H Tanaka. 2001. Conventional diagnosis of C-reactive protein in serum using latex piezoelectric immunoassay. Sensors and Actuators B 76: 173–176.

Albert KJ, NS Lewis, CL Schauer, GA Sotzing, SE Stitzel, TP Vaid and DR Walt. 2000. Cross-Reactive Chemical Sensor Arrays, Chem Rev 100: 2595–2626.

Billah M, HCW Hays and PA Millner. 2008. Development of a myoglobin impedimetric immunosensor based on mixed self-assembled monolayer onto gold. Microchimica Acta 160: 447–454.

Burg TP, M Godin, SM Knudsen, W Shen, G Carlson, JS Foster, K Babcock, and SR Manalis. 2007. Weighing of Biomolecules, Single Cells, and Single Nanoparticles in Fluid Nature 446: 1066–1069

Cho I, E Paek, Y Kim, J Kim and S Paek. 2009. Chemiluminometric enzyme-linked immunosorbent assays (ELISA)-on-a-chip biosensor based on cross-flow chromatography. Analytica Chimica Acta 632: 247–255.

Choi S and J Chae. 2009. A microfluidic biosensors based on competitive protein adsorption for thyroglobulin detection. Biosensors and Bioelectronics 25: 118–123.

Choi S, R Wang, A Lajevardi-Khosh and J Chae. 2010. Using competitive protein adsorption to measure fibrinogen in undiluted human serum. Applied Physics Letters 97: 253701.

Choi S, M Goryll, LYM Sin, PK Wong and J Chae. 2011. Microfluidic-based biosensors toward point-of-care detection of nucleic acids and proteins. Microfluidics and Nanofluidics 10: 231–247.

De M, S Rana, H Akpinar, OR Miranda, RR Arvizo, UHF Bunz and VM Rotello. 2009. Sensing of proteins in human serum using conjugates of nanoparticles and green fluorescent protein. Nature Chemistry 1: 461–465.

Dutra RF, and LT Kubota. 2007. An SPR immunosensor for human cardiac troponin T using specific binding avidin to biotin at carboxymethyldextran-modified gold chip. Clinica Chimica Acta 376: 114–120.

Gervais L and E Delmarche. 2009. Toward one-step point-of-care immunodiagnostics using capillary-driven microfluidics and PDMS substrates. Lab on a chip 9: 3330–3337.

Haab BB. 2003. Methods and applications of antibody microarrays in cancer research. Proteomics 3: 2116–2122.

Haugen B. 2005. Thyroid Neoplasms. Elsevier, Oxford. UK.

Kamahori M, Y Ishige and M Shimoda. 2007. A novel enzyme immunoassay based on potentiometric measurement of molecular adsorption events by an extended-gate field-effect transistor sensor. Biosensors and Bioelectronics 22: 3080–3085.

Kurosawa S, M Nakamura, JW Park, H Aizawa, K Yamada and M Hirata. 2004. Evaluation of a high-affinity QCM immunosensor using antibody fragmentation and 2-methacryloyloxyethyl phosphorylcholine (MPC) polymer. Biosensors and Bioelectronics 20: 1134–1139.

Li Y, J Xiang and F Zhou. 2007. Toward one-step point-of-care immunodiagnostics using capillary-driven microfluidics and PDMS substrates. Plasmonics 2: 79–87.

Lin C, J Wang, H Wu and G Lee. 2010. Microfluidic immunoassays. Journal of the Association for Laboratory Automation 15: 253–274

Lin J. 2008. Thyroglobulin and human thyroid cancer. Clinica Chimica Acta 388: 15–21.

Mohammed M and MPY Desmulliez. 2011. Lab-on-a-chip based immunosensor principles and technologies for the detection of cardiac biomarkers: a review. Lab on a chip 11: 569–595

O'Regan TM, M Pravda, CK O'Sullivan and GG Guilbault. 2002. Development of a disposable immunosensor for the detection of human heart fatty-acid binding protein in human whole blood using screen-printed carbon electrodes. Talanta 57: 501–510.

Rodrigo JP, A Rinaldo, KO Devaney, AR Shaha and A Ferlito. 2006. Molecular diagnostic methods in the diagnosis and follow-up of well-differentiated thyroid carcinoma. Head Neck 28: 1032–1039.

Savin S, D Cvejic, L Mijatovic and SZ Simonovic. 2010. Measuring Thyroglobulin concentrations in patients with differentiated thyroid carcinoma. J Med Biochem 29: 245–253.

Shankaran DR, KV Gobi and N Miura. 2007. Recent advancements in surface plasmon resonance immunosensors for detection of small molecules of biomedical, food and environmental interest. Sensors and Actuators B: Chemical 121: 158–177.

Simon E. 2010. Biological and chemical sensors for cancer diagnosis. Measurement Science and Technology 21: 112002.

Spencer CA and JS LoPresti. 2008. Technology Insight: measuring thyroglobulin and thyroglobulin autoantibody in patients with differentiated thyroid cancer. Nature Clinical Practice 4: 223–233.

Wu G, RH Datar, KM Hansen, T Thundat, RJ Cote and A Majumdar. 2001. Bioassay of prostate-specific antigen using microcantilevers. Nature Biotechnology 19: 856–860.

Wu J, Z Fu, F Yan and H Ju. 2007. Biomedical and clinical applications of immunoassays and immunosensors for tumor markers. Trends in Analytical Chemistry 26: 679–688.

Xu W, S Choi and J Chae. 2010. A contour-mode film bulk acoustic resonator of high quality factor in a liquid environment for biosensing applications. Applied Physics Letters 96: 053703

Yu X, D Xu and Q Cheng. 2006. Label-free detection methods for protein microarrays. Proteomics 6: 5493–5503.

Zheng G, F Patolsky, Y Cui, WU Wang and CM Lieber. 2005. Multiplexed electrical detection of cancer markers with nanowire sensor arrays. Nature Biotechnology 23: 1294–1301.

SECTION 3: TREATMENTS AND ORGANS SPECIFIC APPLICATIONS

17

Optical Biosensors and Applications to Drug Discovery and Development in Cancer Research

Carlo Bertucci[1,a,*] and Angela De Simone[1,b]

ABSTRACT

Optical biosensors are well suited to monitor specific molecular interactions and measure the related binding parameters, which are fundamental for the definition of the mechanism of bio-recognition processes, as well as for their modulation. This analytical technique allows the interactions between analytes and immobilized ligands to be studied without labelling the interacting compounds. Label-free assays are valuable and easy-to-use tools in bio-recognition process monitoring, since they confer higher efficiency, flexibility and lower exposure to experimental artefacts. The sample is observed as close to its native state as possible, thus preventing chemical alteration of the interacting compounds, which could eventually occlude a binding site, interfere with the molecular interaction process and lead to erroneous responses. Nowadays, optical biosensors are applied in several

[1]Department of Pharmaceutical Sciences, University of Bologna, Via Belmeloro 6, 40126–Bologna, Italy.
[a]E-mail: carlo.bertucci@unibo.it
[b]E-mail: angela.desimone2@unibo.it
*Corresponding author

List of abbreviations after the text.

research areas, such as pharmaceutical research, medical diagnostic, environmental monitoring, food safety, and quality control. This chapter reviews the application of optical biosensors to drug discovery and development in cancer research, focusing on target selection and validation, screening of libraries of compounds for their binding to the target, discovery and monitoring of biomarkers. The basic principles of the technique and the experimental set-up for binding assays are discussed, together with the most useful immobilization strategies for target biomolecules.

INTRODUCTION

A biosensor is a device consisting of a biological part on the surface as the recognition element, and a physical transducer that converts the physical parameters of a specific biological interaction into a measurable analytical signal. Many optical biosensor instruments have been developed, most of them based on the surface plasmon resonance (SPR) technology. SPR has the potential to benefit many important research fields, including pharmaceutical research, medical diagnostics, environmental monitoring, and food safety. SPR has a significant role in biomolecular interaction analysis, and is bringing major benefits to drug discovery and development, where the characterization of protein/protein interactions and binding site studies are fundamental to understand the bio-recognition phenomena behind a biological process. SPR allows proteins to be studied in their native state and environment, preserving their native three-dimensional structure, and even associated to membranes: these targets can therefore be studied in conditions relatively close to those *in vivo*. The increasing interest in this analytical technique is due to the advantages of SPR, first of all the lack of labelling requirements. Labelling imposes extra time and cost demands, and may eventually interfere with analysis by occluding a binding site, leading to false negatives. Furthermore, SPR allows real-time interaction studies between immobilized receptors and analytes, a fast collection of kinetic and thermodynamic data, and the detection of analytes over a wide range of molecular weights and binding affinities. This technique allows the quantitation of a bound analyte at equilibrium in the presence of the unbound analyte, while the binding capacity and baseline stability give information about the stability of the immobilized ligand.

For all these reasons, SPR represents a powerful tool in several phases of drug discovery for the efficient, rapid, and easily automated screening of bioactive compounds from synthetic and natural sources. Its wide application in cancer research concerns the discovery and validation of new targets, the discovery of new leads and their development, and the monitoring of biomarkers.

OPTICAL BIOSENSOR TECHNOLOGY AND BIO-SURFACE DERIVATIZATION

Optical biosensing is a relatively novel approach for the label-free detection of molecular interactions. The biomolecule (ligand) is immobilized on a solid surface (affinity surface) where different analytes (ligates) can bind giving rise to a mass migration which can be analyzed to quantify the binding properties of the analytes. The increase (or decrease) of the mass on the affinity surface, due to association (or dissociation) processes, determines a change in refractive index at the sensor/bulk phase interface, which causes reflectivity variations. Measurements are usually carried out under continuous flow of analytes over the sensor surface, which is mounted in a microfluidic system. The flow minimizes the thickness of the diffusion layer, hence maximizing the contact between ligate and immobilized ligand at the sensor surface.

Most optical biosensors are based on the SPR detection principle. This optical phenomenon occurs when light is reflected from a conducting film at the interface between two media with different refractive indices (Fig. 17.1). The sensor chip is the fundamental part of the process: it consists of a thin metal layer (Au or Ag, few hundred angstroms) deposited onto a dielectric prism or grating. The delivery of buffers or sample solutions to the sensor chip surface is controlled by a microfluidic cartridge (IFC), which is a series of precision-cast channels in a hard polymer plate, forming sample loops and flow channels. The light source is a polarized light beam generated by a light-emitting diode working in the near-infrared region. When the light waves are totally reflected, the instrument operates in total internal reflection (TIR) mode. The refraction phenomenon occurs when the direction

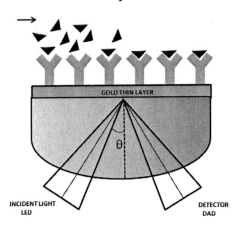

Figure 17.1. SPR detection system.

of a propagating wave changes while crossing the boundary between two media having different refractive indices. The originating evanescent wave propagates into the medium with lower refractive index, and away from the interface. In TIR mode, the response is sensitive to the region near to the sensor surface (few hundred nanometers). The evanescent wave created by TIR interacts with the delocalized surface electrons (plasmons) of the chip metal film at the interface with the low-refractive-index medium. The interaction leads to an amplification of the evanescent wave, due to plasmons excitation with collective resonant oscillation. The incident radiation is then absorbed with a consequent dip in intensity of reflected light, which is monitored by light-sensitive diodes. The response angle is then calculated with high accuracy by real-time computer interpolation.

A biosensor assay can be divided into different steps (Fig. 17.2). The first is the ligand immobilization. The addition of analyte, and subsequent interaction with the immobilized ligand, represents the association phase. This step is followed by the flushing of mobile phase, and the previously formed ligand-ligate complex is dissociated. After the dissociation phase, a regeneration step is needed to recover the surface and the binding characteristic of the ligand. The binding cycle can be repeated using different analytes, or different concentrations of the same analyte. The experiment results are monitored in real-time through a sensorgram, in which the response of the optical biosensor is plotted as a function of time. A typical sensorgram reflects the different phases of the biosensor assay. The first part is related to the passage of the buffer on the immobilized target (baseline); in the second part, an increase in resonance signal is observed due to the analyte binding on the surface (association) and to the consequent increase

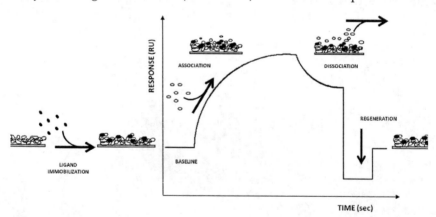

Figure 17.2. Different steps of the biosensor assay: after the ligand immobilization, the binding of analytes to the affinity surface is monitored in real-time through the association and dissociation phases.

in refractive index of the medium adjacent to the sensor surface. In the next step, dissociation, the analyte solution is replaced by the buffer. If the target-analyte complex is not completely removed from the surface, a regeneration solution is required to complete the binding cycle and recover the baseline (Fig. 17.2). The analysis of the sensorgram allows the binding parameters to be determined.

The sensor chip surface is usually composed of a carboxymethylated matrix bound to a gold thin layer. The carboxyl derivatised dextran matrix represents the surface on which bio-assays take place; its hydrophilicity represents a suitable environment for molecular interactions and promotes covalent coupling of ligands. Ligand immobilization is central to the design of biosensor assays. The main features of coupling are stability and the amount of immobilized ligand needed to obtain a stable surface. Two distinct coupling methods for receptor immobilization are available: covalent attachment, which ensures higher stability, and affinity capture of biomolecules. A potential disadvantage of ligand immobilization may be represented by the low capability of controlling ligand orientation. The ligand must maintain its binding properties, so the functional groups involved in the binding process must not be affected by coupling to the sensor chip surface. In the high-affinity capture method, the target binds in the right orientation, because the immobilization tag can be inserted in a specific position in the target structure. On the other hand, this method does not allow in obtaining a highly stable surface; loss of ligand during the assay is therefore more probable, particularly in the regeneration phase.

Covalent Coupling

Several immobilization strategies are allowed for covalent coupling. Amine coupling is the most commonly used: it involves the amino-terminus or lysine residues on the surface of a protein, and is therefore suitable for a heterogeneous population of receptors. The activation of the carboxymethylated surface is obtained by injecting a 1:1 mixture of ethyl-3-(3-dimethylaminopropyl) carbodiimide hydrochloride (EDC) and N-hydroxysuccinimide (NHS). The resulting NHS esters are easily involved in nucleophilic addition. After ligand immobilization, the remaining carboxyl groups, which were not involved in the process, are blocked. Another approach consists in the derivatization of the biosensor surface or the biomolecule itself, obtained by introducing appropriate functional groups to be used in the coupling procedure: this strategy allows the efficient coupling of ligands containing aldehydes or thiol groups. Treatment of the biosensor surface with 2-(2-pyridinyldithio) ethanolamine hydrochloride (PDEA) enables coupling with thiol groups through the formation of disulphide bridges, while treatment with hydrazine enables coupling with aldehyde groups.

Capture Couplings

The alternative coupling method is based on non-covalent interactions that fix the target protein to the chip in order to obtain a more homogeneous population of oriented molecules on the surface. Different strategies are allowed: biotinylated ligands can be captured by streptavidin surfaces, leading to the formation of stable complexes. This capturing method is very useful, since the streptavidin-biotin binding is one of the strongest non-covalent interactions known in nature ($K_a \sim 10^{13}$ M^{-1}), is essentially non-reversible and relatively unaffected by organic solvents or denaturing reagents; an important advantage is represented by the possibility of working in extreme pH conditions. The covalent attachment of monoclonal antibody on the surface by amine coupling allows the interaction with epitope-tagged or fusion proteins which can be directly and reversibly coupled on the surface through antibody-antigen interaction. The nickel-chelation method can be used with histidine-tagged ligands. Iminodiacetic acid (IDA) and nitrilotriacetic acid (NTA) have been widely employed in combination with Ni^{2+}, which displays a moderate affinity for histidine and chelates simultaneously the histidine sextet and the acetic acid residues. The disadvantage of this method is the low-affinity interaction and the consequent decay in the levels of immobilized protein.

CANCER DRUGS DISCOVERY AND DEVELOPMENT

The overexpression of certain proteins in tumour cells is a well-known phenomenon. Some proteins are also secreted into the blood stream and represent tumour markers. The discovery of new markers in body fluids and tissues should allow accurate cancer diagnosis, prognosis, and monitoring of disease progression, regression or recurrence. The development of simple, non-invasive tests for the detection of markers in body fluids is an important goal for the early detection of diseases such as cancer.

Proteomic approaches are based on the use of mass spectrometry methods or affinity methods, such as enzyme-linked immunosorbent assays (ELISA). Affinity methods use fluorescence, radioisotope labelling or enzymatic amplification. Label-based immunoassays need an immobilized antibody on the surface for target-analyte binding from solution, and a secondary antibody used as a label transporter for the visualization of antigen binding. Immunoaffinity biosensors are based on the specific interaction between antigen and antibody for the detection of target-analyte binding. SPR biosensors are preferred to conventional immunoassays such as ELISA for the capability to analyze samples in complex matrices without chemical treatment and with high selectivity.

Several SPR applications emphasize the potentiality of this analytical technique in the early diagnosis of different cancers. The major advantage of SPR is the simplicity of the experiments: the analysis is based on the preparation of the surface by immobilization of an antibody for a specific tumour antigen, followed by the evaluation of the signal in order to determine the presence of tumour markers, since the signal is related to the change in mass on the affinity surface.

SPR represents a useful alternative to immunoassay-based methods. Many studies have been performed to compare SPR to ELISA. These two techniques were compared for the detection of insulin-like growth factor-1 (Guidi et al. 2001), of the antibody against capsid protein of Porcine circovirus type 2 in diluted pig sera (Cho et al. 2006), of fish iridovirus antibody in diluted bream sera (Cho et al. 2007), and of CD166/activated cell leukocyte adhesion molecule (ALCAM) in human sera (Vaisocherovà et al. 2009). Other studies pointed out the capability of SPR in recognizing granulocyte macrophage colony stimulating factor (GM-CSF) antibodies previous than ELISA (Rini et al. 2005). GM-CSF antibodies were induced after administration of yeast expressed GM-CSF products in prostate cancer patients. The differences in antibody detection observed for the two techniques have been related to their technical differences. In SPR, ligand attachment to the layer is based on covalent or capture binding, whereas passive adsorption onto the surface occurs in ELISA. The antigen conformation may be altered during ELISA assays, while immobilization effects on antigen conformation are more predictable in SPR. SPR immobilization allows the detection of different populations of antibodies, including those with rapid dissociation rates or low affinity (Swason et al. 1999; Swason et al. 2002; Wadhwa et al. 2003)

SPR has demonstrated to be preferable to ELISA even in the detection of wild-type and mutant p53 in cell lysates: the total concentration of p53 can be measured through binding to a monoclonal antibody, while the wild-type form can be detected in the same sample through interaction with a consensus double stranded-DNA (Fig. 17.3). The advantages of SPR, with respect to ELISA, are related to the lack of enzymes conjugated with a second antibody, enabling a real-time monitoring of the wild-type p53 expression in normal and cancer cell lysates: p53 gene mutation is in fact followed by an increase in mutant p53 and a decrease in wild-type p53 (Wang et al. 2009).

Other applications of SPR are based on the detection of varying levels of autoantibody biomarkers in human sera samples. The capability of SPR in distinguishing sera samples with overexpressed carcinoembryonic antigen (CEA) autoantibody from healthy samples has been reported; CEA levels are higher in patients affected by colon and ovarian cancer (Ladd et al. 2009).

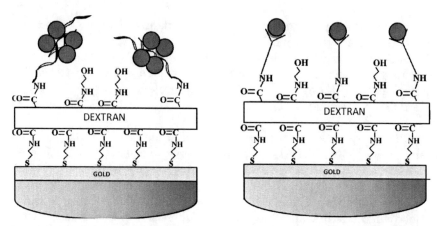

Figure 17.3. SPR detection of wild-type and total p53 proteins by consensus DNA duplexes (left) and monoclonal antibody (right) in two microfl uidic channels. [Adapted and reprinted by permission of the Editor, Wang et al. Anal Chem (2009) 81: 8441–8446].

SPR was also used for the detection of cancer antigen 125 (CA 125), which is another ovarian cancer tumour marker (Suwansa-ard et al. 2009).

SPR was also applied for the identification of different prostate specific antigen (PSA) forms. PSA represents the most useful biomarker for the monitoring and the diagnosis of benign prostatic hyperplasia (BPH) and prostate cancer (PCa) (Stamey et al. 1987; Oesterling 1991). SPR was employed for the characterization of three different forms of PSA, which were previously separated. The three PSA forms were immobilized on the sensor chip surface, and the binding kinetics and affinity for different peptides and monoclonal antibodies were estimated. Since the role of two PSA forms as potential specific markers for BPH was previously reported, those peptides showing higher affinity for these forms could be used as therapeutic drugs for the treatment of different forms of carcinoma (Kumar et al. 2009).

SPR was also applied as an evaluation method for early gastric cancer diagnosis. The optical biosensor was used in immunoassays for the detection of MG7-Ag, a cancer-specific tumour associated antigen, in human sera; the development of this method, based on the immobilization of monoclonal MG7 antibodies on the sensor surface, represents a goal for early diagnosis of gastric cancer. Different samples from MKN45 cancer cell lysate (positive control), and sera from gastric cancer patients and healthy donors were tested, and a difference in MG7-Ag expression intensity was demonstrated (Fang et al. 2010).

Applications of SPR in cancer research extend to anti-cancer drug discovery, due to the advantages previously described and to the capability in obtaining high-throughput screening. Optical biosensors, thanks to the presence of multiple channels on the sensor surface, allow the possibility of screening multiple targets in parallel, detecting actual binding and avoiding non-specific interactions. This application became very useful for the detection of active compounds in complex natural or synthetic matrices. SPR was used to evaluate the activity of some alkaloids, obtained after chromatographic separation of an extract of *Chelidonium majus*. The immobilization of small oligonucleotides on the sensor chip surface revealed the capability of these molecules in intercalating with double stranded nucleic acid (dsDNA) (Fig. 17.4) (Minunni et al. 2005).

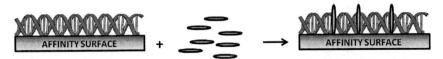

Figure 17.4. Binding of an intercalating analyte to the immobilized DNA. [Adapted and reprinted by permission of the Editor, Minunni et al. Talanta (2005) 65: 578–585].

In a recent study, SPR was used for a fast screening of synthetic peptide fragments in order to evaluate their effects in a more complex biological system. The study focused on a DNA binding protein, MyoD, whose helix-loop-helix (HLH) domain interacts with those of Id1, an inhibitor of DNA binding-proteins. Id proteins are inverse agonists of a family of transcription factors called basic-helix-loop-helix (bHLH), involved in cellular development, proliferation and differentiation. The aim was to synthesize peptide fragments of MyoD capable in binding Id1, in order to prevent the interaction between Id1, MyoD and bHLH, therefore avoiding cancer cell proliferation. The screening of synthetic peptides was carried out immobilizing the Id1 protein on the sensor chip surface. K_D values were determined for each compound, and those with the highest affinity for their target were identified (Chen et al. 2010).

Moreover, SPR represented an optimal tool in fragment screening (Navratilova and Hopkins 2010) against different targets as BACE1 (Kuglstatter et al. 2008), MMP-12 (Nordstrom et al. 2008), thrombin (Hamäläinen et al. 2008) and chymase (Perspicase et al. 2009).

SPR may be also used for a better description of the interaction between a single lead compound and its specific target. Due to the complexity and the different aetiology of cancer, many biological systems have been studied. SPR proved useful for the determination of kinetic constants, rates of association and dissociation and as a proof of the interaction between such promising anti-cancer compounds and their targets. Chen and co-workers tested a Shp2 inhibitor synthesized from a lead compound (NSC-117199).

The protein tyrosine phosphatase (PTP) Shp2 is involved in the mediation of growth factor signalling and its mutations are often correlated with leukaemia. The capability of novel derivatives to bind Shp2 was verified by SPR (Chen 2010).

In another study, the tumour suppressor p53 was immobilized on the sensor chip surface in order to confirm the interaction of two new anti-cancer compounds, GJC29 and GJC30, derived from a docking simulation and a MTT assay on human colon cancer cells, revealing their inhibitory activity against cancer cells proliferation (Okuda et al. 2009).

SPR has been employed to confirm results obtained with different techniques. For example, the binding of non-biotinylated camptothecin (CPT) to the C-20-biotinylated CPT binding site was investigated by quartz-crystal microbalance (QCM) and confirmed by immobilizing the peptide on sensor chip surface (Takakusagi et al. 2005). In another study, Carrasco and co-workers investigated the binding of AT2433-B1, a well-known antitumour agent. Different DNA sequences were immobilized on the sensor chip surface, and AT2433-B1 and its diastereoisomers were found to bind more tightly to GC-rich oligomers rather than AT-rich. This result was confirmed by DNase I footprinting. This important discovery will be very useful for the design of novel suitable compounds addressed to that sequence (Carrasco et al. 2002).

SPR was fundamental to demonstrate the role of paclitaxel (PTX) binding to Bcl-2 in PTX resistant cancer cells. The PTX binding was monitored, and binding parameters were determined (Ferlini et al. 2009). The selectivity of the binding was proved by binding PTX to different targets and binding different analytes to the immobilized Bcl-2. Furthermore, the involvement of the disordered loop domain of Bcl-2 as the binding site for PTX was proved by comparing the binding of PTX to both native Bcl-2 and mutant Bcl-2, where the loop domain was deleted (Fig. 17.5). Interestingly, molecular modelling showed similarities in the binding sites for PTX binding to Bcl-2 and to tubulin, the primary target for taxanes. These results allowed to speculate that PTX could mimic an endogenous peptide ligand (NUR-77), which binds both Bcl-2 and tubulin proteins and, like PTX, changes the function of Bcl-2. This hypothesis was confirmed by Nur77 interacting with both PTX targets (Bcl-2 and β-tubulin), and a peptide sequence mimicking the Nur77 structural region (Fig. 17.6). A new insight was then obtained to understand the down regulation of Bcl-2 in PTX resistant cancer cells, and to design novel anticancer drugs with non-taxane skeleton.

SPR was recently used for the investigation of a nanoparticulate drug delivery system, which may be able to target tumours overexpressing H-ferritin, such as pancreatic and lung cancers. Optical biosensor was

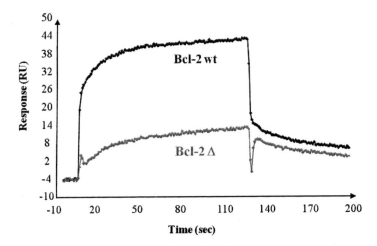

Figure 17.5. Sensorgrams of the kinetic analysis of the selective PTX binding to native Bcl-2 (Bcl-2 wt) as compared to the delete mutant Bcl-2 (Bcl-2 Δ). [adapted and reprinted by permission of American Association for Cancer Research, Ferlini et al. Cancer Research (2009) 69: 6906–6914].

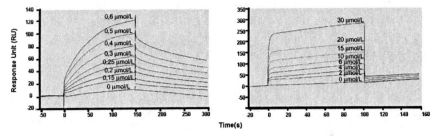

Figure 17.6. Sensorgrams of the interaction between Nur77 with Bcl-2 (left) and tubulin (right). Nur77 and Bcl-2 were analyte and ligand, respectively; Nur77 and tubulin were ligand and analyte, respectively. [Adapted and reprinted by permission of American Association for Cancer Research, Ferlini et al. Cancer Research (2009) 69: 6906–6914].

used for the evaluation of the molecular binding affinity between the monoclonal antibody AMB8LK conjugated to a nanoparticle, and its antigen H-ferritin. The association/dissociation and affinity kinetics values of native monoclonal antibody and AMB8LK immunoNPs were found to be similar. These results point out the capability of conjugated antibody to recognize its antigen (Debotton et al. 2010). Therefore, SPR proved to be useful in the development of a specific drug delivery system in cancer treatment.

KEY FACTS

- Biosensor technology is based on the immobilization of ligands to a modified gold surface. It was introduced in 1991 and is applied to the study of bio-recognition phenomena which take place between an immobilized biological target (ligand) and the analyte. Neither of the interacting compounds needs to be labelled.
- Surface plasmon resonance (SPR) arises when light is reflected under certain conditions from a conducting film at the interface between two media of different refractive indices. SPR is related to the oscillation of free electrons propagating along the film surface. In the 1980's, SPR and related techniques were applied to explore the biological and chemical interactions taking place on thin layers.
- Qualitative information on whether a molecule binds or not to a target may be obtained by SPR, as well as information on the specificity, affinity and kinetics of interaction.
- The monitoring and analysis of molecular recognition processes is a key aspect in drug discovery.
- Optical biosensor technology has a wide range of applications. It can be an optimal tool in different phases of drug discovery as target identification, lead identification, characterization, and early determination of ADME parameters.

DEFINITIONS

- *Biosensor*: a device which incorporates a biologically active layer at the surface as the recognition element and converts the physical parameters of a specific biological interaction into a measurable analytical signal.
- *Surface Plasmon Resonance*: an optical phenomenon which arises when light is reflected from a conducting film at the interface between two media of different refractive indices.
- *Total Internal Reflection*: an operating mode which generates an analytical response, sensitive to a region within a few hundred nanometers of the sensor surface.
- *Integrated Microfluidic Cartridge*: a flexible microfluidics system which allows the continuous flow of an analyte at a controlled flow rate.
- *Ligand*: the interacting molecule which is immobilized on the sensor surface.
- *Analyte*: the interacting molecule which is flushed over the chip surface.

- *Covalent and capture coupling*: the two methods adopted for ligand immobilization. Covalent immobilization involves a chemical reaction between chemical functions on the surface and on the ligand. Capture coupling involves a high-affinity binding through a specific tag on the ligand.
- *Binding cycle*: constituted by several biosensor assay steps (monitoring baseline; association phase; dissociation phase; surface regeneration).

SUMMARY POINTS

- The functioning of optical biosensor instruments is based on the SPR technology. The obtained analytical response is directly proportional to the mass of the analyte, which binds to a sensor chip surface.
- Optical biosensors enable the monitoring of biomolecular interactions in real-time without labelling requirements. SPR can be applied to the study of different biological systems and in many important fields, including pharmaceutical research, medical diagnostics and quality control.
- The development of microfluidic cartridge coupling to appropriate sensor surface allowed the use of this technique. When the immobilized biomolecules are bound by their ligands, an alteration in surface plasmons on the opposite side of the film is created, which is directly proportional to the change in bound, or adsorbed, mass. Binding is measured in terms of changes in refractive index.
- The use of different surfaces enabled the immobilization of different ligands and the study of many biological systems. SPR allowed the development of label-free assays, valuable and easy-to-use as tools in drug discovery, quality control and medical diagnostic. SPR is also involved in the development of simple, non-invasive tests for the detection of cancer biomarkers in body fluids and tissues. In the last decade, SPR represented a valid alternative to immunoassay-based methods, such as ELISA, for antibody detection.
- In optical biosensor experiments, the sample is observed as close to its native state as possible, thus preventing chemical alteration of the interacting compounds, which could eventually occlude a binding site, interfere with the molecular interaction process and lead to erroneous responses, due to false negative or false positive signals and/or background binding.

- Optical biosensors have been applied in cancer research to various biological systems, exploiting different analytical strategies. Due to its high versatility, biosensors are also used in combination with other techniques, including MS. This aspect is relevant in the frame of the high content screening (HCS) approach: in drug discovery and development, the aim is the identification and validation of hits and leads coming from HTS by applying HCS methods.

ABBREVIATIONS

ALCAM	:	Activated Cell Leukocyte Adhesion Molecule
BPH	:	Benign Prostatic Hyperplasia
CA 125	:	Cancer Antigen 125
CEA	:	Overexpressed Carcinoembryonic Antigen
CPT	:	Camptothecin
EDC	:	ethyl-3-(3-dimethylaminopropyl) carbodiimide hydrochloride
ELISA	:	Enzyme-Linked Immunosorbent Assay
GM-CSF	:	Granulocyte Macrophage Colony Stimulating Factor
HLH	:	Helix-Loop-Helix
IDA	:	Iminodiacetic Acid
IFC	:	Integrated micro Fluidic Cartridge
NHS	:	N-hydroxysuccinimide
NTA	:	Nitrilotriacetic Acid
PCa	:	Prostate Cancer
PDEA	:	2-(2-pyridinyldithio) ethanolamine hydrochloride
PSA	:	Prostate Specific Antigen
PTP	:	Protein Tyrosine Phosphatase
QCM	:	Quartz Crystal Microbalance
SPR	:	Surface Plasmon Resonance
TIR	:	Total Internal Reflection

REFERENCES

Carrasco C, M Facompré, JD Chisholm, DL Van Vranken, WD Wilson and C Bailly. 2002. DNA sequence recognition by the indolocarbazole antitumor antibiotic AT2433-B1 and its diastereoisomer. Nucleic Acid Res 8: 1774–1781.

Chen CH, SC Kuo, LJ Huang, MH Hsub and FDT Lunga. 2010. Affinity of synthetic peptide fragments of MyoD for Id1 protein and their biological effects in several cancer cells. J Pept Sci 16: 231–241.

Chen L. 2010. Inhibition of cellular Shp2 activity by a methyl ester analog of SPI-112 Biochem Pharmacol 80: 801–810.

Cho HS and TJ Kim. 2007. Comparison of surface plasmon resonance imaging and enzyme-linked immunosorbent assay for the detection of antibodies against iridovirus in rock bream (Oplegnathus fasciatus). J Vet Diagn Invest 4: 414–416.

Cho HS, TJ Kim, JI Lee and NY Park. 2006. Serodiagnostic comparison of enzyme-linked immunosorbent assay and surface plasmon resonance for the detection of antibody to porcine circovirus type 2. Can J Vet Res 4: 263–268.

Debotton N, H Zer, M Parnes, O Harush-Frenkel, J Kadouche and S Benita. 2010. A quantitative evaluation of the molecular binding affinity between a monoclonal antibody conjugated to a nanoparticle and an antigen by surface plasmon resonance. Eur J Pharm Biopharm 74: 148–156.

Fang X, J Tie, Y Xie, Q Li, Q Zhao and D Fan. 2010. Detection of gastric carcinoma-associated antigen MG7-Ag in human sera using surface plasmon resonance sensor. Cancer Epidemiol 34: 648–651.

Ferlini C, L Cicchillitti, G Raspaglio, S Bartollino, S Cimitan, C Bertucci, S Mozzetti, D Gallo, M Persico, C Fattorusso, G Campiani and G Scambia. 2009. Paclitaxel directly binds to Bcl-2 and functionally mimics activity of Nur77. Cancer Res 69: 6906–6914.

Guidi A, L Laricchia-Robbio, D Gianfaldoni, R Revoltella and G Del Bono. 2001.Comparison of a conventional immunoassay (ELISA) with a surface plasmon resonance-based biosensor for IGF-1 detection in cows' milk. Biosens Bioelectron 16: 971–977.

Hämläinen MD, A Zhukov, M Ivarsson, T Fex, J Gottfries, R Karlsson and M Björsne. 2008. Label-free primary screening and affinity ranking of fragment libraries using parallel analysis of protein panels. J Biomol Screening 13: 202–209.

Kuglstatter A, M Stahl, JU Peters, W Huber, M Stihle, D Schlatter, J Benz, A Ruf, D Roth, T Enderle and M Hennig. 2008. Tyramine fragment binding to BACE-1. Bioorg Med Chem Lett 18: 1304–1307.

Kumar V, MI Hassan, AK Singh, S Dey, TP Singh and S Yadav. 2009. Strategy for sensitive and specific detection of molecular forms of PSA based on 2DE and kinetic analysis: A step towards diagnosis of prostate cancer Clinica Chimica Acta 403: 17–22.

Ladd J, H Lub, AD Taylor, V Goodell, ML Disis and S Jianga. 2009. Direct detection of carcinoembryonic antigen autoantibodies in clinical human serum samples using a surface plasmon resonance sensor. Colloids Surf B: Biointerfaces 70: 1–6.

Minunni M, S Tombelli, M Mascini, AR Bilia, MC Bergonzi and FF Vincieri. 2005. An optical DNA-based biosensor for the analysis of bioactive constituents with application in drug and herbal drug screening. Talanta 65: 578–585.

Navratilova I and AL Hopkins. 2010. Fragment Screening by Surface Plasmon Resonance. ACS Med Chem Lett 1: 44–48

Nordström H, T Gossas, M Hämläinen, P Kälblad, S Nyström, H Wallberg and UH Danielson. 2008. Identification of MMP-12 inhibitors by using biosensor-based screening of a fragment library. J Med Chem 51: 3349–3459.

Oesterling JE. 1991. Prostate specific antigen: a critical assessment of the most useful tumor marker for adenocarcinoma of the prostate. J Urol 145: 907–23.

Okuda Y, HK Nakamura and K Kuwata. 2009. Novel anti-cancer compounds: Structure-based discovery of chemical chaperons for p53 Oncol Rep 22: 739–744.

Perspicase S, D Banner, J Benz, F Müller, D Schlatter and W Huber. 2009. Fragment-based screening using surface plasmon resonance technology. J Biomol Screening 14: 337–349.

Rini B, M Wadhwa, C Bird, E Small, R Gaines-Das and R Thorpe. 2005. Kinetics of development and characteristics of antibodies induced in cancer patients against yeast expressed rDNA derived granulocyte macrophage colony stimulating factor (GM-CSF). Cytokine 29: 56–66.

Stamey TA, N Yang, AR Hay, JE McNeal, FS Freiha and E Redwine. 1987. Prostate-specific antigen as a serum marker for adenocarcinoma of the prostate. N Engl J Med 317: 909–916.

Suwansa-ard S, P Kanatharana, P Asawatreratanakul, B Wongkittisuksa, C Limsakul and P Thavarungkul. 2009. Comparison of surface plasmon resonance and capacitive immunosensors for cancer antigen 125 detection in human serum samples Biosens and Bioelectron 24: 3436–3441.

Swanson SJ, SJ Jacobs, D Mytych, C Shah, SR Indelicato and RW Bordens. 1999. Applications for the new electrochemiluminescent (ECL) and biosensor technologies. Dev Biol Stand 97: 135–147.

Swanson SJ, D Mytych and J Ferbas. 2002. Use of biosensors to monitor the immune response. Dev Biol 109: 71–78.

Takakusagi Y, S Kobayashia and F Sugawaraa. 2005. Camptothecin binds to a synthetic peptide identified by a T7 phage display screen. Bioorg Med Chem Lett 15: 4850–4853.

Vaisocherova H, VM Faca, AD Taylor, S Hanashb and S Jianga. 2009. Comparative study of SPR and ELISA methods based on analysis of CD166/ALCAM levels in cancer and control human sera Biosens Bioelectron 24: 2143–2148.

Wadhwa M, C Bird, P Dilger, R Gaines-Das and R Thorpe. 2003. Strategies for the detection, measurement and characterization of unwanted antibodies induced by therapeutic biologicals. J Immunol Methods 278: 1–17.

Wang Y, X Zhu, M Wu, N Xia, J Wang and F Zhou. 2009. Simultaneous and label-free determination of wild-type and mutant p53 at a single surface plasmon resonance chip preimmobilized with consensus DNA and monoclonal antibody. Anal Chem 81: 8441–8446.

Single-Chain Fragment Variable Recombinant Antibodies and Their Applications in Biosensors for Cancer Diagnosis

Xiangqun Zeng[1],* and Ray Mernaugh[2]

ABSTRACT

Current phage display scFv recombinant antibody technology provides the means to readily select for high affinity scFvs to a multitude of antigens. In this chapter, we describe the use of single chain fragment variable recombinant antibodies (scFv) for use as antigen recognition elements in biosensors. Recombinant scFv can be genetically engineered to self-assemble in the correct orientation at high density on sensor surfaces to produce assays that can specifically detect extremely low concentrations of analytes in complex biological samples such as blood. Methods to refine scFv sensors to reduce biofouling and non-specific binding events are presented. Applications utilizing scFvs to capture

[1]Department of Chemistry, Oakland University, Rochester, MI 48309, USA;
E-mail: zeng@oakland.edu
[2]Department of Biochemistry, School of Medicine, Vanderbilt University, Nashville, TN 37232;
E-mail: r.mernaugh@vanderbilt.edu
*Corresponding author

List of abbreviations after the text.

cells onto sensors or antigens onto nanoparticles are also discussed. The advantage in combining highly sensitive label free transducers (e.g. quartz crystal microbalances or QCM) with highly selective recombinant antibodies is that a wide range of inexpensive, stable, fast, higly sensitive and specific biosensor assays can be developed to detect disease.

INTRODUCTION

Citizens of well-developed nations are living longer than their ancestors. However, as citizens age their chances of developing cancer tend to increase. The costs associated with cancer can be high. These costs are related to cancer patient treatment, symptom relief and recovery, and loss of patient and family member worker productivity and income. Logically, if enough citizens within a nation require cancer care, then the healthcare and financial cost to a nation can become high and economically debilitating.

When diagnosed early, most forms of cancer can be successfully treated at lower cost, or can be rendered less incapacitating or life threatening. Therefore, it is best to diagnose cancer early on to reduce downstream healthcare complications and costs. However, the conventional methods (e.g. mammograms, digital rectal exams, biopsies, etc.) traditionally used to diagnose cancer can be costly, inaccurate or invasive. To overcome these shortcomings, researchers are attempting to develop simple, inexpensive, highly specific and sensitive, non-invasive diagnostic assays (e.g. enzyme-linked immunosorbant assays or ELISAs) to detect cancer biomarkers in human fluids (e.g. serum). Most of these assays use polyclonal, monoclonal IgG, Fab or F(ab')$_2$ fragments, or recombinant antibodies (e.g. recombinant Fab, scFv or Vh fragments) to capture or detect cancer cells or proteinaceous biomarker antigens in serum. Although the approaches taken to develop such assays seem relatively simple and straightforward, they can be fraught with a variety of challenging problems. It is only when problems are identified that measures can be taken to circumvent such problems. The following section will describe some of the various components that may be used to develop cancer diagnostic assays, and the potential advantages and disadvantages these have when used to detect cancer biomarkers in serum.

ANTIBODIES AND ANTIBODY FRAGMENTS AS CANCER BIOMARKER RECOGNITION ELEMENTS

Probably the most difficult component to produce for many of these immunoassays is a high affinity, highly specific antibody that can be used to capture an antigen out of a sample such as serum. An antigen is anything that elicits an immune response. An antigen may display one or more antigenic sites (epitopes) that are around 4–10 or more amino acids in length. Antibodies can bind to linear or conformational epitopes present on an antigen. An antibody to a linear epitope can bind to an antigen even when the antigenic site has been denatured or has lost its shape. An antibody to a conformational epitope can only bind to the antigen if the epitope retains its shape and has not been denatured or distorted. However, antibodies will not bind to linear or conformational epitopes if either is physically buried within an antigen or buried when the antigen is immobilized onto a solid support.

Animals produce antibodies in response to antigenic stimuli. There are five classes (IgA, IgD, IgE, IgG and IgM) of antibodies produced during an animal's humoral immune response. Of these, IgG antibodies or their Fab or F(ab')$_2$ fragments are generally used in assays. For that reason, this chapter will not cover IgA, IgD, IgE and IgM antibodies to any great extent. Each Y-shaped IgG immunoglobulin contains a pair of light (~25 kd) and heavy (~50–55 kd) polypeptide chains. Antigen binding occurs at the top, or amino terminal end, of the Y within the antibody's paratope. The paratope is located within the antibody's idiotype or variable region. The first ~110 amino acids of the light and ~130 amino acids of the heavy chain make up the antibody's variable region (Fig. 18.1).

The amino acids present within the variable region vary from one antigen-specific antibody to another. The variable region amino acids (mainly those within the antibody's complementary determining regions or CDRs) interact with the antigen's amino acids primarily through four forces: hydrogen-bonding, ionic interactions, van der Waal's forces and hydrophobic interactions. These four forces can be perturbed and antigen and antibody binding can be disrupted when the antigen and antibody are exposed, respectively, to extreme changes in pH, salt, temperature or detergent conditions.

The remaining amino acids present within the IgG heavy and light chains represent the antibody's constant regions. There are two different constant region isotypes for antibody light chains [kappa (κ) and lambda (λ)], and five-six different heavy chain isotypes (IgG1, IgG2a, IgG2b, IgG2c, IgG3 and IgG4). The constant region amino acids do not vary appreciably from one antigen-specific antibody isotype to another within the same animal species.

Each B-cell in an animal produces one antibody specific for one antigenic site. If the antigen used to immunize an animal is large and has many unique antigenic sites, then polyclonal antibodies can be produced by many of the animal's B-cell clones (i.e. polyclones) to the large antigen. Generally, polyclonal antibodies are produced by immunizing an animal (e.g. donkey, goat, rabbit, etc.) with an antigen and collecting serum-containing antibodies over a period of weeks or months. Monoclonal antibodies are also produced

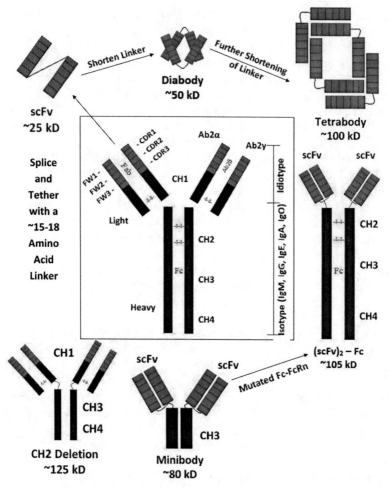

Figure 18.1. ScFv recombinant antibodies. parent antibody and various scFv constructs possible for use in different applications.

Color image of this figure appears in the color plate section at the end of the book.

by immunizing animals (e.g. mice, rabbits, rats, etc.) with antigens. However, once an animal has produced an antigen-specific antibody response, the animals are sacrificied and their spleens, lymph nodes or other lymphatic tissues are removed to obtain the antibody-producing B-cells. Under most cell culture conditions, B-cells only live for a few weeks. However, a long lived myeloma (i.e. cancer) cell can be fused with a single (monoclonal) B-cell using polyethylene glycol or electroporation to produce an immortal hybridoma cell line that produces an antibody specific for just one antigenic site. Depending upon the antigen, monoclonal antibodies can be obtained in

4-26 wk. Polyclonal and monoclonal antibodies can be affinity purified by ion exchange, hydrophobic interaction or size exclusion chromatography, or by antigen, protein A, G or L affinity chromatography. Typically polyclonal and monoclonal antibodies are used as antigen capture elements to develop immunoassays. However, since antibodies can bind to different antigens that display cross reactive epitopes, monoclonal rather than polyclonal antibodies are generally used as capture elements to reduce the chances that an irrelevant antigen will be captured and detected in an assay to produce a false positive signal.

Enzymes can be used to fragment IgG into smaller antigen-binding fragments. This approach is taken to remove parts of an antibody that may be responsible for creating an assay background problem. The enzyme papain digests an antibody above the hinge region where the top of the Y-shaped antibody meets the bottom. The Fab (fragment antibody binding) fragments (~50kd) obtained through papain digestion can be separated away from the bottom or Fc (fraction crystallizeable) fragment of the Y-shaped antibody using, in most cases, Fc-binding reagents like protein A or G, bound to beads to remove the Fc domains. The enzyme pepsin can digest IgG just below the hinge region to produce $F(ab')_2$ fragments (~110kd). Whereas the Fab fragments only consist of one of the upper arms of the Y-shaped IgG, the $F(ab')_2$ consist of two Fab fragments held together by sets of antibody heavy interchain disulfide bonds. As such, each Fab displays one while each $F(ab')_2$ fragment displays two paratopes (Fig. 18.1).

Antibodies can be expressed as recombinant proteins in bacteria, yeast or other cells in one of several formats. Antibodies can be expressed as recombinant Fab fragments and will exhibit most of the features exhibited by Fab fragments produced through papain digestion of IgG. Single chain fragment variable (scFv) recombinant antibodies (~27 kd) are composed of the variable heavy (Vh) and variable light (Vl) chain regions (i.e. the idiotype) of an antibody genetically linked together with a short stretch of amino acids (e.g. glycine and serine) to form a single chain. The linker amino acids used to join Vh and Vl chains can be varied from 0 to 15 or more amino acids to vary scFv valency from monomers, to dimers, tetramers, etc.. Nanobodies are smaller than scFv and are composed of just the Vh region of an antibody. ScFv can also be genetically linked to an antibody constant heavy chain region (e.g. the CH3 region) to create minibodies (Fig. 18.1). Many recombinant antibodies are selected from large (>1 billion member) phage (i.e. bacterial virus), yeast or ribosome-displayed recombinant libraries. As with all of these systems, the antibody and its respective genes are joined together as a single unit. Therefore, the antibody's genes accompany the antibody wherever the antibody goes and binds to an antigen. The antibody-encoding genes can eventaully be transferred to a host cell to make large quantities of the recombinant antibodies that bound to the antigen. The advantages in using recombinant antibody libraries are that no animals are needed, and the libraries can be used to select for antigen-specific antibodies (even to poorly immunogenic molecules) within a few weeks (Engberg et al. 2001). The expression of the selected recombinant antibodies can be carried out in prokaryotes (mainly *E. coli*), or if glycosylation is needed, in eukaryotes (e.g. yeast, insect cells, plant cells, and mammalian cells) (Engberg et al. 2001). Recombinant antibodies can be purified in several ways. They can be engineered to display a hexahistidine or His-tag and semi-purified using an immobilized metal affinity chromatography (IMAC), or can be engineered to display a peptide tag (e.g. c-myc, HA, Flag, E-tag, etc.) and affinity-purified using columns containing antibodies specific for the tags. Purified recombinant antibodies can be directly labeled with biotin and can be used to capture antigens using avidin/streptavidin/neutravidin bound to solid supports (e.g. piezoimmunosensor surfaces). Alternatively, amino acids (e.g. those present within the linker of an scFv) can be changed through site-directed mutagenesis to cysteines, histidines or arginines to directly couple scFv onto sensor (e.g. gold) surfaces. As shown in Section 4 below, scFv (e.g. A10B) engineered to contain linker bearing cysteine or arginine amino acids retain antigen-binding specificity and have been successfully used in piezoimmunosensor assays (Shen et al. 2005a; Shen et al. 2005b). Essentially, scFv obtained from a phage-displayed antibody library are quite flexible and will retain antigen binding activity when biotinylated or genetically engineered for immobilization onto streptavidin, gold or derivatized sensor (e.g. QCM) surfaces.

The type of antibody or antibody fragment to use in an immunoassay is dependent upon its affinity, avidity or antigen-binding specificity. An antibody's affinity represents the antigen-binding strength between a single paratope (e.g. a Fab fragment) and a single epitope. High affinity antibodies can bind (associate) faster and let go (dissociate) of an antigen slower than a low affinity antibody, and are more suited for detecting trace amounts of antigens in assays.

Avidity is similar to affinity. Whereas affinity measures the binding strength between one paratope and one epitope, avidity measures the cumulative binding strength that occurs between multiple paratopes on one antibody (e.g. the 10 paratopes on one IgM) with multiple repeating epitopes in one particle (e.g. a virus). If a single paratope-bearing scFv demonstrates low affinity for a virus, it can be re-engineered as a dimer (two paratopes), trimer (three paratopes), etc. (Fig. 18.1). Each additional paratope will stabilize antigen/antibody interactions by reducing antibody dissociation rates to enhance the antibody's ability to bind to and detect antigens in assays.

The antigen-binding specificity of an antibody represents the antibody's ability to bind to the target antigen only, amongst all other components present in a sample. Generally, mouse monoclonal antibodies are used as immunorecognition elements in many assays. However, since human serum can contain heterophilic antibodies that bind to mouse antibodies, the heterophilic antibodies can also bind to the mouse capture and detection antibodies to produce a false positive assay signal, whether the antigen is present or not (Persselin and Stevens 1985). Human Fab antibodies can be used as immunorecognition elements to overcome problems associated with heterophilic antibodies. However, human serum can also contain antibodies that react with human Fab fragments to produce false positive assay signals. Therefore, use of Fab as immunorecognition elements may be limited (Persselin and Stevens 1985). Recombinant scFv fragments have been used to overcome problems associated with mouse IgG and Fab fragments and may be more suitable as capture agents in human serum-based assays (Shen et al. 2005a).

BIOSENSORS AND THEIR APPLICATIONS IN CANCER DIAGNOSIS

A wide variety of sensor techniques have been utilized and developed to detect some of the most promising cancer biomarkers (Rasooly and Jacobson 2006). Some of the most common protein biomarkers associated with cancer are prostate specific antigen (prostate cancer), cancer antibody CA 15-3 (breast cancer), carcinoembryonic antigen (liver, colon, pancreatic, and ovarian cancer), alpha-fetoprotein (liver and testicular cancers) and CA 125 (breast cancer). A more thorough list is shown in Table 18.1 (Tothill 2009). In many cases a threshold limit has been established for these biomarkers and is used in clinical applications. However, many of the known biomarkers are not all that useful in diagnostics because they are not present until later on in the disease. Instead, most biomarkers are either used to assign risk factors or determine disease prognosis.

Cancer biomarker antigens in samples are traditionally detected using quantitative assays such enzyme-linked immunosorbant assays (ELISAs) or qualitative assays such as Western blots, immunofluorescence (IF) and immunohistochemistry (IHC). Immunofluorescence and IHC assays are used to detect antigens in cell or tissue (e.g. biopsy) samples. Optical sensors such as the BIAcore, ProteOn XPR36 (BioRad), Epic (Corning) and Octet (Forte Bio) can use a single antibody, immobilized onto a gold-coated glass or waveguide sensor surface, to capture an antigen from solution. Antigen binding to antibodies can then be measured using light refractive index

Table 18.1. Cancer biomarkers.

Cancer Type Disease	Biomarker
Prostate	PSA, PAP
Breast	CA 15-3, CA 125, CA 27.29, CEABRCA1, BRCA2, MUC-1, CEA, NY-BR-1, ING-1
Leukaemia	Chromosomal Abnormalities
Testicular	α-Fetoprotein (AFP), β-Human Chorionic Gonadatropin, CAGE-1,ESO-1
Ovarian	CA 125, AFP, hCG, p53, CEA
Any Solid Tumor	Circulating tumor cells in biological fluids, expression of targeted growth factor receptors
Colon and Pancreatic	CEA, CA 19-9, CA 24-2, p53
Lung	NY-ESO-1, CEA, CA 19-9, SCC, CYFRA 21-1, NSE
Melanoma	Tyrosinase, NY-ESO-1
Liver	AFP, CEA
Gastric Carcinoma	CA 72-4, CEA, CA 19-9
Esophagus Carcinoma	SCC
Trophoblastic	SCC, hCG
Bladder	BAT, FDP, NMP22, HA-Hase, BLCA-4, CYFRA 21-1

List of many of the identified cancer biomarkers associated with different cancer types (Tothill 2009).

or surface plasmon resonance (SPR) changes on sensor surfaces to detect antigen binding events. SPR sensors have been used to detect CA 15-3, CEA, CA 125, and methylated DNA sequences (Chang et al. 2010; Ladd et al. 2009; Suwansa et al. 2009; Pan et al. 2010). Other methods such as opto-fluidic ring resonators (Suter et al. 2010) and AIN FBAR (Lee and Song 2010) have been successfully developed to detect cancer biomarkers. The advantages in using optical sensor platforms are that they consume small amounts of sample and can be used to measure antigen/antibody binding in real-time. The disadvantages are that the instruments and consumables (e.g. sensor surfaces) can be quite expensive, any microfluidic devices used can become blocked during operation, and the design and optimization of assays can be time-consuming and technically demanding. Micro-cantilever sensors bearing antibodies can be used to detect antigens in solution. The micro-cantilever deflects or bends when the mass of the sensor changes upon antigen binding. The advantage in using micro-cantilevers is that these sensors can be used to develop very sensitive assays. The disadvantage in using these sensors is that changes (noise, light, ambient pressure, etc.) in the environment can interfere with and create background problems in assays (Backmann et al. 2005). A surface acoustic wave (SAW) sensor has been designed by Gruhl et al. to detect the breast cancer marker HER-2/neu (Gruhl et al. 2010). Electrochemical methods have also been used to quantify biomarkers such as PSA (Sarkar et al. 2002; Lin et al. 2008), AFP (Du et al. 2010) , CA 125 (He et al. 2003) and DNA methylation (Goto et al. 2010).

RECOMBINANT ANTIBODIES AS RECOGNITION ELEMENTS FOR IMPROVED IMMUNOSENSOR PERFORMANCE

Our laboratories have successfully developed a very simple scFv based-recombinant antibody piezoimmunosensor technology for use in the detection and quantification of a unique antibody in serum samples and proteins in breast cancer cells (Shen et al. 2005a; Shen et al. 2005b; Shen et al. 2007; Shen et al. 2008). Piezoimmunosensor technology uses a quartz crystal microbalance (QCM) to measure the interactions between a QCM surface-bound scFv and an antigen or antibody present in a sample. QCM is a mass sensor in which a foreign mass (i.e. scFv) is strongly coupled to the resonator. Interfacial mass changes related to changes in the QCM oscillation frequency are represented by Sauerbrey's equation: $\Delta f = -2\Delta mnf_0^2$ / $[A(\mu_q\rho_q)^{1/2}]$, where n is the overtone number, μ_q is the shear modulus of the quartz (2.947×10^{11} g/(cm·sec²) and ρ_q is the density of the quartz (2.648 g/cm³). Antigen binding to a sensor surface changes its mass and electronic vibrational frequency which can be recorded to determine antigen presence. Unlike traditional immunoassay platforms, only one antibody (e.g. an scFv) is needed to carry out piezoimmunosensor assays and no wash steps are required. The ligand/surface (i.e. scfv/sensor surface) in pezoimmunsensors can, unlike traditional immunoassays (e.g. ELISAs), be readily interrogated to accurately determine ligand density. As such piezoimmunosensor assays can be more easily reproduced and quality-controlled to reduce inter-assay variation. A summary of scFv and their uses as recognition elements is presented in Table 18.2. The low cost, one-step readout of non-labeled QCM transducers and the high specificity of antigen-antibody recognition represent one of the most promising biosensor technologies for near or real-time analysis of cancer biomarkers in clinical samples.

Engineered scFv for Piezoimmunosensor Use

Antibody (i.e. scFv) immobilization on sensor surfaces represents a critical step in biosensor development. It is important to immobilize a sufficient amount of properly oriented scFv on the sensor surface to specifically capture and detect trace amounts of antigen.

A model scFv antibody/antigen system was used to determine which scFv amino acids were best suited for scFv immobilization on the gold sensor surface. The scFv (designated A10B) was developed using the antibody genes of a monoclonal antibody-producing hybridoma cell line.

Table 18.2. Current scFv based sensors.

Analyte	Antibody Form	Transducer
Disease		
HIV-1 virion infectivity factor	scFv (VH and VHD)	Piezoelectric
L. *monocytogenes*	scFv	SPR
SARS virus	scFv	Imaging Ellipsometry
L. *monocytogenes*	scFv (phage bound)	Amperometric
Her2 (human epidermal growth factor receptor 2)	scFv	Piezoelectric microcantilever
Her2 (human epidermal growth factor receptor 2)	scFv	Optofluidic ring resonator
Foot and mouth disease virus	SD6 scFv	ELISA
Biowarfare		
Venezuelan equine encephalitis virus	scFv	Potentiometric
B. *anthracts* S-layer protein	scFv	Resonant Mirror
Haptens		
Morphine-3-glucuronide	scFv	SPR
Contaminants		
Aflatoxin B1	scFv (mono- and dimeric)	SPR
Parathion (insecticide)	scFv	Piezoelectric

List of currently developed scFv based sensors for the detection of various analytes (Alcala et al. 2002; Capobianco et al. 2008; Conroy et al. 2009; Gohring et al. 2010; Backmann et al. 2005).

The cell line produces an IgG1 antibody (designated A10B) that binds to rabbit IgG (the antigen). Monoclonal A10B Fab fragments (obtained by papain digestion) and the genetically engineered A10B scFv recombinant antibodies all specifically bind rabbit IgG (Shen et al. 2008). The peptide linker connecting Vh and Vl domains in scFv joins the A10B Vh and Vl domains. Generally, the 15 amino acid (GGGGS)$_3$ peptide is used as an scFv peptide linker. This linker was re-engineered to contain different metal binding amino acids [(e.g. cysteine (A10B-cys) or histidines (A10B -his)] (Table 18.3, Figs. 18.2–18.3). Modified scFv directly self-assemble onto the gold surface (via strong adsorption of cysteine or histidine to gold) with optimum density and orientation. It is important to note that the location of the cysteine within the scFv was important for immobilization as cysteines within the linker are more available to bind with gold than those present in the scFv framework region (Shen et al. 2005a). Bacterial protein expression can be problematic when cysteines amino acids are components of the protein. To circumvent this problem, positively charged arginine (R) amino acids were used in lieu of cysteine to immobilize A10B scFv (RG3) onto an anionic charged template surface [(11-mercaptoundecanoic acid (MUA) or poly(sodium 4-styrenesulfonate) (PSS)].

Table 18.3. Linker amino acids in A10B scFv constructs.

A10B Rs	(GGGGS)$_3$
A10B Cys	(CGGGS) (GGGGS)$_2$
A10B His	SHGGH GGGGG GGGGS
A10B RG3	RGRGRGRGRSRGGGGS
A10B ZnS4	VISNHAGSSRRL
A10B Cds6	PWIPTPRPTFTG

Amino acid sequences used in the linker proteins for the various A10B scFv constructs.

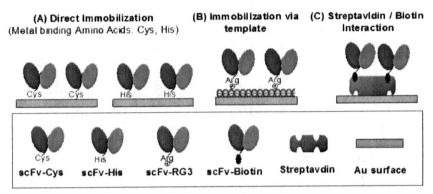

Figure 18.2. Methods for coupling of scFvs to Au sensor surface.

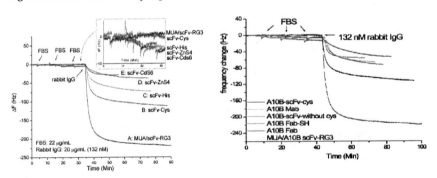

Figure 18.3. Comparison of IgG, Fab and various scFv immunorecognition elements for selectivity and sensitivity; **(left)** MUA/scFv-RG3, scFv-Cys, scFv-His, scFv-ZnS4, scFv-CdS6; **(right)** IgG, Fab, scFv and scFv-cys. FBS 22μg/mL (permission from ACS).

Color image of this figure appears in the color plate section at the end of the book.

The A10B scFv-RG3 sensor exhibited the greatest assay sensitivity in comparison to whole A10B IgG, Fab, non-specifically adsorbed A10B scFv (i.e. A10B scFv without cys) and A10B scFv bearing a linker-containing cysteine (Fig. 18.3) (Shen et al. 2005a; Shen et al. 2005b).

IgG, Fab and scFv Comparisons for Use in Piezoimmunosensors

We compared the specificity and sensitivity of piezoimmunosensors for serum-based assays using A10B IgG, Fab and scFv recognition elements. In comparison to A10B IgG and Fab fragments, assay sensitivity and specificity in the presence of serum was greatest for the A10B scFv-cys modified sensor (Fig. 18.3). Additionally, the A10B scfv-cys sensor exhibited nanomolar sensitivity and was able to measure IgG concentration in fresh drawn rabbit blood serum yielding results comparable to an ELISA (Shen et al. 2005a).

When A10B was engineered to contain different linker amino acids, our results demonstrated that the anionic charged SAM template facilitated the oriented immobilization of A10B scFv-RG3 on the sensor surface and apparently reduced A10B scFv-RG3 protein denaturation (Shen et al. 2007; Shen et al. 2008). A 42-fold improvement in assay sensitivity was obtained using MUA/A10B scFv-RG3 (200pM assay sensitivity) in comparison to an A10B Fab antibody sensor and a five-fold improvement in comparison to an A10B scFv-cys sensor (Fig. 18.3). With 20 amino acids to choose from, engineered recombinant scFv in combination with SAM technology represents an emerging strategy for the development of highly sensitive, specific and stable scFv based immunosensors.

Piezoimmunosensor Determination of Antibody Affinity

The rabbit IgG/scFv binding association constant (K_a) and concentration of antigen bound in nanograms (ΔM) can be obtained from the relationship of time versus frequency change at various rabbit IgG antigen concentrations according to Equation (1).

$$[\text{rabbit IgG}]+[\text{scFv}] \underset{\text{Koff}}{\overset{\text{Kon}}{\rightleftharpoons}} [\text{rabbit IgG-scFv complex}] \tag{1}$$

Based on Langmuir adsorption isotherm, the association (K_a) and dissociation (K_d) constants for rabbit/scFv binding can be described using Equation (2):

$$\frac{[\text{rabbit IgG}]}{\Delta M} = \frac{[\text{rabbit IgG}]}{\Delta M_{max}} + \frac{1}{\Delta M_{max} K_a} \tag{2}$$

In Equation (2), ΔM_{max} is the maximum amount of rabbit IgG that can be bound. ΔM (the amount of rabbit IgG bound at equilibrium) is a function of the rabbit IgG concentration and will not change with time; and [rabbit IgG] is the original concentration of rabbit IgG. A representative plot of [rabbit IgG]/ΔM vs. [rabbit IgG] was obtained. According to Equation (2), the ratio of the slope to the intercept yields the association constant (Ka). Dissociation constant (Kd) was calculated as 1/Ka. The association constant (Ka) of A10B scFv-Cys with rabbit IgG was determined to be 1.9 $\times 10^7$ M^{-1} which is consistent to the (2.2$\pm$1.5)$\times 10^7$ M^{-1}, measured by Biacore SPR (Tang et al. 2006).

ScFv-based Piezoimmunosensor Assay Sensitivity Enhancement

(a) Amplification of the antigen mass

QCM is a mass sensor, thus, the sensitivity of a piezoimmunosensor depends on the scFv (e.g. A10B scFv bound to the sensor) as well as the mass of the analyte (e.g. rabbit IgG) captured from a sample. The scFv engineering strategies previously described allow for scFv immobilization with optimum orientation to increase assay specificity and sensitivity. Potentially, the increase in sensitivity is due to an increase in the density of scFvs (i.e. paratopes) immobilized onto the sensor surface. Theoretically, this leads to an artificial increase in scFv/sensor avidity and a real increase in assay sensitivity. QCM assay sensitivity can also be increased through the use of gold nanoparticles (NPs) conjugated to secondary recognition elements (e.g. protein A). The NPs can bind to the antigen (e.g. rabbit IgG) captured onto the scFv (e.g. A10B) surface to increase sensor mass, assay signal and sensitivity. As depicted in Fig. 18.5, pure Au NP and protein A coated Au NP show little non-specific binding to the scFv immobilized on the sensor surface. However, the protein A coated gold nanoparticles (15nm) bind to the rabbit IgG which further amplified the mass of the rabbit IgG target. This method increased the limits of detection to 8pM. Additionally, QCM sensitivity can be improved by varying the sensor surface (e.g. adjusting surface roughness using non-polished vs. polished QCM crystals) and electronic oscillation frequency. QCM sensitivity increases with the square of the fundamental oscillation frequency (f_0) and linearly with n (overtone number). Thus by working with crystals of higher f_0, or at higher harmonics, higher sensitivities can be obtained. We observed close to a five-fold increase in signal intensity experimentally when a 25 instead of a 10 MHz quartz crystal was used.

(b) Blocking piezoimmunosensor non-specific interactions

BSA has been traditionally used to block non-specific binding reactions in assays. Several studies show that polyethylene glycol compounds are effective blocking agents (Wang et al. 2009). We have tested carbohydrates

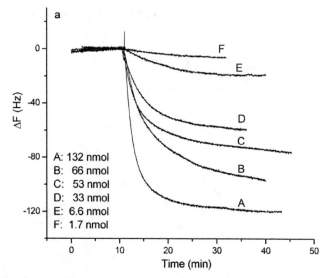

Figure 18.4. Binding of IgG with scFv-cys (permission from ACS).

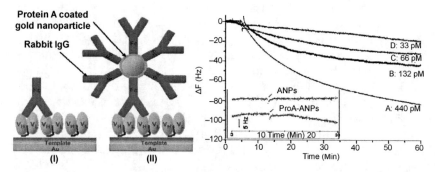

Figure 18.5. ScFv –AuNP; **(left)** binding of rabbit IgG without (I) or with Protein A coated Au NP (II), A-D; **(right)** the addition of Au NP or protein A coated Au NP to scFv immobilized surfaces (permission from ACS).

Color image of this figure appears in the color plate section at the end of the book.

in combination with other blocking agents (e.g. BSA) to reduce nonspecific binding on sensor surfaces (Fig. 18.6). Six carbohydrate monomers were synthesized and derivatized with a sulfur (-SH) functional group. As shown in Fig. 18.6 (top curves), glucose, galactose and sialic acid SAMs can block the non-specific adsorption of human serum effectively. More importantly, A10B scFv-cys on a sensor surface blocked with BSA and sialic acid specifically detected antigen in human serum with little background assay signal (Fig. 18.6 - bottom curves).

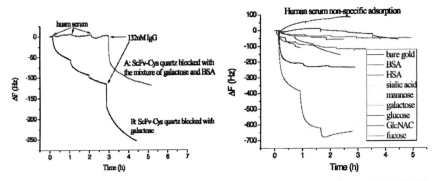

Figure 18.6. Blocking effect of BSA, HSA and different carbohydrate; **(left):** at 0.2%, 0.5%, 1% and 2% human serum final concentrations; **(right):** scFv-cys piezoimmunosensor sensitivity and specificity when blocked with galactose only or with the mixture of galactose and BSA (final human serum concentrations: 0.2%, 0.5%, 1% with 132nM rabbit IgG) (Permission from ACS).

Color image of this figure appears in the color plate section at the end of the book.

Multiple ScFv Piezoimmunosensor Arrays

Human serum contains biomolecules that can bind non-specifically to recognition elements (e.g. scFv) on sensor surfaces to produce false positive assay results. ScFv specific for different antigens (e.g. CYP1B1, CYP1A1, etc.) coupled to different QCM sensors can be used to detect non-specific binding events in assays. If an antigen (e.g. CYP1B1) is present in a sample, binding will occur only with the positive (e.g. anti-CYP1B1 scFv) but not the negative (e.g. anti-rabbit IgG) sensor surface. If binding occurs on both sensors, then the presumption is that sample non-specific binding is occurring. CYP1B1 is a P450 enzyme that is involved in the metabolism of many endogenous and exogenous compounds, including carcinogens. Because of its microsomal location in the cell, CYP1B1 cannot be measured directly using existing methods, but can be measured indirectly via the determination of its catalytic products. Three CYP1B1-specific scFv antibodies (designated B66, D23, L21) were obtained using a phage-displayed recombinant antibody library, purified, labeled with biotin and used to develop piezoimmunosensors (Fig. 18.7). We observed quantitative detection of CYP1B1 in model solutions of normal and malignant (e.g. T47D breast cancer) cell lysates. The scFv-QCM biosensors produced similar results (Fig. 18.4) and showed excellent sensitivity (limit of detection 2.2 ± 0.9 nM) and specificity with different anti-CYP1B1 scfvs producing similar dissociation constants [scFv D23: (1.59 ± 0.91) x 10^{-7} M, scFv B66: (1.52 ± 0.34) x 10^{-7} M, scFv L21: (1.52 ± 0.68) x 10^{-7} M].

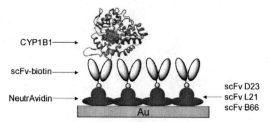

Figure 18.7. Schematic representation of scFv-QCM based CYP1B1 measurements.

Anti-CYP1B1 scFv-QCM sensor specificity in the presence of contaminants was ascertained by adding proteins [rabbit IgG, fetal bovine serum (FBS), CYP1A1 (a eukaryotic P450 similar but not identical to CYP1B1), BMV-3 (a P450 from the bacterium *Bacillus megatarium*)], lipids, detergents or fractionated microsomes to the anti-CYP1B1 scFv QCM assay (Fig. 18.8). Minimal or no non-specific adsorption was detected when CYP1A1 (Curve A), P450 BMV3 (Curve B), microsomes devoid of CYP1B1 (Curve C), rabbit IgG and FBS (Curve D), lipids and detergents (Curve E) were added to the anti-CYP1B1 QCM sensor. Less than 10 Hz signal was observed showing

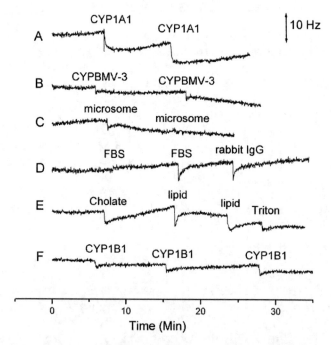

Figure 18.8. Selectivity of scFv-B66 QCM sensor. **A**: 60 nM CYP1A1; **B**: 30 nM P450 BMV-3; **C**: 2.4 μg/mL microsome without CYP1B1; **D**: 14.4 μg/ml FBS and 130 nM rabbit IgG; **E**: 0.01% cholate, 0.02% Triton, and 6.43 x 10⁻⁵ M lipid (1,2-Dilauroyl-sn-glycero-3-phosphocholone); **F**: A10B scFv-Cys QCM sensor was exposed to 60 nM CYP1B1 (Permission from ACS).

insignificant cross reactivity of the CYP1B1 piezoimmunosensors for CYP1A1 and P450 BMV-3. Our results demonstrated that an anti-CYP1B1 scFv-based QCM assay could be used to detect and quantify CYP1B1 in cell samples. Results from this study suggest that CYP1B1 enzymes are over expressed in some tumor cell lysates (Hela, HCC, and 4T1). The anti-CYP1B1 scFv-based QCM assay can potentially be used to determine the stage of tumor development (e.g. when P450s are up-regulated) and may be useful in identifying the endogenous function(s) of P450 in tumor cells. Compared to traditional methods like ELISA and CO-difference spectrometry, scFv-QCM assays produce higher selectivity and specificity and therefore show promise as a possible way to clarify questions relevant to cancer diagnosis, monitoring and treatment.

OTHER APPLICATIONS OF SCFV SENSORS

It is apparent that recombinant antibodies can be used to develop a wide range of biosensors with diagnostic potential. The discussion below describes other assays in which scfv have been used.

(a) scFv-based Nanoparticle Immunoassay

The anti-rabbit IgG scFv (designated A10B cys-scFv) used for piezoimmunosensor development was conjugated to gold NPs and used to develop colorimetric immunoassays. Assay readout was based on the unique phenomenon in which gold NPs change color upon aggregation. When rabbit IgG was added to A10B cys-scFv on gold NPs, the gold NPs aggregated to produce a visible red-shift color change (Fig. 18.9). The assay,

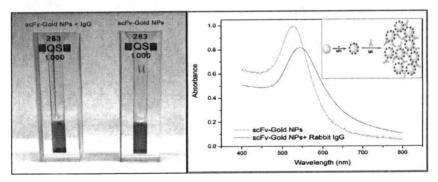

Figure 18.9. AuNP-scFv colorimetric assay; **(left):** visible difference in color change with IgG biding; **(right):** absorbance spectrum showing shift in peak absorbance with IgG binding (permission from Elsevier).

Color image of this figure appears in the color plate section at the end of the book.

which was used to visualize the interaction of rabbit IgG with A10B cys-scFv on gold NPs, had a detection limit of 1.7 nM (Fig. 18.9) (Liu et al. 2009). This unique optical feature makes small (<60 nm) gold NPs useful for detecting biomolecular interactions using a simple optical readout at ~520 nm. Since gold NPs exhibit extremely high extinction coefficients, they can be used to develop scFv-based assays that are more sensitive than traditional (e.g. fluorescence dye-based) assays (Liu et al. 2009).

(b) ScFv as a Template for Fc Sensors

The A10B scFv-RG3 (Table 3) was immobilized onto a pre-formed functionalized self-assembled monolayer (SAMs) template surface (Fig. 18.10). The monomeric ScFv can bind to the CH1 region of any rabbit IgG to form a highly oriented IgG layer with the IgG Fc region pointing toward the solution phase. This results in a highly oriented Fc sensor that can be used to study the thermodynamics and kinetics of binding between the Fc portion of immunoglobulins and cell surface Fc receptors (FcR), an important area of the immune system. The Fc sensor was used to study the binding between *Staphylococcus aureus* (*S. aureus*) and Macrophage bearing Fc receptors (Fig. 18.10) (Yan et al. 2011). The results demonstrated that non-labeled scFv-based QCM sensors could be used to detect interactions between whole cells and immobilized molecules on a sensor surface. Potentially, this approach can be used to monitor cell binding, in real time, to molecules that stimulate cancer cell activity; and as such, may represent a useful approach for drug discovery, cancer diagnostics, monitoring and treatment.

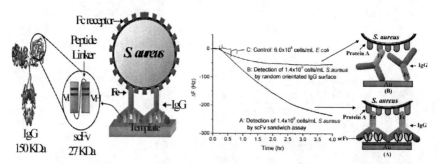

Figure 18.10. Fc sensor for the detection of cell's surface Fc receptor; QCM results for the detection of *S. aureus*. **(A)** Acid treated *S. aureus* were added to MUA/scFv-RG3/IgG surface; **(B)** Acid treated *S. aureus* were added to random oriented IgG surface; (C) Negative control: *E. coli* were added to MUA/scFv-RG3/IgG surface (permission from ACS).

Color image of this figure appears in the color plate section at the end of the book.

APPLICATION TO OTHER AREAS OF HEALTH AND DISEASES

Recombinant scFv-based sensors represent promising assay platforms to explore and detect cancer, infectious diseases, etc. Recombinant scFv can be genetically engineered to self-assemble on sensor surfaces at high density and in the correct orientation to produce highly sensitive and specific assays to detect analytes in very complex mixtures such as blood. A wide variety of sensing technologies are available for use and can be fabricated for high throughput to detect multiple analytes in a single sample (Jin et al. 2009).

KEY FACTS

- Most immunoassays use an antibody bound to a bead, sensor, solid support, etc. to capture an antigen out of a sample solution.
- The captured antigen is then detected using a labeled antibody that binds to another site on the captured antigen.
- The label can be a dye, enzyme, quantum dot or isotope that, when present, produces a signal that can be measured and recorded.
- The strength of the signal correlates with and is used to determine the antigen concentration in a sample.
- This assay format in which the antigen is sandwiched between capturing and detecting antibodies is presently used to detect prostate specific antigen (PSA) and diagnose prostate cancer in men (Terness et al. 1995; Healy et al. 2007).

DEFINITIONS

- *Biomarker*: a characteristic that is objectively measured and evaluated as an indicator of normal biologic processes, pathogenic processes, or pharmacologic responses to a therapeutic intervention.
- *Immunoassay*: a biochemical test that uses antibody to measure the presence or concentration of a substance that is usually in a complex mixture of substances (i.e. blood).
- *ScFv (single chain fragment variable)*: a type of recombinant antibody that only consists of the variable heavy and light chains linked together by a linker peptide.
- *Variable Heavy (Vh)*: the portion of the heavy chain of an antibody that is responsible for binding to the antigen.
- *Variable Light (Vl)*: the portion of the light chain of an antibody that is responsible for binding to the antigen.

SUMMARY POINTS

- Antibodies are Y-shaped immunglobulins produced by animal or human B-cells in response to an antigenic stimulus. Antibodies contain two or more pairs of heavy and light chain polypeptides. The five classes of antibodies are IgA, IgD, IgE, IgG and IgM.
- Polyclonal antibodies can be obtained directly from the serum of animals immunized with an antigen, or from hybridoma cell lines producing monoclonal antibodies in tissue culture. Recombinant antibodies can be obtained from bacteria yeasts or mammalian cells genetically engineered to express antibodies or antibody Fab, scFv, Vh, etc. fragments.
- Antibodies bind to antigens through hydrogen bonds, van der Waals's, ionic and hydrophobic forces. Antigen/antibody interactions are dependent upon the nature of the amino acids that make up the antigen and the variable/idiotype region of an antibody.
- Antibodies or antibody fragments can be bound or conjugated to beads, biotin, fluorescent dyes, enzymes, or surfaces and used to capture or detect antigens in assays.
- Antibodies or antibody fragments (e.g. scFv) can be used in ELISA, Western blot, immunohistochemistry, immunofluorescence endpoint immunoassays or in surface plasmon resonance, microcantilever or piezoimmunosensor/QCM assays to detect antigens or to study biomolecular interactions in real-time.

ACKNOWLEDGEMENT

We thank Michael Kerry for help with the literature summary, the support of Oakland University, Vanderbilt University Institute of Chemical Biology and NIH (R21EB000672-01, R33EB000672 and R21EB009513).

ABBREVIATIONS

CYP1B1	:	Cytochrome P450, family 1, subfamily B, polypeptide 1
ELISA	:	enzyme-linked immunosorbant assays
Fab	:	antibody-binding region
IF	:	immunofluorescence
IgG	:	Immunoglobulin G
IHC	:	immunohistochemistry
NP	:	Nanoparticle
QCM	:	Quartz Crystal Microbalance

ScFv   :   Single-Chain Fragment Variable Recombinant
                        Antibodies
SPR   :   Surface Plasma Resonance
Vh   :   variable heavy chain of Immunoglobulin G
Vl   :   variable light chain of Immunoglobulin G

REFERENCES

Alcala P, NF Miralles, JX Feliu and A Villaverde. 2002. Co-activator of antibody responsive, enzymatic sensors by a recombinant scFv antibody fragment produced in *E-coli*. Biotechnology Letters 24: 1543–1551.

American Cancer Society. What's new in prostate cancer research and treatment? Revised 10/27/2010. http://www.cancer.org/Cancer/ProstateCancer/DetailedGuide/prostate-cancer-new-research.

Backmann N, C Zahnd, F Huber, A Bietsch, A Pluckthum, HP Lang, HJ Guntherodt, M Hegner and C Gerber. 2005. A label-free immunosensor array using single-chain antibody fragments. Proceedings of the National Academy of Sciences of the United States of America 102: 14587–14592.

Breitling F and S Dubel. 1999. Antibody Engineering, Recombinant Antibodies. John Wiley &Sons, Inc and Spektrum Akademischer Verlag.

Capobianco JA, WY Shih, QA Yuan, GP Adams and WH Shih. 2008. Label-free, all electrical, in situ human epidermal growth receptor 2 detection. Review of Scientific Instruments 79: 76–101.

Chang CC, NF Chiu, DS Lin, YC Su, YH Liang and CW Lin. 2010. High sensitivity detection of cancer antigen 15-3 using a gold/zinc oxide thin film surface plasmon resonance based biosensor. Analytical Chemistry 82: 1207–1212.

Conroy PJ, S Hearty, P Leonard and RJ O'Kennedy. 2009. Antibody production, design and use for biosensor-based applications. Seminars in Cell & Developmental Biology 20: 10–26.

Du D, Z Zou, Y Shin, J Wang, H Wu, MH Engelhard, J Liu, IA Aksay and Y Lin. 2010. Sensitive immunosensor for cancer biomarker based on dual signal amplification strategy of graphene sheets and multienzyme functionalized carbon nanospheres. Anal Chem 82: 2989–2995.

Engberg J, B Jensen Liselotte, F Yenidunya Ali, K Brandt and E Riise. 2001. Phage—display Libraries of Murine Antibody Fab Fragments. p 65. *In:* R Kontermann and S Dubel (eds.) Springer –Verlag Berlin Heidelberg.

Goto K,. D Kato, N Sekioka, A Ueda, S Hirono and O Niwa. 2010. Direct electrochemical detection of DNA methylation for retinoblastoma and CpG fragments using a nanocarbon film. Analytical Biochemistry 405: 59–66.

Gohring JJ, PS Dale and X Fan. 2010. Detection of HER2 breast cancer bioimarker using the opto-fluidic ring resonator biosensor. Sensors and Actuators B 146: 226–230.

Gruhl FJ, M Rapp and K Lange. 2010. Label-free detection of breast cancer marker HER-2/neu with an acoustic biosensor. Procedic Engineering 5: 914–917.

He Z, N Gao and W Jin. 2003. Determination of tumor marker CA 125 by capillary electrophoretic enzyme immunoassay with electrochemical detection. Analytica Chimica Acta. 497: 75–81.

Healy DA, CJ Hayes, P Leonard, L McKenna and R O'Kennedy. 2007. Biosensor developments: application to prostate-specific antigen detection. Trends in Biotechnology 25: 125–131.

Jin X, Y Huang, A Mason and X Zeng. 2009. Multichannel Monolithic Quartz Crystal Microbalance Gas Sensor Array. Analytical Chemistry 81: 595–603.

Ladd J, H Lu, AD Taylor, V Goodell, ML Disis and S Jiang. 2009. Direct detection of carcinoembryonic antigen autoantibodies in clinical human serum samples using surface plasmon resonance. Colloids and Surfaces B: Biointerfaces 70: 1–6.

Lee TY and JT Song. 2010. Detection of carcinoembryonic antigen using AlN FBAR. Thin solid films 518: 6630–6633.

Lin S, X Zhang, Y Wu, Y Tu and L He. 2008. Prostate-specific antigen detection by using a reusable amperometric immunosensor based on reversible binding and leasing of HRP-anti PSA from phenylboronic acid modified electrode. Clinica Chimica Acta 395: 51–56.

Liu Y, Y Liu, RL Mernaugh and X Zeng. 2009. Single chain fragment variable recombinant antibody functionalized gold nanoparticles for a highly sensitive colorimetric immunoassay. Biosensors and Bioelectronics 24: 2853–2857.

Pan S, J Xu, Y Shu, F Wang, W Xia, Q Ding, T Xu, C Zhao, M Zhang, P Huang and S Lu. 2010. Double recognition of oligonucleotide and protein in the detection of DNA methylation with surface plasmon resonance biosensors. Biosensors and Bioelectronics 36: 850–853.

Persselin JE and RH Stevens. 1985. Anti-Fab antibodies in humans: predominance of minor immunoglobulin G subclasses in rheumatoid arthritis. J Clin Invest 76: 723–730.

Rasooly A and J Jacobson. 2006. Development of biosensors for cancer clinical testing. Biosensors and Bioelectronics 21: 1851–1858.

Sarkar P, PS Pal, D Ghosh, SJ Setford and IE Tothill. 2002. Amperometric biosensors for detection of the prostate cancer marker (PSA). International Journal of Pharmaceuticals 238: 1–9.

Shen Z, GA Stryker, RL Mernaugh, L Yu, H Yan and X Zeng. 2005a. Single-chain fragment variable antibody piezoimmunosensors. Anal Chem 77: 797–805.

Shen Z, RL Mernaugh, H Yan, L Yu, Y Zhang and X Zeng. 2005b. Engineered recombinant single-chain fragment variable antibody for immunosensors. Anal Chem 77: 6834–42.

Shen Z, H Yan, F Parl, RL Mernaugh and X Zeng. 2007. Recombinant antibody piezoimmunosensors for the detection of cytochrome P450 1B1. Anal Chem 79: 1283–9.

Shen Z, H Yan, Y Zhang, RL Mernaugh and X Zeng. 2008. Engineering peptide linkers for scFv immunosensors. Anal Chem 80: 1910–7.

Suter JD, DJ Howard, J Shi, CW Caldwell and X Fan. 2010. Label-free DNA methylation analysis using opto-fluidic ring resonators. Biosensors and Bioelectronics 26: 1016–1020.

Suwansa S, P Kanatharana, P Asawatreratanakul, B Wongkittisuksa, C Limsakul and P Thavarungkul. 2009. Comparison of surface plasmon resonance and capacitive immunosensors for cancer antigen 125 detection in human serum samples. Biosensors and Bioelectronics 24: 3436–3441.

Tang Y, R Mernaugh and X Zeng. 2006. Nonregeneration Protocol for Surface Plasmon Resonance: Study of High-Affinity Interaction with High-Density Biosensors. Anal Chem 78: 1841–1848.

Terness P, I Kohl, G Hubener, R Battistutta, L Moroder, M Welschof, C Dufter, M Finger, C Hain, M Jung and G Opelz. 1995. The natural human IgG anti-F(ab')$_2$ antibody recognizes a conformational IgG1 hinge epitope. J Immunol 154: 6446–6452.

Tothill IE 2009. Biosensors for cancer markers diagnosis. Seminars in Cell & Developmental Biology 20: 55–62.

Wang Y, K El-Boubbou, H Kouyoumdjian, B Sun, X Huang and X Zeng. 2009. Lipoic Acid Glyco-Conjugates, a New Class of Agents for Controlling Nonspecific Adsorption of Blood Serum at Biointerfaces for Biosensor and Biomedical Applications. Langmuir 26: 4119–4125.

Yan H, Z Shen, R Mernaugh and X Zeng. 2011. Single Chain Fragment Variable Recombinant Antibody as a Template for Fc Sensors. Analytical Chemistry 83: 625–630.

19

DNA Biosensor for Rapid Detection of Anticancer Drugs

Sigen Wang[1,*] and Ruili Wang[2]

ABSTRACT

Cancer continues to be a worldwide killer. By 2020, the world population is expected to have increased to 7.5 billion; of this number, approximately 15 million new cancer cases will be diagnosed, and 12 million cancer patients will die. Many people who have cancer will use anticancer drugs as part of the course of their treatment. Anticancer drugs are powerful medicines that destroy cancer cells and keep cancer from spreading to other areas of the body. Analytical tools are needed for screening and routine analysis of anticancer drugs in their discovery and pharmaceutical development processes. Many anticancer drugs have a tendency to interact with DNA causing changes in its structure and base sequence, which results in disturbing the DNA cross linking reaction. As such, the development of DNA biosensors has attracted great interest in the detection of anticancer drug-DNA interaction. In this chapter, we will briefly review the recent development of the electrochemical DNA biosensors for detection of anticancer drug–DNA

[1]Department of Radiation Oncology & Department of Physics and Astronomy, University of North Carolina, 101 Manning Drive, CB# 7512, Chapel Hill, NC 27599-7512, USA; E-mail: sgwang@email.unc.edu and sgwang88@yahoo.com
[2]Division of Pharmacotherapy and Experimental Therapeutics, School of Pharmacy, University of North Carolina, 311 Pharmacy Lane, CB# 7569, Chapel Hill, NC 27599-7569, USA; E-mail: rlwang@email.unc.edu and wangruili@hotmail.com
*Corresponding author

List of abbreviations after the text.

interaction. We will focus on reviewing the biosensor technology development and its application in some anticancer drug detection such as cyclophosphamide, daunomycin, etc. The detection of the pre- and post-electrochemical signals of DNA or anticancer drug interaction provides good evidence for the interaction mechanism to be elucidated. This interaction can also be used for the quantification of these anticancer drugs and for the determination of new anticancer drugs targeting DNA. The electrochemical DNA biosensors enable us to detect, evaluate and predict anticancer drugs with DNA interaction and further understand the interaction mechanism between anticancer drugs and DNA.

INTRODUCTION

Cancer is a term used for diseases in which abnormal cells divide without control and are able to invade other tissues. All cancers begin in cells. Cancerous cells are also called malignant cells. Cancer cells can spread to other parts of the body through the blood and lymph systems. Cancers are primarily an environmental disease with 90–95% of cases due to environmental factors and 5–10% due to genetics (Anand et al. 2008). Cancer is not just one disease but many diseases. There are more than 100 different types of cancer. Most cancers are named for the organ or type of cell in which they start. Cancer continues to be a worldwide killer, despite the enormous amount of research and rapid developments seen during the past decade. According to recent statistics, cancer accounts for around 23% of the total deaths in the USA and is the second most common cause of death after heart disease. Death rates for heart disease, however, have been steeply decreasing in both older and younger populations in the USA from 1975 through 2002. In contrast, no significant decrease in death rates for cancer has been observed in the United States (Knudson 2001). In 2010, estimated new cases and deaths from cancer were 1,529,560 (not including nonmelanoma skin cancers) and 569,490 in the United States, respectively. By 2020, the world population is expected to have increased to 7.5 billion; of this number, approximately 15 million new cancer cases will be diagnosed, and 12 million cancer patients will die (Bray and Moller 2006).

Many people who have cancer will use anticancer drugs as part of the course of their treatment (cancer treatment is commonly a combination of treatment including anticancer drugs as well as complementary and alternative cancer therapies). The first use of drugs to treat cancer, however, was in the early 20th century, although it was not originally intended for that purpose. Anticancer drugs are powerful medicines that destroy cancer cells and keep cancer from spreading to other areas of the body. The roles associated with the use of the most commonly-used anticancer drugs are : (a) to damage the deoxyribonucleic acid (DNA) of the affected cancer cells; (b) to inhibit the synthesis of new DNA strands to stop the cell from replicating, because the replication of the cell is what allows the tumor to grow; and (c) to stop mitosis or the actual splitting of the original cell into two new cells since stopping mitosis stops cell division (replication) of the cancer and may ultimately halt the progression of the cancer. The majority of anticancer drugs (or chemotherapeutic drugs) can be divided into alkylating agents, antimetabolites, anthracyclines, plant alkaloids, topoisomerase inhibitors, and other antitumor agents (Pazdur et al. 2009).

Analytical tools are needed for screening and routine analysis of anticancer drugs in their discovery and pharmaceutical development processes. Many anticancer drugs have a tendency to interact with DNA causing changes in its structure and base sequence, which results in disturbing the DNA cross linking reaction. As such, the development of DNA biosensors has attracted great interest in detection of anticancer drugs and their interaction with DNA (Wang et al. 1998; Oliveira Brett et al. 2002; Erdem and Ozsoz 2002; Rauf et al. 2005; Wang et al. 2009). In this chapter, we briefly review the recent development of the electrochemical DNA biosensors for detection of anticancer drugs such as cyclophosphamide, daunomycin, etc. The detection of the pre- and post-electrochemical signals of DNA or anticancer drug interaction provides good evidence for the interaction mechanism to be elucidated. This interaction could also be used for the quantification of these anticancer drugs and for the determination of new anticancer drugs targeting DNA. Electrochemical DNA biosensors enable us to evaluate (detect) and predict anticancer drugs with DNA interaction and further understand the interaction mechanism between anticancer drugs and DNA.

DNA BIOSENSOR

Biosensors are small devices that combine a biological component with a detector component. Typical biosensors are comprised of three components, as shown in Fig. 19.1: (a) the sensitive elements (biologically-derived material); (b) the transducer or detector element that transforms the detected signal in a readable and quantified output and (c) the signal processor (an amplification/processing element), that displays the transformed signal in a user-friendly way. Different methods can be used to transduce the generated signals such as electrochemical or electrical transduction, optical transduction, thermal transduction and piezoelectric transduction.

Electrochemical DNA biosensors comprise a nucleic acid recognition layer, which is immobilized over an electrochemical transducer. The role of the nucleic acid recognition layer is to detect the changes occurring in the DNA structure during interaction with DNA-binding molecules. The signal transducer will determine the change that has occurred at the recognition

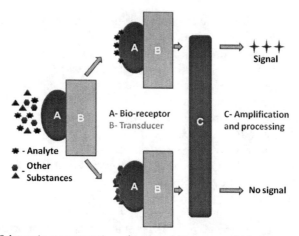

Figure 19.1. Schematic representation of a typical biosensor which is comprised of three components: a biorecognition layer (bioreceptor), a signal transducer and amplification/ processing element. One compound (7 point star) of a mixture of substances specifically interacts with the biological part of the sensor. The resulting biological signal is converted into a physical signal by a transducer. Substances which are not capable of interacting with the biological component will not produce any signal (unpublished).

layer and convert this into an electronic signal which can then be relayed to the end user.

The detection of anticancer drugs by the DNA biosensor is through observing the electrochemical signal related to anticancer drug-DNA interactions. This signal is generated during interaction in the drug action (Rauf et al. 2005; Wang et al. 2009).

DEVELOPMENT OF DNA BIOSENSORS FOR DETECTION OF ANTICANCER DRUG-DNA INTERACTION

Anticancer drugs interact with DNA in several different ways such as intercalation, non-covalent groove binding, covalent binding/cross-linking, DNA cleaving and nucleoside-analog incorporation. This is a result of complex formation occurring between DNA and drug. The typical methods of interaction are as follows: (a) the drug–DNA interaction is through control of transcription factors and polymerases, in which drug interacts with proteins that bind to DNA; (b) the drug–DNA interaction through RNA binding either to the DNA double helix to form nucleic acid triple helix structures or to exposed DNA single strand forming DNA–RNA hybrids that may interfere with transcriptional activity; and (c) the drug–DNA interaction involves the binding of small aromatic ligand molecules to DNA double helical structures (Graves and Velea 2000; Erdem and Ozsoz 2002; Rauf et al. 2005).

The detection of anticancer drug–DNA interaction by using electrochemical DNA biosensors is mainly based on the electrochemical behavior of the anticancer drug in the absence or presence of DNA. In recent years, different DNA biosensors have been developed for detection of anticancer drugs with DNA. The difference includes using different immobilization techniques (materials), different electrochemical techniques, and different types of modified electrodes (solutions).

Immobilization Techniques (materials)

As mentioned in Section 2, in electrochemical DNA biosensors, the recognition layer (biomolecules or biological component) is immobilized over an electrochemical transducer surface. Immobilization can be achieved by a variety of techniques and is one of the key steps in biosensor development. The requirements for this process are: (a) immobilization should give a stable layer of biomolecules; (b) the biocomponent should not be destroyed by the procedure; (c) activity of biocomponent (or analyte) and its binding capacity should not be significantly reduced; and (d) substrate specificity of the biocomponent must not change. If the chosen immobilization procedure fails on one of these points, the method has to be changed (Guilbault 1988; Keusgen 2002).

Different immobilization techniques for biological components have been developed for biosensor construction in recent years. The typical immobilization methods include: (a) biological elements are bound by physical or chemical adsorption with a high affinity for the solid support; (b) biological elements are trapped in polymer matrices (gel structure) and (c) biological elements are covalently coupled to a solid support.

The selection of DNA immobilization materials is a critical issue since DNA immobilization material plays a role in both DNA immobilization and signal transduction. It directly affects the overall performance of the biosensor since it will dictate the accessibility of the DNA to drugs in solution and hence can influence the affinity of drug binding and electron transfer. Different types of immobilization materials have been explored for electrode modification for the investigation of the interaction between anticancer drugs and DNA, these electrodes include carbon nanotube (CNT) electrode (Wang et al. 2009), carbon paste electrode (Gherghi et al. 2003; Wang et al. 2009), glassy carbon electrode (Oliveira Brett et al. 2002; Chu et al. 1998; Kalanur et al. 2008; Hajian et al. 2009), hanging mercury drop electrode (Gherghi et al. 2003), gold electrode (Yau et al. 2003), pencil graphite electrode (Karadeniz et al. 2003), and pyrolytic graphite electrode (Vacek et al. 2009).

Electrochemical Techniques

In the study of the interaction between anticancer drugs and DNA by using electrochemical DNA biosensors, different electrochemical techniques have been used, such as differential pulse voltammetry (DPV) (Kalanur et al. 2008; Wang et al. 2009), cyclic voltammetry (Wang et al. 1998; Oliveira Brett et al. 2002), square wave voltammetry (Oliveira Brett et al. 1998), and chronopotentiometry (Vacek et al. 2009).

A three-electrode setup (system) which consists of a working electrode, a reference electrode (an Ag/AgCl or saturated calomel electrode) and an auxiliary electrode (also called counter electrode) is used to measure the electrochemical signals in all electrochemical procedures (Wang et al. 2009). In the three electrode system, the auxiliary electrode, along with the working electrode, provides circuit over which current is either applied or measured. Here, the potential of the auxiliary electrode is usually not measured and is adjusted so as to balance the reaction occurring at the working electrode. This configuration allows the potential of the working electrode to be measured against a known reference electrode without compromising the stability of that reference electrode by passing current over it. Auxiliary electrodes are often fabricated from electrochemically inert materials such as gold, platinum, or carbon.

Interaction Study Approaches

Three strategies have mainly been used for the detection study of anticancer drugs-DNA interaction including the use of DNA modified electrode, the use of drug-modified electrode or the use of solution with (or without) DNA and anticancer drug.

The DNA modified electrode method involves DNA being immobilized on the surface of the electrode with covalent attachment, electrostatic attraction or entrapment within a polymer layer. As mentioned in Section 3.1, the immobilization materials include CNTs (Wang et al. 2009), carbon paste electrode (Gherghi et al. 2003; Wang et al. 2009), glassy carbon electrode (Oliveira Brett et al. 2002; Chu et al. 1998; Kalanur et al. 2008; Hajian et al. 2009), hanging mercury drop electrode (Gherghi et al. 2003), gold electrode (Yau et al. 2003), pencil graphite electrode (Karadeniz et al. 2003), or pyrolytic graphite electrode (Vacek et al. 2009). The key criteria for DNA immobilization is that the DNA is maintained at the electrode interface, that the DNA is accessible to binding of the target molecule in solution and that the method of immobilization is compatible with the method of transduction. Our group used the DNA modified electrode method to detect the anticancer drug of cyclophosphamide (Wang et al. 2009).

The anticancer drug-modified electrode approach involves the target of the anticancer drug being immobilized on the surface of the electrode. During the electrochemical process, the changes in the electrochemical signals of the anticancer drug are monitored and recorded when the anticancer drug interacts with DNA. Oliveira-Brett et al. used this method for detection of *in situ* adriamycin (Oliveira-Brett et al. 2002).

In contrast to the DNA modified electrode and drug-modified electrode methods, the solution method involves placing the anticancer drug and DNA in the same solution. The interaction of anticancer drug with DNA can be detected through monitoring and comparing the electrochemical signal changes of the anticancer drug–DNA complex in the solution with or without DNA (drugs). Xia et al. (Xia et al. 1999) used this method to study the interaction mechanism of anticancer drug pharmorubicin to DNA.

APPLICATIONS OF DNA BIOSENSOR FOR ANTICANCER DRUG DETECTION

Many anticancer drugs have been known to interact with DNA to exert their biological activities. In general, DNA-acting anticancer drugs can be classified into three categories. Drugs in the first category form covalent linkages with DNA; drugs in the second one form noncovalent complexes with DNA by either intercalation or groove-binding; drugs in the final category cause DNA backbone cleavages.

An electrochemical DNA-biosensor is a receptor-transducer that commonly employs double stranded DNA (dsDNA) immobilized onto the surface of an electrochemical transducer as the molecular recognition element. The interaction of an analyte (anticancer drugs) with dsDNA may lead to the rupture of hydrogen bonds and consequential opening of the double helix resulting in increased accessibility to the constituent bases. The extent of DNA damage can be determined by monitoring the oxidation of the exposed bases by voltammetric methods, etc.

We will review several examples of electrochemical DNA biosensor applications in detection of anticancer drugs, with a focus on the detection of anticancer drugs of cyclophosphamide and daunomycin.

Detection of Anticancer Drug of Cyclophosphamide

Cyclophosphamide (a cytostatic drug) is an alkylating agent used singly or as part of a combination to treat a wide variety of neoplastic diseases. Its structure is shown in Fig. 19.2. Among the anticancer drugs, cyclophosphamide has been one of the most effective anticancer agents for the treatment of malignant and non-malignant disorders in oncology for

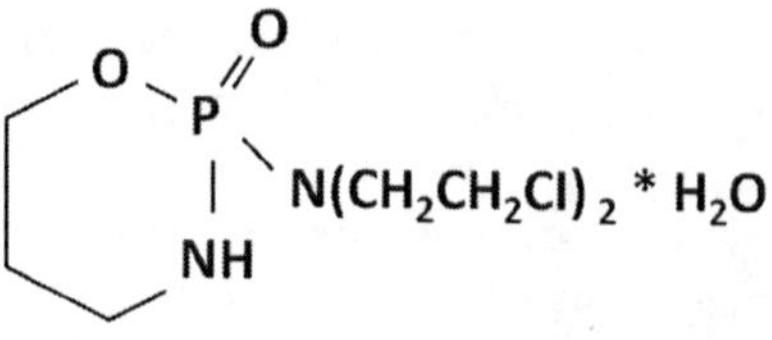

$$O - P \overset{O}{\underset{NH}{\parallel}} N(CH_2CH_2Cl)_2 * H_2O$$

Figure 19.2. Structure of cyclophosphamide (unpublished).

over 40 yr. It has been documented that the cyclophosphamide is effective in the treatment of burkitt's lymphoma, bladder cancer, bone cancer, cervical cancer, endometrial cancer, lung cancer, prostate cancer, testicular cancer, breast cancer and cancer of the adrenal cortex. The mechanism is that the cyclophosphamide creates fragmented DNA, prevents DNA synthesis via cross-linking of DNA, and creates mutations in nucleotides.

Several techniques are reported for analysis of the cyclophosphamide, such as gas chromatography (Huitema et al. 2001), liquid chromatography–tandem mass spectrometric assay (DiFrancesco et al. 2007), and high-performance liquid chromatography (Rustum and Hoffman 1987). These approaches can achieve more specificity of the drug. However, these methods are time-, labor- and cost-consuming; therefore, it will be difficult for a high throuput drug screening and *in situ* analysis.

Our group developed a carbon nanotube based electrochemical DNA biosensor for rapid detection of cyclophosphamide. Figure 19.3 shows the study procedure. A new material of CNTs is used as DNA immobilization material and differential pulse voltammetry is used to detect the interaction

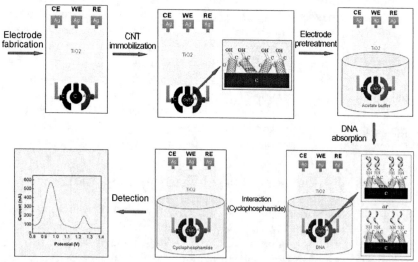

Figure 19.3. Schematic illustration of the experimental procedure. (with permission from [Wang et al. 2009]).

of dsDNA with cyclophosphamide based on the changes of guanine and adenine oxidation signals. The three-electrode system consisted of a CNT (or carbon paste) modified screen-printed electrode as the working electrode, a Ag/AgCl screen-printed electrode as the reference electrode and a carbon paste electrode as the counter electrode.

Carbon nanotubes as immobilization material

Different types of immobilization materials, especially carbon based materials, have been used for DNA immobilization to investigate the interaction between anticancer drugs and DNA, including carbon paste, glassy carbon, and pencil graphite, etc. Screen-printing is becoming a simple and fast method for the mass production of disposable electrochemical sensors. However, both glassy carbon and pencil graphite are not compatible with screen-printing technology. CNTs are a relatively new type of carbon material which can be considered as the result of folding graphene layers into carbon cylinders. CNTs have been recognized as one of the most promising electrode materials since the first electrode application in the oxidation of dopamine in 1996 (Britto et al. 1996). There has been an increase in the use of CNTs as an immobilization material in electrochemical biosensor development because CNT can also promote electron transfer. The study of glucose and DNA biosensors based on CNTs demonstrates that their performance is much superior to those based on other carbon materials in terms of reaction rate, reversibility, reproducibility, sensitivity and hybridization efficiency (Wang et al. 2003, 2004). Additionally, like carbon paste, CNTs are also well compatible with screen-printing technology. Figure 19. 4 shows the scanning electron microscopy (SEM) and transmission electron microscopy (TEM) images of the CNTs used (Wang et al. 2009).

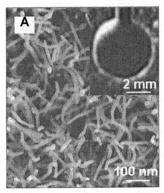 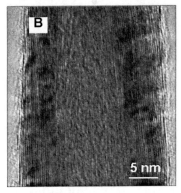

Figure 19.4. (A) SEM image of the CNTs used, inset: image of a completed CNT modified screen-printed electrode, and **(B)** TEM image of the CNTs (with permission from [Wang et al 2009)].

Preparation of screen printed electrodes

The electrodes were prepared on a polyvinyl chloride (PVC) membrane with a thickness of 25 µm by using a DEK 248 screen-printing machine. The electrode structure and fabrication steps are shown in Fig. 19.5. A portion of working electrodes was modified with CNTs. The process is described as follows. After CNT growth, the CNTs were ball milled to shorten their length and then soaked in an aqueous nitric acid (HNO_3) solution to remove the residues of Ni catalyst and to introduce carboxylic acid groups to the nanotubes. After soaking in HNO_3 solution, peaks at around 1742 cm^{-1} and 3000 cm^{-1}, corresponding to the C=O and OH stretch bands of the carboxylic groups, were detected using fourier transform infrared spectroscopy (FTIR), indicating that carboxylic acid groups were present on the surface of the CNTs (Wang et al. 2003, 2004, 2009). 2 mg of CNTs were dispersed in 200 ml of doubly distilled water. The CNT suspension was subsequently cast on the disc area of the working electrodes. After the water was evaporated, CNT modified screen-printed electrodes were fabricated.

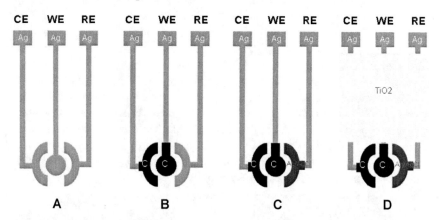

Figure 19.5. Structure and fabrication procedure of screen-printed electrodes. **(A)** After printing silver (Ag) base layer on PVC film; **(B)** after printing carbon paste (C) layer for the counter-electrode (CE) and the working electrode (WE), **(C)** after printing Ag/AgCl layer for the reference electrode (RE); and **(D)** after printing TiO$_2$ insulating layer on the area with silver connection lines (with permission from [Wang et al 2009]).

Immobilization of DNA and absorption of cyclophosphamide

Double stranded (ds) calf thymus DNA (from Sigma) was used. Prior to immobilization of DNA to the CNT surface, the electrode was pretreated by applying a potential of +1.6 V (vs. Ag/AgCl) for 120 s and +1.8 V (vs. Ag/AgCl) for 60 sec under stirred conditions in a 0.25 M acetate buffer solution (pH 4.75). This helped to oxidize the impurities and create a more favorable hydrophilic surface for DNA immobilization, whilst also strengthening CNT adhesion to the electrode surface. The electrode was then transferred into the 0.25 M acetate buffer solution (pH 4.75) containing dsDNA and a potential of +0.5 V (vs. Ag/AgCl) was applied for 5 min. The dsDNA concentration used was optimized so that the DNA can cover the electrode surface completely. The optimization was performed by measuring the peak current of the characteristic guanine of dsDNA in relation to the increasing concentration of dsDNA at the electrode surface. Figure 19.6 illustrates the different peak heights obtained by varying the DNA concentration at the CNT and carbon paste modified electrodes. It can be seen that the current increases with higher DNA concentration and then levels off. This observation is in agreement with the report by Gherghi et al (Gherghi et al 2003). The points at which the curve plateaus are at around 35 mg/L for both CNT and carbon paste modified electrodes. This indicates that the electrode surface was completely covered. The concentration of 35 mg/L was therefore selected for absorption of DNA to the electrodes (Wang et al 2009).

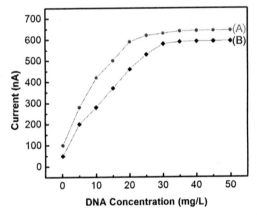

Figure 19.6. Dependence of peak current of the characteristic guanine peak of dsDNA in relation with increasing concentration of dsDNA at **(A)** CNT and **(B)** carbon paste modified electrode (with permission from [Wang et al. 2009]).

After immobilization of DNA, the electrode was immersed into a 0.25 M acetate buffer solution (pH 4.75) containing different concentrations of cyclophosphamide (from Sigma) under stirred conditions for 180 sec by applying a potential of +0.5 V (vs. Ag/AgCl). After the absorption of cyclophosphamide, the electrode was gently rinsed with doubly distilled water for 10 sec to remove the cyclophosphamide which was not immobilized. No cyclophosphamide was immobilized on the samples which were only used for the detection of the oxidation signals of guanine and adenine. The inset of Fig. 19.4(A) shows an image of a completed CNT modified screen-printed electrode.

Detection of cyclophosphamide–DNA interaction and its reproducibility

In order to identify the peaks that occur after interaction of cyclophosphamide with dsDNA, an interaction measurement of cyclophosphamide with a bare CNT and a carbon paste modified electrode (in the absence of dsDNA) was conducted in the potential range of +0.8 ~ +1.4 V. The data are shown in Figs. 19.7(A) and 19.8(A); it can be seen that no pronounced peaks were detected, indicating that cyclophosphamide was electrochemically inactive to the bare CNT and carbon paste modified electrodes.

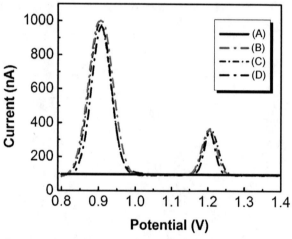

Figure 19.7. Differential pulse voltammograms for the interaction of cyclophosphamide with **(A)** a bare CNT modified electrode, **(B)**, **(C)** and **(D)** dsDNA immobilized at CNT modified electrodes (with permission from [Wang et al. 2009]).

Figure 19.7(B)~(D) shows typical DPV results obtained from the interaction of cyclophosphamide with dsDNA at the CNT modified electrode in the potential range of +0.8~ +1.4 V. Two peaks at around +0.9 V and +1.2 V, corresponding to guanine and adenine, were detected. Compared to the electrochemical signals of dsDNA before the interaction with the drug, shown in Fig. 19.6, it can be seen that the interaction of dsDNA with the drug increased the guanine oxidation signal. This can be attributed to the following mechanism: the cyclophosphamide may cleave dsDNA helix so that the opening of the double helix can make the guanine bases and adenine bases more available to the oxidation. In order to examine the detection reproducibility, a series of samples were measured using DPV

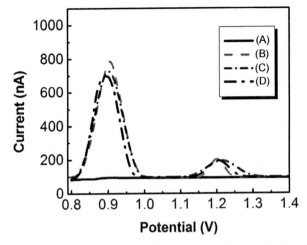

Figure 19.8. Differential pulse voltammograms for the interaction of cyclophosphamide with **(A)** a bare carbon paste modified electrode, **(B), (C)** and **(D)** dsDNA immobilized at carbon paste electrodes (with permission from [Wang et al. 2009]).

under the same conditions. Figure 19.7(B)~(D) shows three typical DPV results. By employing CNT modified electrodes, little change is observed among guanine peaks in DPVs. The relative standard deviation based on the guanine signal was calculated to be 2.0%. For comparison, a similar measurement was also performed in the potential range of +0.8 ~ +1.4 V using the carbon paste modified electrode, as shown in Fig. 19.8(B)~(D). Similar to the results obtained from the CNT modified electrode, only two peaks at around +0.9 V and +1.2 V corresponding to guanine and adenine, were detected. The relative standard deviation based on the guanine signal was 5.8%. This indicates that the use of CNT-based biosensors resulted in a higher detection reproducibility.

The experimental results show that both the CNT- and carbon paste-based biosensors can be used to detect the cyclophosphamide-DNA interaction. Interestingly, the CNT-based biosensor has a faster response and higher detection reproducibility, which can be attributed to the special structure of the CNT modified electrodes. As shown in Fig. 19.4, CNTs have a tiny tubal structure with a diameter of 20 nm. Some ends of CNTs were vertically aligned. This increased both the immobilization area for the DNA absorption and the spacing between the absorbed DNA, thereby increasing the accessibility of DNA to the drug target of cyclophosphamide. In contrast, for carbon paste modified electrode, DNA was absorbed on a flat electrode surface. Some oxidizable groups of electroactive bases such as guanine and adenine were shielded, reducing the accessibility of DNA to the cyclophosphamide. In addition, CNTs have the ability to promote electron transfer. As a result, a faster response was produced from the CNT modified electrode. On the other hand, FTIR measurement indicated that carboxylic acid groups were present on the CNT surface. Large immobilization sites with carboxylic acid groups present at the CNT surface can lead to an effective and strong absorption of DNA on the CNT surface, increasing the uniformity and stability of the DNA film on CNTs, resulting in a higher detection reproducibility of DNA with cyclophosphamide at CNT modified electrode samples.

The study indicates that the DNA biosensors based on CNT screen-printed electrodes can be used as a screening device for rapid detection of the anticancer drug of cyclophosphamide (Wang et al 2009).

Detection of the Anticancer Drug of Daunomycin

Daunomycin (trade name is cerubidine) is an anticancer (antineoplastic or cytotoxic) chemotherapy drug. This medication is classified as an anthracycline antitumor antibiotic which is commonly used to treat acute myelogenous leukemia and acute lymphoblastic leukemia.

DNA biosensors were developed for the detection of the anticancer drug daunomycin–DNA interaction. Wang et al. (Wang et al. 1998) reported a study of the interaction of antitumor drug daunomycin with dsDNA in solution and at the electrode surface by cyclic voltammetry and constant current potentiometric stripping analysis (CPSA) with carbon paste electrode. As a result of intercalation of daunomycin between the base pairs in dsDNA, the CPSA daunomycin peak area decreased and a new more positive shoulder (peak) appeared at the potential from +0.79 to +0.81V. This shoulder was attributed to the oxidation of the drug intercalated in DNA. They suggested that interactions of daunomycin with surface-confined DNA may take place even *in vivo* in cancer patient cells. Differences in the way of drug interactions with DNA in solution and at surfaces might be important for the efficiency of the administered drug.

Chu et al. (Chu et al. 1998) studied the interaction of daunomycin with DNA using rotating disk electrode. They calculated the binding constant K ($K = 2.35 \times 10^5 M^{-1}$) and binding site size n_s of the daunomycin–DNA interaction ($n_s = 6$) by titration curve and non-linear regression analysis. This means that daunomycin covered six base pairs of DNA after intercalation. Their study forms a theoretic guide for the design of new anticancer drugs and chemical treatment of tumor and virus.

Hajian et al. (Hajian et al. 2009) explored interaction of the daunorubicin with calf thymus DNA to study the binding mechanism. The apparent binding constant K of daunorubicin with DNA has been found to be 7.8×10^4 L.mol^{-1}. Their observation indicates an intercalation mechanism between daunorubicin and DNA. They suggest that understanding how the structure of molecules affects their binding mode and binding affinity to DNA will help to design new drugs, with biological and antitumor activity.

Detection of Other Anticancer Drugs

Besides the above mentioned examples, the detection of interaction of some other anticancer drugs including adriamycin (Oliveira Brett et al. 2002; Vacek et al. 2009), mitoxantrone (Hajihassan and Rabbani-Chadegani 2009), Actinomycin D (2-Aminophenoxazine-3-one) (Li et al. 2008), mitomycin C (Erdem et al. 2008; Marin et al. 1998), Tarabine PFS (Cytosar-U) (El-Hady et al. 2004), pharmorubicin (Xia et al. 1999), etc., has also been reported. Limited by the length of the chapter, we cannot extensively review these works. But the reported work demonstrated the feasibility of DNA biosensors for detection of the anticancer drugs. The DNA biosensor provides a convenient, sensitive and rapid approach for the detection of anticancer drugs and the study of their interaction mechanism with DNA.

APPLICATION TO OTHER AREAS OF HEALTH AND DISEASE

DNA biosensors are, by definition, small sensing devices comprising a biological component intimately connected to a physical transducer. It permits a quantitative study of the interaction between an anticancer drug compound and an immobilized biocomponent (DNA).

It has been demonstrated that DNA biosensor provides a convenient and sensitive approach for detection of many types of anticancer drugs. DNA biosensors are unique and innovative tools that may provide complementary data and information on anticancer drugs. Their use opens up new paths into anticancer drug screening, design and discovery.

The DNA biosensors have also potential for detection of toxic compounds, this makes the DNA biosensors a sensitive, rapid and portable tool for applications in clinical chemistry, in environmental and in food analysis.

KEY FACTS OF DNA BIOSENSOR FOR ANTICANCER DETECTION

- Cancer continues to be a worldwide killer. By 2020, the world population is expected to have increased to 7.5 billion; of this number, approximately 15 million new cancer cases will be diagnosed, and 12 million cancer patients will die.

- Many people who have cancer will use anticancer drugs as part of the course of their treatment. Anticancer drugs are powerful medicines that destroy cancer cells and keep cancer from spreading to other areas of the body.
- DNA biosensor is an analytical tool for screening and routine analysis of anticancer drugs in their discovery and pharmaceutical development processes.
- It has been demonstrated that DNA biosensors can be used to detect quite a few anticancer drugs such as cyclophosphamide, daunomycin, adriamycin, etc.

DEFINITIONS

- *Cancer*: Cancer is a term used for diseases in which abnormal cells divide without control and are able to invade other tissues. All cancers begin in cells. Cancerous cells are also called malignant cells. Cancers are primarily an environmental disease with 90–95% of cases due to environmental factors and 5–10% due to genetics.
- *Anticancer drug*: Anticancer or antineoplastic drugs are used to treat malignancies, or cancerous growths. Drug therapy may be used alone, or in combination with other treatments such as surgery or radiation therapy.
- *DNA*: DNA or Deoxyribonucleic acid is a nucleic acid that contains the genetic instructions used in the development and functioning of all known living organisms (with the exception of RNA viruses). The main role of DNA molecules is the long-term storage of information.
- *Biosensor*: Biosensors are small devices that combine a biological component with a detector component. Typical biosensors are comprised of three components, (a) the sensitive elements (biologically-derived material); (b) the transducer or detector element that transforms the detected signal in a readable and quantified output and (c) the signal processor (an amplification/processing element), that displays the transformed signal in a user-friendly way. Electrochemical DNA biosensors comprise a nucleic acid recognition layer.
- *Cyclophosphamide*: Cyclophosphamide is an alkylating agent used singly or as part of a combination to treat a wide variety of neoplastic diseases. It has been one of the most effective anticancer agents for the treatment of malignant and non-malignant disorders in oncology for over 40 yr.
- *Carbon nanotube*: Carbon nanotube is a relatively new type of carbon material and can be considered as the result of folding graphene

layers into carbon cylinders. They can be composed of a single shell—single-walled nanotubes or several shells—multi-walled nanotubes. CNTs have been recognized as one of the most promising electrode materials since it can also promote electron transfer.

SUMMARY AND FUTURE DIRECTION

- Cancer, second only to heart disease, is the leading cause of death in the United States. However, progress has been made in the early detection of cancer and in improvements of cancer therapies. But no significant decrease in death rates for cancer has been observed in the United States. This indicates that fighting cancer is much more complicated than expected.
- Anticancer drugs are powerful medicines that destroy cancer cells and keep cancer from spreading to other areas of the body. The majority of anticancer drugs (or chemotherapeutic drugs) can be divided into alkylating agents, antimetabolites, anthracyclines, plant alkaloids, topoisomerase inhibitors, and other antitumor agents.
- Progress has recently been made in the development of new DNA biosensor techniques to detect and study many kind of anticancer drugs–DNA interaction.
- DNA biosensors can be used to determine the anticancer drug–DNA interaction and can contribute to drug discovery and effective treatment for cancer through providing knowledge regarding the efficacy of candidate drug binding with DNA and through providing information of the mechanism of the DNA–drug interaction.
- On the other hand, DNA biosensor technologies, while promising, still need to bridge the gap between experimental status and the harder reality of applications in pharmaceutical industry and healthcare.
- In view of the developments in DNA biosensor techniques for the determination of anticancer drug–DNA interaction, DNA biosensors would be available to be used for anticancer drug screening and development in the near future.

ABBREVATIONS

CE	:	Counter electrode
CNT	:	Carbon nanotube
CPSA	:	Constant current potentiometric stripping analysis
DNA	:	Deoxyribonucleic acid

dsDNA	:	Double stranded DNA
DPV	:	Differential pulse voltammetry
FTIR	:	Fourier transform infrared spectroscopy
PVC	:	Polyvinyl chloride
RE	:	Reference electrode
SEM	:	Scanning electron microscopy
TEM	:	Transmission electron microscopy
WE	:	Working electrode

REFERENCES

Anand P, AB Kunnumakara, C Sundaram, KB Harikumar, ST Tharakan, OS Lai, B Sung and BB Aggarwal. 2008. Cancer is a preventable disease that requires major lifestyle changes. Pharmaceutical Research 25(9): 2097–2116.

Bray F and B Moller. 2006. Predicting the future burden of cancer. Nature Reviews Cancer 6: 63–74.

Britto PJ, KSV Santhanam and PM Ajayan. 1996. Carbon nanotube electrode for oxidation of dopamine. Biosensors & Bioelectronics 41: 121–125.

Chu X, GL Shen, JH Jiang, TF Kang, B Xiong and RQ Yu. 1998. Voltammetric studies of the interaction of daunomycin anticancer drug with DNA and analytical applications. Analytica Chimica Acta 373: 29–38.

DiFrancesco R, JJ Griggs, J Donnelly and R DiCenzo. 2007. Simultaneous analysis of cyclophosphamide, doxorubicin and doxorubicinol by liquid chromatography coupled to tandem mass spectrometry. Journal of Chromatography B 852: 545–553.

El-Hady DA, MI Abdel-Hamid, MM Seliem, V Andrisano and NA El-Maali. 2004. Osteryoung square wave stripping voltammetry at mercury film electrode for monitoring ultra trace levels of Tarabine PFS and its interaction with ssDNA. Journal of Pharmaceutical and Biomedical Analysis 34: 879–890.

Erdem A and M Ozsoz. 2002. Electrochemical DNA biosensors based on DNA–drug interactions. Electroanalysis 14: 965–974.

Erdem A, H Karadeniz, A Caliskan and A Vaseashta. 2008. Electrochemical DNA sensor technology for monitoring of drug-DNA interations. NANO 3(4): 229–232.

Gherghi IC, ST Girousi, AN Voulgaropoulos and R Tzimou-Tsitouridou. 2003. Study of interactions between actinomycin D and DNA on carbon paste electrode (CPE) and on the hanging mercury drop (HMDE) surface. Journal of Pharmaceutical and Biomedical Analysis 31: 1065–1078.

Graves DE and LM Velea. 2000. Intercalative binding of small molecules to nucleic acids. Curr Org Chem 4: 915.

Guilbault GG. 1988. Enzyme electrode probes. Methods Enzymol 137: 14–29.

Hajian R, N Shams and A Parvin. 2009. DNA-binding studies of daunorubicin in the presence of methylene blue by spectroscopy and voltammetry techniques. Chinese Journal of Chemistry 27: 1055–1060.

Hajihassan Z and A Rabbani-Chadegani. 2009. Studies on the binding affinity of anticancer drug mitoxantrone to chromatin, DNA and histone proteins. Journal of Biomedical Science 16: 31.

Huitema ADR, C Reinders, MM Tibben, S Rodenhuis and JH Beijnen. 2001. Sensitive gas chromatographic determination of the cyclophosphamide metabolite 2-dechloroethyl cyclophosphamide in human plasma. Journal of Chromatography B 757: 349–357.

Kalanur SS, J Seetharamappa, GP Mamatha, MD Hadagali and PB Kandagal. 2008. Electrochemical behavior of an anti-cancer drug at glassy carbon electrode and its determination in pharmaceutical formulations. Int J Electrochem Sci 3: 756–767.

Karadeniz H, B Gulmez, F Sahinci, A Erdem, GI Kaya, N Unver, B Kivcak and M Ozsoz. 2003. Disposable electrochemical biosensor for the detection of the interaction between DNA and lycorine based on guanine and adenine signals. Journal of Pharmaceutical and Biomedical Analysis 33: 295–302.

Keusgen M. 2002. Biosensors: new approaches in drug discovery. Naturwissenschaften 89: 433–444.

Knudson AG. 2001. Two genetic hits (more or less) to cancer. Nature Reviews Cancer 1(2): 157–162.

Li XM, HQ Ju and SS Zhang. 2008. Investigation of the interaction between ssDNA and 2-aminophenoxazine-3-one and development of an electrochemical DNA biosensor. Oligonucleotides 18: 73–80.

Marin D, P Perez, C Teijeiro and E Palecek. 1998. Interactions of surface-confined DNA with acid-activated mitomycin C. Biophysical Chemistry 75: 87–95.

Oliveira Brett AM, TRA Macedo, D Raimundo, MH Marques and SHP Serrano. 1998. Voltammetric behaviour of mitoxantrone at a DNA-biosensor. Biosensors & Bioelectronics 13: 861–867.

Oliveira Brett AM, M Vivan, IR Fernandes and JAP Piedade. 2002. Electrochemical detection of *in situ* adriamycin oxidative damage to DNA. Talanta 56: 959–970.

Pazdur R, LD Wagman and KA Camphausen. 2009. Cancer management: A multidisciplinary approach. 11th edn. CMP United Business Media New York.

Rauf S, JJ Gooding, K Akhtar, MA Ghauri, M Rahman, MA Anwar and AM Khalid. 2005. Electrochemical approach of anticancer drugs–DNA interaction. Journal of Pharmaceutical and Biomedical Analysis 37: 205–217.

Rustum A and N Hoffman. 1987. Determination of cyclophosphamide in whole-blood and plasma by reversed-phase high-performance liquid-chromatography. Journal of Chromatography-Biomedical Applications 422: 125–134.

Vacek J, L Havran and M Fojta. 2009. Ex situ voltammetry and chronopotentiometry of doxorubicin at a pyrolytic graphite electrode: Redox and catalytic properties and analytical applications. Electroanalysis 21(19): 2139–2144.

Wang J, M Ozsoz, X Cai, G. Rivas, H Shiraishi, DH Grant, M Chicharro, J Fernandes and E Palecek 1998. Interactions of antitumor drug daunomycin with DNA in solution and at the surface. Bioelectrochemistry and Bioenergetics 45: 33–40.

Wang SG, Q Zhang, RL Wang and SF Yoon. 2003. A novel multi-walled carbon nanotube-based biosensor for glucose detection. Biochemical and Biophysical Research Communications 311: 572–576.

Wang SG, RL Wang, PJ Sellin and Q Zhang. 2004. DNA biosensors based on self-assembled carbon nanotubes. Biochemical and Biophysical Research Communications 325: 1433–1437.

Wang SG, RL Wang, PJ Sellin and S Chang. 2009. Carbon nanotube based DNA biosensor for rapid detection of anti-cancer drug of cyclophosphamide. Current Nanoscience 5(3): 312–317.

Xia C, GL Shen, JH Jiang and RQ Yu. 1999. Intercalation of pharmorubicin anticancer drug to DNA studied by cyclic voltammetry with analytical applications. Analytical Letters 32(4): 717–727.

Yau HCM, HL Chan and MS Yang. 2003. Electrochemical properties of DNA-intercalating doxorubicin and methylene blue on n-hexadecyl mercaptan-doped 5'-thiol-labeled DNA-modified gold electrodes. Biosensors and Bioelectronics 18: 873–879.

20

Using UV Light to Engineer Biosensors for Cancer Detection: The Case of Prostate Specific Antigen

Maria Teresa Neves-Petersen,[1,2,*] Antonietta Parracino[3] and Steffen B. Petersen[1,4,5]

ABSTRACT

The demand for new biosensors for early disease diagnostics has increased and the scientific community has intensified their research into developing a new generation of biosensors. Here it is shown that light assisted molecular immobilization (LAMI), a novel photonic immobilization technology, leads to the successful creation of a biosensor for the detection of prostate specific antigen (PSA), a prostate

[1]International Iberian Nanotechnology Laboratory (INL), P-4715-310, Braga, Portugal; E-mail: teresa.petersen@inl.int
[2]Nanobiotechnology Group, Department of Biotechnology, Chemistry and Environmental Sciences, University of Aalborg, Sohngaardsholmsvej 57, DK-9000 Aalborg, Denmark; E-mail: m.parracino@yahoo.it
[3]Nanobiotechnology Group, Department of Physics and Nanotechnology, University of Aalborg, Sohngaardsholmsvej 57, DK-9000 Aalborg, Denmark; E-mail: sp@hst.aau.dk
[4]Nanobiotechnology Group, Department of Health Science and Technology, Aalborg, University, Frederik Bajers Vej 7 D2, Aalborg, Denmark; E-mail: sp@hst.aau.dk
[5]University at Buffalo, The State University of New York Buffalo, The Institute for Lasers, Photonics and Biophotonics, NY 14260-3000, USA.
*Corresponding author

List of abbreviations after the text.

and breast cancer biomarker. Our work has focused on the discovery and application of new engineering principles inspired by the properties of biological systems to the design, analysis, and manipulation of biological systems. We have created prostate specific antigen (PSA) and Fab anti-PSA biosensor arrays using UV light assisted molecular immobilization, aiming at the detection and quantification of PSA, a cancer marker. LAMI technology proved successful in immobilizing biomedical relevant molecules while preserving their activity, highlighting that insight into how light interacts with biomolecules may lead to new biomedical devices. The new photonic technology involves formation of free, reactive thiol groups upon UV excitation of aromatic residues located in spatial proximity of disulphide bridges, a conserved structural feature in both PSA and Fab molecules. The created thiol groups bind onto thiol reactive surfaces leading to oriented, covalent protein immobilization. Protein activity was confirmed carrying out immunoassays. The UV light induced mechanism is expected to be applicable to about 50% of all proteins, since about half of all proteins contain both aromatic residues as well as one or more disulphide bridges. Interestingly, UV light based therapy may also hold promise in cancer treatment.

INTRODUCTION

Human health is a result of a complex blend of hereditary, environmental and lifestyle factors. Whereas the society in general is committed to treating human disease, such actions come at a cost. The current demographic trend in most western societies is that the number of retirees grows rapidly, while the fraction of the population that is working declines. Since health care costs escalate late in life, the demographic trends represent a serious problem for western societies. Human ingenuity has led to the development of a plethora of advanced diagnostics and therapeutic approaches that cure or improve the life span of the patient. Human beings are approaching the limit beyond which health care costs cannot be carried by the society alone. Cancer, for example, is one of the major causes of mortality worldwide, being the cause of death for approximately 30% of the population. New approaches for securing human health and life quality will be in high demand. Novel approaches to diagnostics as well as therapeutics are expected to emerge at the interface between nanobiotechnology, biophotonics, materials science, molecular biology, and protein science.

One new technology relevant for biosensor and drug delivery is light assisted molecular immobilization (LAMI). The new photonic technology uses UV light in order to achieve covalent and uniform oriented coupling of biomolecules onto thiol reactive surfaces. The technology uses knowledge derived from protein bioinformatic studies, protein science, biophysics, biophotonics, and materials science. The technique of UV light assisted immobilization of disulfide containing proteins has been used in order to functionalize surfaces with biomolecules according to any desired pattern, including protein microarrays. Since light is used in order to immobilize biomolecules, the area onto which they are immobilized is limited to the focal area of the UV beam. The result is a new simple and inexpensive way of creating high density protein arrays with feature sizes down to a few hundred nanometers, which represents an improvement of at least 10 fold over existing commercially available high density protein arraying methods.

We hereby present the application of light assisted molecular immobilization in cancer diagnostics, specifically in the detection of prostate specific antigen (PSA), a valuable biomarker for prostate cancer screening. Quantification of PSA levels has been a common medical practice since elevated PSA levels in blood is correlated with the development of prostate cancer and breast cancer (Black et al. 2000; Mannello and Gazzanelli 2001). Free PSA and PSA-ACT (PSA complexed alpha-1-antichymotrypsin, a proteinase inhibitor) are the two dominant forms of PSA contributing to the total PSA serum concentration. PSA belongs to the kallikrein, serine-protease family. Kallikreins are peptidases (enzymes that cleave peptide bonds in proteins), a subgroup of the serine protease family. In men, PSA is expressed by prostate gland cells. In women it is secreted in the periurethal gland (Lilja et al. 1991) as well as in the breast. PSA is released into breast secretion and in the amniotic fluid (Borchert et al. 1997), a process which is hormone regulated (Kim and Coetzee 2004). PSA levels in female breast tissue are generally quite low, increasing during the onset of benign diseases. PSA levels rise during the onset of prostate cancer or other disorders involving PSA secreting organs. The higher a man's PSA level is, the more likely the chances of prostate cancer. Identifying cancer in an earlier stage could result in a better prognosis, thus increasing life expectancy. Currently, a blood test for PSA level measurement is the most effective method for early prostate cancer detection. It is believed that if PSA concentration is 0–2.5 ng/ml the risk of developing the disease is low. Prostate cancer has been found in men with PSA levels below 4 ng/ml. The review by Healy et al. highlights the performance of current and novel technologies used for PSA detection, done using antibodies specific for the different forms of PSA and for the different PSA epitopes. The detection limit of commercially available biosensors used to monitor PSA concentration in blood is 4 ng/ml or 0.16 nM (Healy et al. 2007).

Light assisted immobilization of free PSA and Fab anti-PSA onto thiol functionalized optical flat slides (slides polished to atomic surface smoothness $< \pm 20$ angstroms over 1.0 μm^2) leading to high-density functional protein arrays is reported in the present chapter. The specific Fab anti-PSA is an antibody fragment that recognizes an epitope of free PSA molecule. Immobilized PSA was detected upon incubation with Fab anti-PSA and immobilized Fab anti-PSA was detected upon incubation with free PSA. Both immunoassays were successful. LAMI technology allows for the creation of microarrays of biomarkers of pharmaceutical importance such as PSA and Fab anti-PSA, rendering the immobilized proteins active. pM concentration of immobilized PSA has been detected with immunoassays. LAMI is a competitive technology in terms of sensitivity, specificity, density, high signal to noise and reproducibility (Duroux et al. 2007). The working principle of LAMI technology as well as its potential application will be addressed in this chapter.

Interestingly, the reaction mechanism triggered by UV light in proteins containing aromatic residues and disulphide bridges (Neves-Petersen et al. 2009a) has also been used in order to modulate the function of the epidermal growth factor receptor (EGFR), a receptor protein most abundant in several types of cancer cells, as addressed below. Therefore, the same technology can be used both for diagnosis and potentially for the treatment of some cancers.

BIOPHOTONICS AND MICROARRAYING TECHNOLOGY FOR MEDICAL DIAGNOSTICS

The current trend in demographic data shows that the retiree population is growing rapidly while the working population is declining. This trend means that the society will have an urgent need to diagnose, treat or prevent the outbreak of diseases. One of the tools in the fight against disease will be advanced, next generation biosensors. Protein microarrays are becoming increasingly important for medical diagnostics in order to achieve high-throughput analysis systems. Miniaturization of biological and chemical experiments or assays demands a precise measurement of the smallest amounts of reagents, e.g. on microarray sensor surfaces. Pin dispensing, piezoelectric injectors and laser direct write techniques are successfully used to dispense tiny amounts of liquids in the form of either simple spots or larger microarrays (Ringeisen et al. 2002; Strobl et al. 2004; Hsieh et al. 2004; Gutmann et al. 2004; Gutmann et al. 2005). The most obvious attempt is for the downscaling of common fluid handling systems, to reduce the amount of analytes required, minimize fabrication and analysis costs. However, one of the drawbacks of microfluidic systems is the high risk of contamination and the potential for clogging the lumen of the miniaturized tubes. The photonic immobilization technology allows for the creation of microarrays of PSA and Fab anti-PSA overcome these problems, as will be addressed below. Classical immobilization methods for proteins and peptides have relied on adsorption onto the surface non-covalently (Angenendt et al.

2003) or through covalent modes of attachment to surfaces chemically modified with aldehydes, activated esters or epoxide crosslinkers (Liu et al. 2000). All of these modes of attachment lead to random orientation of the immobilized proteins, which can result in the loss of protein activity, thus impairing sensitivity of detection and poor control of the density of immobilized molecules (MacBeath and Schreiber 2000; Haab et al. 2001). LAMI technology has been described by Jonkheijm et al. as the key chemical strategy for generating covalent and oriented protein immobilization onto biochips (Jonkheijm et al. 2008). This technology involves formation of free, reactive thiol groups upon UV excitation of protein aromatic residues located in spatial proximity of disulphide (SS) bridges, a conserved structural feature in proteins. If light-induced cleavage of SS bonds occurs at or close to a thiol reactive surface, such as a glass, quartz or gold surfaces, the protein is immobilized onto the surface (Fig. 20.1).

A   B

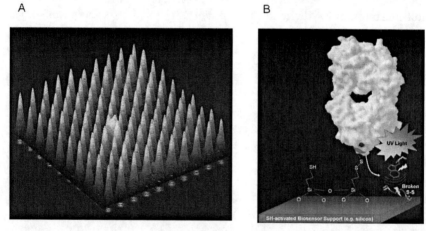

Figure 20.1. Light Assisted Molecular Immobilization (LAMI) photonic technology. (A) Protein microarray engineered with LAMI using 280nm laser light focused to a spot size of five micron. The displayed array has five micron spots, 10 micron pitch leading to an array density equivalent to 10^4 spots per $1mm^2$ of sensor surface. (B) The principle of light induced immobilization sketched with tryptophan near a disulphide bridge in a protein molecule. UV illumination of aromatic residues leads to disulphide bridge (SS) opening and to the formation of free SH groups, which will react to thiol reactive surfaces.

Since this happens where the UV photons are present, the size of the focal spot determines the spatial location and extent of the immobilization. If suitable optical elements are used, the focal spot can be constricted to a few micrometer diameter size. The process is fast (ms), and is determined by physicochemical parameters as well as the photon fluency. The pattern of immobilized molecules on the surface can be controlled by shaping the pattern of the UV light used for molecular immobilization (Petersen et al.

2010). This novel technology bypasses the use of micro-dispenser techniques and associated technical difficulties and avoids the use of thermochemical/ chemical steps common to traditional immobilization methods, which can compromise the structure and/or function of the bound protein. The immobilized proteins maintain their activity (Parracino et al. 2010).

Several sensor biomolecules have already been immobilized using LAMI followed by successful detection of the protein's catalytic activity or binding capacity such as cutinase (an esterase), alkaline phosphatase and lysozyme (Neves-Petersen et al. 2006), Fab chlorotoxin (Duroux et al. 2007), major histocompatibility complex (MHC, Snabe et al. 2006), immunoglobulins' Fab fragments (Neves-Petersen et al. 2006 and Parracino et al. 2010), prostate specific antigen (PSA, Parracino et al. 2010), and bovine serum albumin (BSA, Parracino et al. 2011). We have previously reported that MHC immobilized with LAMI proved to be more active than non-immobilized MHC: the level of bound W6/32 mAb conjugate per MHC molecule immobilized with LAMI on the slide surface is more than 2x larger than on the surface not exposed to UV-light (Snabe et al. 2006). This indicates that LAMI preserved protein structure/function and lead to correctly oriented MHC molecules onto the surface. Loss of protein activity is only felt when the protein is excited with UV light for prolonged time periods much longer than the illumination time needed for immobilization using LAMI technology (Neves-Petersen et al. 2006; Olsen et al. 2007) or when an intact disulphide bridge is critical for activity. LAMI requires that the proteins are excited with UV laser light for ~100ms (power in the sub mW) in order to achieve protein immobilization. In the mentioned studies we have used a UV laser beam with 0.9mW average power in order to create the protein microarrays. Immobilization has also been achieved with much lower power (nW) using a Xenon lamp, as reported in Neves-Petersen et al. (Neves-Petersen et al. 2009b).

High Density Protein Micro Arrays

With LAMI technology, proteins will only be immobilized in the regions where UV light excites the protein film on a surface, allowing the creation of patterns of immobilized protein molecules with diffraction limited resolution (Skovsen et al. 2009; Petersen et al. 2010). This has been achieved when the technique of UV-light-assisted immobilization of disulfide containing proteins has been combined with the Fourier-transforming properties of lenses as well as with a simple millimeter scale feature size spatial mask. The result is a new simple and inexpensive way of creating high-density protein arrays with feature sizes down to a few hundred nanometers, which represents an improvement of 10-fold over existing commercially available high density protein arraying methods. This allows us to increase the array density to 10^6 spots/mm². When using a focused laser beam in order to immobilize the proteins, the density of the micro arrays can be increased by tighter focusing of the laser beam (Parracino et al. 2010).

BIOPHOTONICS IN NEW CANCER THERAPY

As mentioned above, UV excitation (~260–295nm) of aromatic residues in proteins containing disulphide bridges (SS) leads to the disruption of the SS bonds. This knowledge has been used in the development of a new cancer therapy. Pulses of UV light have been used to modulate the structure and function of the epidermal growth factor receptor (EGFR), stopping the proliferation of cancer cells and inducing apoptosis. EGFR is a protein rich in aromatic residues in close spatial proximity to disulphide bridges, which renders the protein extremely sensitive to UV light. Bioinformatics studies reveal that for a protein the size of EGFR, we would expect the average fraction of disulphide bridges to be around 0.2%. However, human EGFR does not fit this picture and the observed fraction of disulphide bridges is 11% (Petersen et al. 2008). Because of the high number of both disulphide bridges as well as tryptophan/tyrosine residues in spatial proximity to SS bonds, EGFR fulfills all basic criteria for being able to respond to UV light by opening one or more disulphide bridges. If excited with UV light for sufficiently long time period (min), the induced photochemical reaction will lead to structural changes in this protein which impair its function. This hypothesis has been successfully confirmed in two different skin-derived cancer cell lines. Laser-pulsed UV illumination of the two cell lines, which over expresses the EGF receptor, had led to the arrest of the EGFR signaling pathway and to apoptosis (Olsen et al. 2007).

THE POTENTIAL OF NANOPARTICLES IN BIOPHOTONICS

The recent technological advances in optical components, hardware and laser systems have paved the way for the development of bionanophotonics, which merges biomedical science, technology and nanophotonics. Fluorescence spectroscopy and confocal microscopy nowadays provide high sensitivity and unprecedent optical resolution. The use of nanoparticles for optical bio-imaging, optical diagnostics and light guided and activated therapy are examples of new areas within bionanophotonics. Of special interest is the use of nanoparticles for intracellular diagnostics and targeted drug-delivery. Using fluorescence confocal microscopy it is possible to monitor *in vivo* the drug nanocarrier into cellular components. Biophotonics and nanofabrication of biological systems are two of the front running and promising fields of science that offer new possibilities in the areas of protein-based diagnostics, therapeutic areas, bio-imaging, and protein based nanocarriers and biomarker identification.

Knowledge on nanoparticles' fabrication allows us to restrict their size down to a few nanometer (< 20nm), this way being compatible for human applications without leading to occlusion of blood vessels. Very interesting classes of molecules that can be immobilized onto nanoparticles are peptide hormones and chemotherapeutical drugs. The exciting properties of new nanomaterials have brought to nanomedicine innovative possibilities, such as the development of new drug-delivery systems (Fig. 20.2). The use of nanoparticles for optical bio-imaging and diagnostics, and light guided, activated therapies are examples of new applications within bionanophotonics.

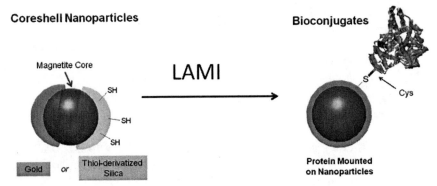

Figure 20.2. Bio-functionalization of nanoparticles using LAMI. The surface of nanoparticles and core-shell nanoparticles can be functionalized with biomolecules using light assisted molecular immobilization technology, engineering this way active drug-delivery systems and/or biosensors.

APPLICATIONS TO OTHER AREAS OF HEALTH AND DISEASE

Diagnosis and Therapy in One Procedure

Nanotechnology provides new possibilities both in diagnosis and therapy. Nanoparticles are excellent systems for the development of biosensors and drug-delivery systems to be used in the human body. Nanoparticles can be constructed in different ways, e.g. gold particles, silica particles, super paramagnetic particles or core–shell particles, with, e.g. a magnetic core and a silica/gold shell. Each particle can be decorated with a protein that may have diagnostic or therapeutic properties. Thus one may construct nanoparticles that can diagnose, e.g. the presence of cancer in a tissue. Conversely, nanoparticles may also attain a therapeutic role. Nanoparticles in the size range from 20–100 nm have a very high surface/volume ratio such that both diagnostic and therapeutic substances can be linked to the same particle. One can envision functionalized nanoparticles with Fabs targeted towards cancer cell antigens. If those particles are also loaded with cytotoxic compounds, then the basic idea is that the Fab molecules will guide the nanoparticle towards cellular antigens. While bound to the cell the cytotoxic component will be released and interfere with the cell metabolism in some detrimental way. Our group has also biofunctionalized gold and core-shell nanoparticles with medically relevant proteins using LAMI (Parracino et al. 2011).

Localized Tumor Therapy

The above mentioned light based photonic therapy can be implemented for destroying localized tumors even if located inside the human or other animal's body since light can be guided through the use of optical fibers anywhere in the body.

ARRAYING PROSTATE SPECIFIC ANTIGEN (PSA) AND FAB ANTI-PSA WITH LAMI TECHNOLOGY

LAMI requires the presence of aromatic residues and disulphide bridges in the protein to be immobilized. The 3D structure of PSA (1pfa.pdb) can be seen in Fig. 20.4, where the disulphide bridges and aromatic residues in PSA are highlighted. The catalytic Ser 195, His 57, Asp 102 is highlighted in a large ball and stick. Trp residues are highlighted in a small ball and stick. Tyr and Cys residues are highlighted as sticks. The shortest distance between an atom in Trp 20 and Cys 157 is 5.3 Å. The close proximity of disulphide bridges to the aromatic residues is a feature that makes this protein a good candidate for LAMI technology. In Fab fragments, the two Cys residues which form an intra-domain disulphide bridge between the two faces of the β-sheet are located nearby a Trp residue (see Fig. 20.1). It has been shown that these residues are conserved in more than 60 different Fabs (Ioerger et al. 1999), which makes Fab fragments excellent candidate for LAMI as well.

Optical Setup for Arraying PSA and Fab Anti-PSA Using LAMI

In Fig. 20.3 the optical setup is displayed and is used to illuminate the protein film placed on the optically flat slide held by the computer controlled stage. Optically flat quartz slides were thiolated as previously described (Neves-Petersen et al. 2006). Detailed description of the illumination setup has been previously described (Duroux et al. 2007). Near UV light at 280nm was used to illuminate each protein film. A bitmap of an array is loaded into the computer. The surface is illuminated according to the bitmap, i.e. light will hit the surface reproducing the image in the bitmap. Molecules will only be immobilized on the surface if they have been illuminated. The fluorescence of the immobilized molecules can then be observed after washing the slide in order to remove the non-immobilized protein molecules (the ones that have never been illuminated).

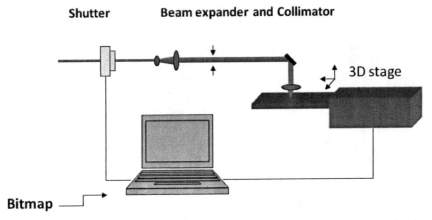

Figure 20.3. Optical setup and LAMI. Optical setup used to carry out light assisted molecular immobilization using laser light at 280nm.

Array Imaging

After immobilization of the proteins with LAMI technology the slides were washed and imaged with a Tecan LS 200 scanner which was used in order to visualize immobilized proteins with 6µm resolution as previously described (Parracino et al. 2010). MATLAB 2009b was used to develop a software package (BNIP-Pro) allowing for advanced analysis of microarray images (Parracino et al. 2010). Full PSA and Fab microarrays were imaged with

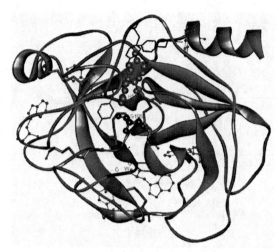

Figure 20.4. Prostate Specific Antigen 3D structure. 3D representation of PSA (1pfa.pdb). Catalytic Ser 195, His 57, Asp 102 is highlighted in a large ball and stick. Trp are highlighted in a small ball and stick. Tyr is highlighted as sticks. Cys are highlighted as sticks.

the Tecan LS 200 scanner (Figs. 20.5A and 20.5B, respectively). Figure 20.5A displays the intensity of light scattered by 4x5 arrayed PSA-FITC. Figure 20.5B clearly confirms light induced immobilization of Fab fragments: a 7x7 array of immobilized Fab is displayed. Reasonably uniform intensity profiles along the axes of both arrays are observed. Spots are well resolved since non-illuminated protein has been washed away from slide regions that have not been illuminated. LAMI proved to be a powerful technique for the creation of PSA and Fab microarrays, allowing for rapid, covalent immobilization of proteins onto biosensor surfaces. The smaller size of the

A   B

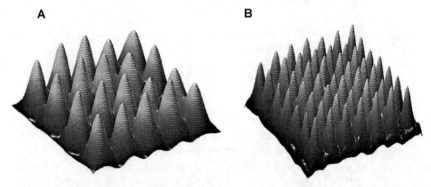

Figure 20.5. PSA and Fab anti-PSA Microarrays created with LAMI. (A) 3D visualization of the intensity of light scattered by arrayed PSA-FITC; **(B)** 3D visualization of the fluorescence intensity emitted by arrayed Fab-AF647 5A10 anti-PSA. With permission from Wiley Blackwell, Protein Science vol. 19, page 1753.

Fab fragments compared to antibodies can be advantageous since smaller MW is likely to lead to an increase in the number of immobilized molecules per square area.

LAMI allows for the creation of ultra high density arrays, where the distance between spots (pitch) is of the order of a few micrometers. In order to observe such arrays one has to use high quality, high resolution microscopy, where sub-micrometer features can be resolved.

Immunoassays

The reactivity of the immobilized PSA was detected upon incubation with Fab anti-PSA and immobilized Fab anti-PSA was detected upon incubation with free PSA according to the protocol previously described (Parracino et al. 2010). Figures 20.6A and 20.6B depict the strategy for Fab immobilization followed by recognition of PSA and the strategy for PSA immobilization followed by Fab recognition, respectively. Negative control experiments have been previously described (Parracino et al. 2010). After the immunoassay the slides were washed and a Tecan LS 200 scanner was used in order to visualize the proteins (Parracino et al. 2010). Figure 20.7

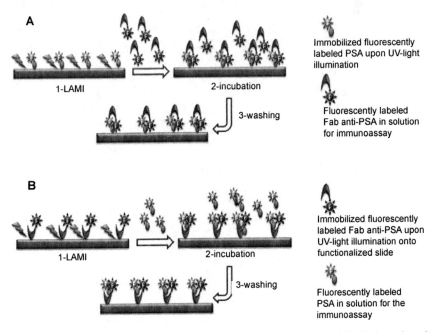

Figure 20.6. Work Flow for microarray fabrication with LAMI. (A) Light-induced immobilization of PSA followed by immunoreaction with Fab anti-PSA; **(B)** Light-induced immobilization of Fab anti-PSA followed by immunoreaction with PSA. With permission from Wiley Blackwell, Protein Science vol.19, page 1754.

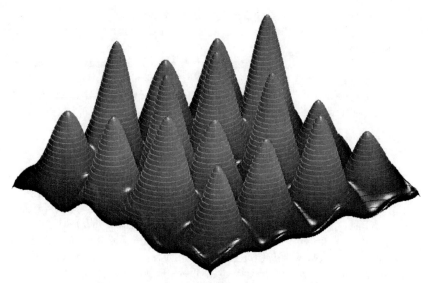

Figure 20.7. **Fab anti-PSA cross reacts with immobilized PSA.** 3D visualization of the fluorescence intensity of Fab-AF647 anti PSA-5A10 after cross reaction with immobilized PSA-FITC. With permission from Wiley Blackwell, Protein Science vol 19, page 1755.

displays the fluorescence emission intensity of Fab-AF647 anti-PSA after cross-reacting with immobilized PSA-FITC. The activity of immobilized Fab-AF647 anti-PSA has also been detected upon incubation with PSA-AF555 (Parracino et al. 2010). Fluorescence immunoassays confirmed the binding capacity of immobilized PSA and Fab fragments after LAMI (Fig. 20.6). This proves that after LAMI the conformation of PSA's epitope and the Fab anti-PSA's binding site remains intact, rendering them active. Negative controls confirmed the specificity of the immunoreactions (Parracino et al. 2010).

KEY FACTS ON LIGHT ASSISTED MOLECULAR IMMOBILIZATION TECHNOLOGY

Prompers et al. reported in 1999 that UV excitation of cutinase lead to the reduction of disulphide bonds in the protein. Early in 2000 Neves-Petersen et al. published a model that correctly fitted the observed photophysical process and showed that the light triggered reaction leading to the formation of free thiol groups in the protein could be used to immobilize biomolecules onto surfaces. The team has illustrated the principle and its applications in a series of papers (Neves-Petersen et al. 2002; Neves-Petersen et al. 2006; Duroux et al. 2007; Neves-Petersen et al. 2009a,b; Skovsen et al. 2009; Parracino et al. 2010; Parracino et al. 2011).

- The protein candidate for LAMI needs aromatic residues and disulphide bridges, a preserved feature in proteins throughout evolution (Petersen et al. 1999). UV excitation leads to the formation of reactive thiol groups which attach the biomolecule onto thiol reactive surfaces. LAMI achieves covalent and oriented protein immobilization while classical immobilization methods, e.g. chemisorption lead to random immobilization.
- LAMI is expected to work well on 50% of all proteins.
- LAMI allows for the creation of protein microarrays with sub-micrometer and nanometer resolution. Multi photon excitation allows LAMI to be carried out with e.g. IR light.
- LAMI has been used to array functional biomolecules of medical and industrial interest. Antibodies or Fab molecules can be coupled to activated surfaces.
- Ultra high density biosensors with a spot density of 10^6 spots/mm^2 can be achieved.
- Multipotent biosensors can be constructed as well as nanoparticles based drug delivery systems.

DEFINITIONS

- *PSA*: Prostate Specific Antigen, a cancer mark associated with the progression of prostate and breast cancer.
- *Fab*: fragment of antigen binding. This is a fragment of an antibody which contains regions that specifically recognize the antigen to which they specifically bind.
- *LAMI*: Light Assisted Molecular Immobilization, a new photonic technology that uses UV light (260–295nm) in order to achieve covalent immobilization of, e.g. protein molecules onto a thiol reactive surface.
- *UV light*: ultraviolet light, which is light with wavelengths ranging from 100–400nm. This UV range may be further subdivided into to UV-A (315–400 nm), UV-B (280–315nm), and UV-C (200–280nm) and the vacuum UV range (100–200nm).
- *Optically flat quartz slides*: microarray substrates that offer a polished atomically smooth glass surface (±20 angstrom over 1.0 μm^2) superior covalent coupling efficiency and low background. Homogenous SiO_2 groups provide superior silane reactivity.
- *MHC*: Major Histocompatibility Complex—A part of the cellular immune response relies on complex formation of antigenic peptides with MHC molecules, followed by presentation of the MHC complex to T cells which activate the required immune response. There are two types of MHC molecules—class I and class II. MHC-I is found

in most cells where they recognize and bind peptides with large specificity (peptides which are derived from cytosolic proteins produced by, for example, intracellular vira). MHC-II is only found in specialized antigen presenting cells that continuously search for unknown proteins.

- *mAb*: monoclonal antibody, are monospecific antibodies that are the same because they are made by identical immune cells that are all clones of a unique parent cell.
- *W6/32*: is a monoclonal antibody (mAb) that recognizes an epitope (part of the antigen recognized by the immune system) expressed on human MHC.

SUMMARY

- A highly conserved structural motif in proteins (aromatic residues in close proximity of disulphide bridges) can be activated by light (~260–295nm) leading to covalent immobilization of biomolecules (Light Assisted Molecular Immobilization or LAMI, Fig. 20.1).
- LAMI leads to the creation of new engineered bio-conjugated sensors/carriers to be used in diagnosis and therapeutics (Figs. 20.1, 20.2).
- LAMI allows the biofunctionalization of surfaces with resolution below 1 micrometer. Biofunctionalized nanoparticles can now be used as drug-delivery systems or biosensors (Fig. 20.2)
- LAMI allows the creation of protein microarrays with a density equivalent to 10^6 spots inside 1mm^2 sensor when combined with Fourier optics and a spatial mask (Skovsen et al. 2009).
- LAMI has been used to create microarrays for the detection of the cancer marker PSA. Protein activity was confirmed carrying out immunoassays (Figs. 20.6 and 20.7). LAMI proved successful in immobilizing biomedically relevant molecules (Fig. 20.5) while preserving their activity.
- LAMI is competitive in terms of sensitivity, specificity, density, high signal to noise and reproducibility (Duroux et al. 2007).
- The reaction mechanism behind LAMI also led to a new light based cancer therapy (Olsen et al. 2007; Petersen et al. 2008).

ABBREVIATIONS

ACT	:	antichymotrypsin, a protease inhibitor that binds PSA
AF	:	Alexa Fluor fluorescent dye
BSA	:	Bovine Serum Albumin

Cys	:	Cysteine
Fab	:	fragment of antigen binding
FITC	:	Fluorescein isothiocyanate fluorescent dye
LAMI	:	Light Assisted Molecular Immobilization
MHC	:	Major Histocompatibility Complex
mAb	:	monoclonal antibody
PSA	:	Prostate Specific Antigen
Tyr	:	Tyrosine
Trp	:	Tryptophan
UV light	:	ultraviolet light
W6/32	:	is a monoclonal antibody that recognizes an epitope expressed on human MHC

REFERENCES

Angenendt P, J Glokler, KZ Onthur, H Lehrach and DJ Cahill. 2003. 3D protein microarrays: performing multiplex immunoassays on a single chip. J Anal Chem 75: 4368–4372.

Black MH, M Giai, R Ponzone, P Sismondi, H Yu and EP Diamandis. 2000. Serum Total and Free Prostate-specific Antigen for Breast Cancer Diagnosis in Women. Clinical Cancer Research 6: 467–473.

Borchert GH, DN Melegos, G Tomlinson, M Giai, R Roagna, R Ponzone, L Sgro and EP Diamandis. 1997. Molecular forms of prostate-specific antigen in the serum of women with benign and malignant breast diseases. Br J Cancer 76(8): 1087–1094.

Duroux M, E Skovsen, MT Neves-Petersen, L Duroux, L Gurevich and SB Petersen. 2007. Light-induced immobilisation of biomolecules as a replacement for present nano/micro droplet dispensing based arraying technologies. Proteomics 7(19): 3491–3499.

Gutmann O, R Kuehlewein, S Reinbold, R Niekrawietz, CP Steinert, B de Heij, R Zengerle and M Daub. 2004. Highly parallel nanoliter dispenser for microarray fabrication. Biomed. Microdevices 6: 131–137.

Gutmann O, R Kuehlewein, S Reinbold, R Niekrawietz, CP Steinert, B de Heij, R Zengerle and M Daub. 2005. Fast and reliable protein microarray production by a new drop-in-drop technique. Lab Chip 5: 675–681.

Haab BB, MJ Dunham and PO Brown. 2001. Protein microarrays for highly parallel detection and quantitation of specific proteins and antibodies in complex solutions. Genome Biol 2: 1–13.

Healy DA, CJ Hayes, P Leonard, L McKenna and R O'Kennedy. 2007. Biosensor developments: application to prostate-specific antigen detection. Trends in Biotechnology 25(3): 125–131.

Hsieh HB, J Fitch, D White, F Torres, J Roy, R Matusiak, B Krivacic, B Kowalski, R Bruce and S Elrod. 2004. Ultra-high throughput microarray generation and liquid dispensing using multiple disposable piezoelectric ejectors. J Biomol Screen 9: 85–94.

Jonkheijm P, D Weinrich, H Schröder, CM Niemeyer and H Waldmann. 2008. Chemical Strategies for Generating Protein Biochips Angew Chem Int Ed 47: 9618–9647.

Ioerger TR, C Du and DS Linthicum. 1999. Conservation of cys-cys trp structural triads and their geometry in the protein domains of immunoglobulin superfamily members. Mol Immunol 36: 373–386.

Kim J and GA Coetzee. 2004. Prostate specific antigen gene regulation by androgen receptor. J Cell Biochem 93(2): 233-41.

Lilja H, A Christensson, U Dahlén, MT Matikainen, O Nilsson, K Pettersson and T Lövgren. 1991. Prostate-specific antigen in serum occurs predominantly in complex with a1-antichymotrypsin. Clin Chem 37(9): 1618–25.

Liu ZH, HK Wang, JN Herron and GD Prestwich. 2000. Photopatterning of antibodies on biosensors. Bioconjug Chem 11: 755–761.

MacBeath G and SL Schreiber. 2000. Printing proteins as microarrays for high-throughput function determination. Science 289: 1760–1763.

Mannello F and G Gazzanelli. 2001. Prostate-specific antigen (PSA/hK3): a further player in the field of breast cancer diagnosis. Breast Cancer Res 3(4): 238-43.

Neves-Petersen MT, Z Gryczynski, J Lakowicz, P Fojan, S Pedersen, E Petersen and SB Petersen. 2002. High probability of disrupting a disulphide bridge mediated by an endogenous excited tryptophan residue. Protein Science 11: 588–600.

Neves-Petersen MT, T Snabe, S Klitgaard, M Duroux and SB Petersen. 2006. Photonic Biosensors: UV light induced molecular switch allows sterically oriented immobilisation of biomolecules and the creation of protein nanoarrays. Protein Science 15: 343–351.

Neves-Petersen MT, S Klitgaard, E Skovsen, T Pascher, T Polivka, SB Petersen, A Yartsev and V Sundström. 2009a. Flash photolysis of cutinase: identification and decay kinetics of transient intermediates formed upon UV excitation of aromatic residues: Flash photolysis studies of cutinase. Biophysical Journal 97(1): 211–226.

Neves-Petersen MT, M Duroux, E Skovsen, L Duroux and SB Petersen. 2009b. Printing novel architectures of nanosized molecules with micrometer resolution using light. Journal of Nanoscience and Nanotechnology 9(6): 3372–3381.

Olsen BB, MT Neves-Petersen, S Klitgaard, OG Issinger and SB Petersen. 2007. UV light blocks EGFR signalling in human cancer cell lines. International Journal of Oncology 30(1): 181–185.

Parracino A, MT Neves-Petersen, AK di Gennaro, K Pettersson, T Lövgren and SB Petersen. 2010. High density microarrays for biomarkers detection: arraying prostate specific antigen and Fab anti-PSA using UV light. Protein Science 19(9): 1751–1759.

Parracino A, GP Gajula, AK di Gennaro, M Correia, MT Neves-Petersen, J Rafaelsen and SB Petersen. 2011. Photonic immobilization of BSA for nanobiomedical applications: creation of high density microarrays and superparamagnetic bioconjugates. Biotechnology and Bioengineering 108(5): 999–1010.

Petersen MTN, PH Jonson and SB Petersen. 1999. Amino acid neighbours and detailed conformational analyses of cysteines in proteins. Protein Engineering 12(7): 535–548.

Petersen SB, M. Neves-Petersen and B Olsen. 2008. The EGFR family of receptors sensitizes cancer cells towards UV light. Proc. SPIE 6854, 68540L; doi:10.1117/12.760510

Petersen SB, AK di Gennaro, MT Neves-Petersen, E Skovsen and A Parracino. 2010. Immobilization of biomolecules onto functionalized surfaces according to UV Diffraction Patterns Applied Optics 49(28): 5344–5350.

Prompers JJ, CW Hilbers and HAM Pepermans. Tryptophan mediated photoreduction of disulfide bond causes unusual fluorescence behaviour of Fusarium solani pisi cutinase. Febs Letters 456(3): 409–416.

Ringeisen BR, PK Wu, H Kim, A Pique, RY Auyeung, HD Young, DB Chrisey and DB Krizman. 2002. Picoliterscale protein microarrays by laser direct write. Biotechnol Prog 18: 1126–1129.

Snabe T, GA Røder, MT Neves-Petersen, SB Petersen and S Buus. 2006. Oriented Coupling of Major Histocompatibility Complex (MHC) to Sensor Surfaces using Light Assisted Immobilisation Technology. Biosens Bioelectron 21: 1553–1559.

Skovsen E, A Kold, MT Neves-Petersen and SB Petersen. 2009. Photonic Immobilization of High Density Protein Arrays Using Fourier Optics. Proteomics 9: 1–4.

Strobl CJ, Z Von Guttenberg and A Wixforth. 2004. Nano- and pico-dispensing of fluids on planar substrates using SAW. IEEE Trans. Ultrason. Ferroelectr. Freq Control 51: 1432–1436.

Index

About the Editors

Victor R. Preedy BSc, PhD, DSc, FIBiol, FRCPath, FRSPH is a Professor at King's College London and also at King's College Hospital. He is attached to both the Diabetes and Nutritional Sciences Division and the Department of Nutrition and Dietetics. He is also Director of the Genomics Centre and a member of the School of Medicine. Professor Preedy graduated in 1974 with an Honours Degree in Biology and Physiology with Pharmacology. He gained his University of London PhD in 1981. In 1992, he received his Membership of the Royal College of Pathologists and in 1993 he gained his second doctoral degree, for his outstanding contribution to protein metabolism in health and disease. Professor Preedy was elected as a Fellow to the Institute of Biology in 1995 and to the Royal College of Pathologists in 2000. Since then he has been elected as a Fellow to the Royal Society for the Promotion of Health (2004) and The Royal Institute of Public Health (2004). In 2009, Professor Preedy became a Fellow of the Royal Society for Public Health. In his career Professor Preedy has carried out research at the National Heart Hospital (part of Imperial College London) and the MRC Centre at Northwick Park Hospital. He has collaborated with research groups in Finland, Japan, Australia, USA and Germany. He is a leading expert on the science of health. He has lectured nationally and internationally. To his credit, Professor Preedy has published over 570 articles, which includes 165 peer-reviewed manuscripts based on original research, 90 reviews and over 40 books and volumes.

Dr Vinood B. Patel, PhD is currently a Senior Lecturer in Clinical Biochemistry at the University of Westminster and honorary fellow at King's College London. Dr Patel obtained his degree in Pharmacology from the University of Portsmouth, his PhD in protein metabolism from King's College London in 1997 and carried out post-doctoral research at Wake Forest University School of Medicine, USA where he developed novel biophysical techniques to characterise mitochondrial ribosomes. He presently directs studies on metabolic pathways involved in fatty liver disease, focussing on mitochondrial energy regulation and cell death. Dr Patel has published over 150 articles, including books in the area of nutrition and health prevention.

Color Plate Section

Chapter 8

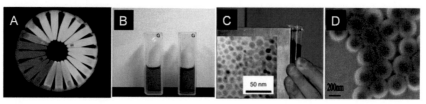

Figure 8.2. Commonly used nanomaterials. Pictures of typical nanomaterials: **(A)**, quantum dots; **(B)**, gold nanoparticles; **(C)**, nano-γ-Fe$_2$O$_3$; **(D)**, polymer.

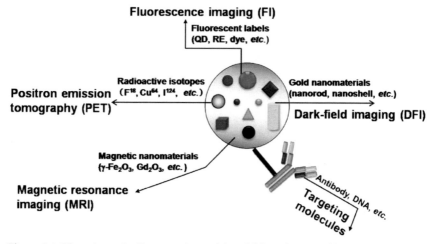

Figure 8.4. The schematic diagram of a multimodal imaging nanobiosensor. Schematic diagram of a multimodal imaging nanobiosensor fabricated by integrating optical tags, radioactive isotopes, magnetic nanoparticles, and targeting molecules. Here, QD refers to quantum dot and RE refers to rare earth.

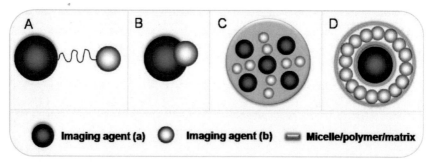

Figure 8.5. The schematic diagram of the fabrication strategy of multimodal imaging nanbiosensor. Schematic diagram for the fabrication of multimodal imaging nanbiosensor by different methods: **(A)**, covalent bonding; **(B)**, epitaxial growth; **(C)**, encapsulation/embedding; **(D)**, self-assembly.

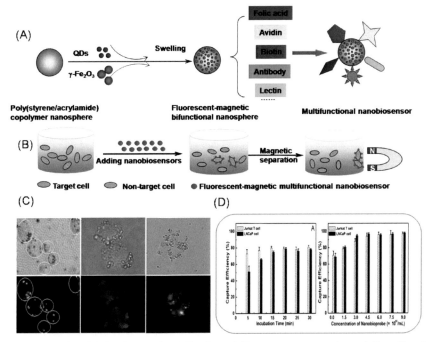

Figure 8.6. The fabrication and application of fluorescent-magnetic multifunctional nanobiosensor. Schematic diagrams for **(A)** fabrication of a fluorescent-magnetic multifunctional nanobiosensor and; **(B)** separation of cells with fluorescent-magnetic multifunctional nanobiosensors; **(C)** Capture and imaging of human breast cancer cells (left panel), human leukaemia cells (middle panel), and human prostate carcinoma cells (right panel). The top row for bright field images; the bottom row for fluorescent images. **(D)** The efficiency of fluorescent-magnetic multifunctional nanobiosensors to capture target cells. QDs: quantum dots. Reproduced with permission from References (Xie et al. 2005; 2007; Song et al. 2011). Copyright 2005 Wiley-VCH Verlag GmbH & Co. KGaA and copyright 2011 American Chemical Society.

Chapter 18

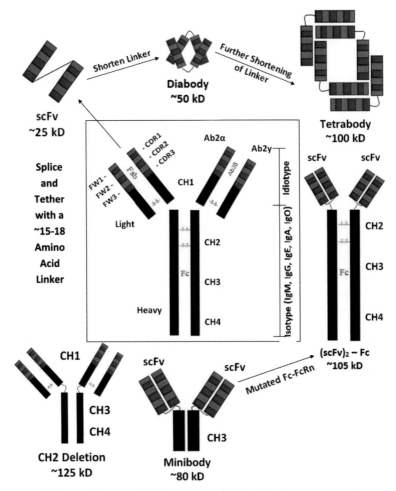

Figure 18.1. ScFv recombinant antibodies. parent antibody and various scFv constructs possible for use in different applications.

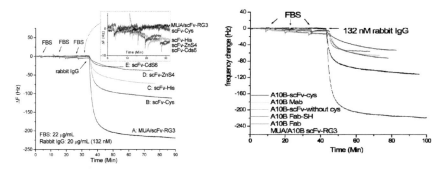

Figure 18.3. Comparison of IgG, Fab and various scFv immunorecognition elements for selectivity and sensitivity; **(left)** MUA/scFv-RG3, scFv-Cys, scFv-His, scFv-ZnS4, scFv-CdS6; **(right)** IgG, Fab, scFv and scFv-cys. FBS 22µg/mL (permission from ACS).

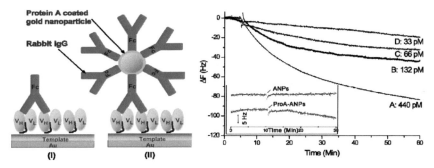

Figure 18.5. ScFv –AuNP; **(left)** binding of rabbit IgG without (I) or with Protein A coated Au NP (II), A-D; **(right)** the addition of Au NP or protein A coated Au NP to scFv immobilized surfaces (permission from ACS).

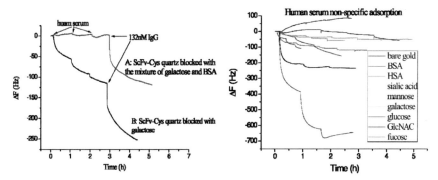

Figure 18.6. Blocking effect of BSA, HSA and different carbohydrate; **(left):** at 0.2%, 0.5%, 1% and 2% human serum final concentrations; **(right):** scFv-cys piezoimmunosensor sensitivity and specificity when blocked with galactose only or with the mixture of galactose and BSA (final human serum concentrations: 0.2%, 0.5%, 1% with 132nM rabbit IgG) (Permission from ACS).

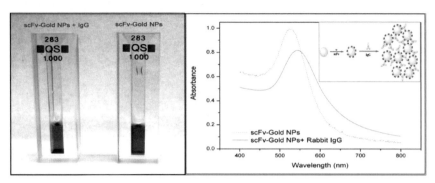

Figure 18.9. AuNP-scFv colorimetric assay; **(left):** visible difference in color change with IgG biding; **(right):** absorbance spectrum showing shift in peak absorbance with IgG binding (permission from Elsevier).

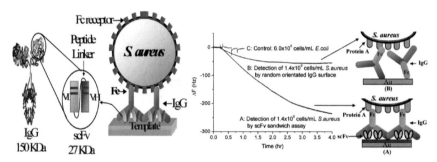

Figure 18.10. Fc sensor for the detection of cell's surface Fc receptor; QCM results for the detection of *S. aureus*. **(A)** Acid treated *S. aureus* were added to MUA/scFv-RG3/IgG surface; **(B)** Acid treated *S. aureus* were added to random oriented IgG surface; (C) Negative control: *E. coli* were added to MUA/scFv-RG3/IgG surface (permission from ACS).

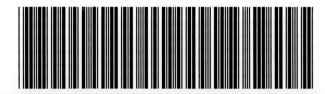